ALAM S. KHAN,
M.B, FRCP(c)
'78
CALGARY, CANADA

AUSCULTATION
OF THE HEART

Auscultation
of the Heart

THIRD EDITION

ABE RAVIN, M.D., F.A.C.C., F.A.C.P.

Clinical Professor of Medicine
University of Colorado Medical Center, Denver
Former Director, Cardiology Division
General Rose Memorial Hospital, Denver

LANE D. CRADDOCK, M.D., F.A.C.C.

Associate Clinical Professor of Medicine
University of Colorado Medical Center, Denver
Director, Cardiology Division
General Rose Memorial Hospital, Denver

PHILLIP S. WOLF, M.D., F.A.C.C., F.A.C.P., F.C.C.P.

Associate Clinical Professor of Medicine
University of Colorado Medical Center, Denver
Associate Director, Cardiology Division
General Rose Memorial Hospital, Denver

DAVID SHANDER, M.D., F.A.C.C., F.A.C.P., F.C.C.P.

Assistant Clinical Professor of Medicine
University of Colorado Medical Center, Denver
Associate Director, Cardiology Division
General Rose Memorial Hospital, Denver

YEAR BOOK MEDICAL PUBLISHERS, INC.
Chicago • London

Reprinted, October 1959
Reprinted, October 1962
Second Edition, 1967
Reprinted, July 1970
Reprinted, July 1973
Third Edition, 1977

Library of Congress Catalog Card Number: 76-53227
International Standard Book Number: 0-8151-7101-3

Preface to the Third Edition

THE THIRD EDITION of this book needs no justification and little introduction. The first two editions brought clinical auscultation to an advanced level. As further advances are made, and
they continuously are being made, updating is necessary.
Thus, this third edition expands old material, introduces new
interpretations of some already known phenomena, and attempts to include new findings in light of maturing clinical
understanding of certain important cardiac problems. The latter findings include refinements in bedside evaluation of left
ventricular outflow obstruction, the click-murmur syndrome
and ischemic heart disease, as well as new descriptions of
postoperative auscultatory findings. A chapter on nonauscultatory phenomena is included to sharpen those findings that
complement auscultation. The overall purpose continues to
be as stated in the first edition, that is, to show that very little
happens to a heart that does not give some auscultatory clue to
the trained observer.

Echocardiography has contributed a more detailed knowledge of mechanical events and has helped to pinpoint certain
valvular positions in sequence. The well-known dynamics of
muscular subaortic stenosis, the click-murmur syndrome, mitral leaflet flutter in the Austin Flint phenomenon, and precise
measurement of valve motion in mitral stenosis have all been
better elucidated by this method. We take advantage of this in
an attempt to illustrate dynamics and the reflected auscultatory phenomena more clearly.

Those of us who have received our training in more recent

v

years are fortunate. We were handed a rich legacy, not least of which is the assurance that clinical auscultation is a powerful tool. Along with that, however, goes the unspoken obligation to further refine an art-science already elegant and to teach the novice from that vantage point.

Much is said of the first heart sound and, we hope, with due accuracy. At least as much is yet unknown. We are quite certain that future studies will add greatly to its usefulness in clinical auscultation such that, as with the second heart sound, it may be introduced at an early stage of training.

As in previous editions, no attempt is made to give individual credit to "original" work. We agree that, by and large, it is frequently inaccurate if not downright hazardous. We also gratefully acknowlege all the many workers in the field whose contributions have been incorporated here and whose identities may be gleaned only from the expanded bibliography.

In the preparation of the third edition we wish to thank the following: Diane Yacovetta for having typed the entire manuscript and for serving as general manager with great equanimity; Dorothy Bailey for searching the literature repeatedly; and Sheldon Luper, Sara Gustafson, Peggy Perlmeter and Dennis Collier for preparing the new illustrations. Our thanks also go to our colleagues for their encouragement and to our students for their stimulation. Most of all, to Abe Ravin for having the idea and doing the work in the first place and for possessing that indefinable quality that always makes for a better world, medical and otherwise.

Lastly, to a close association of three men for surviving this revision.

LANE D. CRADDOCK

PHILLIP S. WOLF

DAVID SHANDER

Preface to the First Edition

FEW PHASES of physical examination as important and as universally used as cardiac auscultation are done with so little confidence. All doctors, except for a small number of specialists, have occasion to listen to the heart, and yet few have learned to perform a skillful auscultation and to interpret properly the results. To be sure, some persons cannot adequately hear sounds and distinguish rhythms and consequently cannot listen satisfactorily to a heart. But I believe that with an understanding of the basic principles of auscultation and with moderate experience, most doctors can get the information made available by this procedure — and with the simplest of instruments.

Auscultation often yields the first and only evidence of heart disease. It is the most valuable means of recognizing valvular damage and enables the doctor to anticipate future changes in the heart and to treat the patient accordingly. Most of the common arrhythmias can be recognized by auscultation alone, although the electrocardiogram often must give the final answer. Congenital heart deformities, a failing myocardium, pericarditis, abnormal vascular pressures, all give important auscultatory signs that supplement data obtained by other methods of examination. Very little happens to a heart that does not give some auscultatory clue to the trained observer.

A more recent upsurge in interest in cardiac auscultation has resulted from phonocardiography and cardiac surgery. Marked improvement in instruments for recording heart sounds and murmurs, together with improved methods for correlating these with other cardiac phenomena, has advanced our knowledge of auscultation. The advent of surgery of congenital and acquired heart disease has led to important advances in our knowledge of auscultation. The ability to correlate what is heard with the pathologic findings at an operation instead of at autopsy has been of inestimable value. The knowledge thus obtained has made cardiac auscultation the single most important guide to surgery of acquired valvular disease.

The purpose of this book is to indicate what constitutes skillful auscultation and to describe the normal and abnormal auscultatory findings insofar as the trained ear can recognize them. Fortunately, the trained ear is probably still the best instrument for recognition of most murmurs. In the field of the heart sounds, extra sounds, and gallop rhythms, phonocardiography often gives information not available to the ear; however, an attempt will be made to describe only what the ear can recognize. Theory will be given only insofar as it makes more understandable the auscultatory findings. The information contained in this book represents the work of numerous people, absorbed and digested by the author over many years; with few exceptions, however, I have made no attempt to give the credit that is due. I fully realize my debt to these individuals and gratefully acknowledge their help.

For help in the preparation of this book, I wish to thank the following: Drs. A. A. Luisada, A. Lanari, S. G. Blount, M. Wassermil, C. R. Hawes, and A. J. Stone, for reading the manuscript and offering many valuable suggestions; Marjorie Kimmerle, for checking the grammar; Glenn Mills and William Wheeler, for the photography; Ruth Kantor, for many of the illustrations; Jan Ellzey, for typing the manuscript; and Dr. Rose Ravin, my wife, for everything.

A.R.

Table of Contents

1. **Sound** 1
   Some Properties of Sound 1
   Transmission of Sound 3

2. **The Stethoscope** 5
   Description 5
   Amplifying Stethoscopes 10
   Phonocardiography 10
   Use of the Stethoscope 11

3. **Graphic Recording of Auscultation** 19

4. **Heart Sounds** 27
   Timing of Heart Sounds 27
   First Heart Sound 28
   Second Heart Sound 39
   Third Heart Sound 51

5. **Abnormal and Extra Heart Sounds** 53
   Fourth Sound 56
   Ejection Sounds 62
   Systolic Clicks 67
   Opening Snap of the Mitral Valve 69
   Third Heart Sound 75
   Summation Sounds (Summation Gallop) 78

6. **Murmurs: General Considerations** 82
   Production 82
   Regurgitation and Stenosis 84

ix

Description of Murmurs 85
Transmission of Murmurs 93
Relation of Murmurs and Thrills 94

7. Systolic Murmurs 96
The Systolic Murmur of Mitral Regurgitation 96
Conditions Producing Mitral Regurgitation 102
The Systolic Murmur of Tricuspid Regurgitation 107
The Systolic Murmur of Aortic Stenosis and Aortic
    Valvular Deformity 109
The Basal Systolic Murmur Associated with
    Arteriosclerosis and/or Hypertension 114
Subaortic Stenosis 116
Innocent Systolic Murmurs 120
Cardiopulmonary Murmur 125

8. Diastolic Murmurs 126
The Diastolic Murmur of Mitral Stenosis 126
The Diastolic Murmur of Tricuspid Stenosis 134
The Diastolic Murmur of Aortic Regurgitation 136
Apical Diastolic Murmurs Not Associated with Organic
    Mitral Stenosis 140
The Diastolic Murmur of Pulmonary Regurgitation . . . 145
Other Causes of Diastolic Murmurs 147

9. Pericardial Friction Rub; Venous Hum; Extracardiac
    Auscultation 148
Pericardial Friction Rub 148
Venous Hum 150
Extracardiac Auscultation 152

10. Cardiac Arrhythmias 158
Regular Rhythms with Rapid Heart Rate 161
Regular Rhythms with Normal Heart Rate 165
Regular Rhythms with Slow Heart Rate 166
Rhythmically or Transiently Irregular Rhythms with
    Normal Heart Rate 166
Transiently Irregular Rhythms with Rapid Heart Rate . . 168
Transiently Irregular Rhythms with Slow Heart Rate . . 168
Absolutely Irregular Rhythms 168

11. Congenital Heart Disease 171
Patent Ductus Arteriosus 171
Ventricular Septal Defects 177

Atrial Septal Defects 180
Valvular, Discrete Subvalvular and Supravalvular Aortic
    Stenosis 184
Coarctation of the Aorta 185
Pulmonary Valvular Stenosis with an Intact Ventricular
    Septum 187
Tetralogy of Fallot 189
Other Congenital Heart Lesions 190

12. **Auscultatory Phenomena in Rheumatic Heart Disease** . . **192**
Acute Rheumatic Carditis 192
Mitral Valve Involvement 193
Aortic Valve Involvement 203
Selection of Patients with Valvular Involvement for
    Cardiac Surgery 206

13. **Arteriosclerosis and Ischemic Heart Disease** **209**
General Arteriosclerosis 209
Acute Myocardial Ischemia 211
Acute Myocardial Infarction 213

14. **Auscultatory Phenomena in Various Conditions** **216**
Myocardial Failure 216
Cardiac Tumors 217
Cardiomyopathy 218
Hypertension and Hypertensive Heart Disease 218
Marfan's Syndrome 219
Pectus Excavatum and Straight Back Syndrome 220
Thyrotoxicosis 220
Cardiovascular Syphilis 221
Endocarditis 222
Pulmonary Embolism 222
Carcinoid Syndrome 223
Ankylosing Spondylitis 224
Rheumatoid Arthritis 224
Systemic Lupus Erythematosus (SLE) 224
Methysergide-Induced Endocarditis 225

15. **Postsurgical Sounds** **226**
Prosthetic Valves 226
Pacemakers 229
Valve Surgery 229
Congenital Heart Surgery 230

Coronary Revascularization 231
Aneurysm Resection 231
Idiopathic Hypertrophic Subaortic Stenosis 232
Other Prosthetic Devices 232

16. Nonauscultatory Findings in Cardiovascular Disease . . 233
Blood Pressure and Pulse 237
Venous Pressure and Pulsations 241

17. Use of Physiologic and Pharmacologic Maneuvers in
Auscultation 245
Physiologic Maneuvers 245
Pharmacologic Maneuvers 250

18. Eponyms 258

Selected Bibliography 260
Index 273

CHAPTER 1

_____

Sound

Some Properties of Sound

SOME CONCEPTION of the production, characteristics and transmission of sound is essential for the intelligent discussion of heart sounds and murmurs. Only features pertinent to the present discussion will be covered.

Vibrations of a certain frequency range and intensity, when they reach the ear, give the impression of sound. Sounds differ from one another in three respects: *pitch, quality* and *loudness.*

① PITCH. — The frequency of the vibration determines the pitch of the sound, and the lower the frequency the lower the pitch. If the vibrations are less frequent than 20 per second or more than 20,000 per second, they cannot be heard by the human ear. The pitch of many of the sounds emitted by the heart is in the lower range of human audibility; thus, 80% of the energy of the first and second heart sounds is in frequencies below 70 vibrations per second, and most sounds and murmurs are composed of frequencies below 500 per second. Frequency components over 650 are of little importance in auscultation. Physicians differ in their capacity to hear sounds at the upper and lower limits of audibility, and the ability to hear low-frequency vibrations is a great advantage. This may possibly be improved by training.

② QUALITY. — A sound consisting of a single fundamental frequency gives the impression of a tone or note, and the frequency of vibration determines the pitch of the note. Most notes have, in addition, higher-frequency vibrations, called

1

overtones, which determine the quality. Thus, the same note has different overtones when produced by a piano, violin or trumpet; the resulting difference in quality permits one to recognize the note as coming from the respective instrument.

Sounds consisting of many different fundamental frequencies give the impression of noise, and most of the sounds heard on auscultation are noises. It is the spectrum of frequencies that gives a murmur its quality. Thus, if a sound consists of a narrow band of frequencies clustered around 400 vibrations per second, the impression obtained is that of the high-pitched, blowing, systolic murmur of mitral regurgitation. If the frequencies below 400 are added and all the frequencies from 180 to 400 are present, the murmur takes on a harsh character similar to the murmur of aortic stenosis. Quality as used in auscultation, therefore, depends on frequency makeup rather than on overtones.

③ LOUDNESS AND INTENSITY. — Intensity, in a strict sense, refers to the physical aspect of the sound, whereas loudness refers to the subjective aspect. The intensity of a sound is proportional to the amplitude of the vibration and is independent of the ear. Loudness corresponds to the degree of sensation produced and is dependent both on the intensity of the sound and on the sensitivity of the ear to that particular sound. The ear is most sensitive to sounds in the frequency range between 500 and 5,000. Below a frequency of 500, the sensitivity of the ear decreases rapidly. A sound with a frequency of 500 vibrations per second will be louder to the ear than a sound of 100 vibrations per second, even if the two sounds have the same intensity. Since many of the sounds encountered in auscultation have frequencies below 100 vibrations per second, and most sounds are below 500, the ear is, unfortunately, at its poorest in the range where the main portion of the heart sounds and murmurs occurs.

Although loudness and intensity are thus, in a strict sense, not the same, in general and throughout this book the term *intensity* is used in the same sense as *loudness.*

Associated with intensity is the phenomenon of "masking" — a reduction in the ability of the ear to hear certain sounds in the presence of other sounds. The ear adjusts itself to the intensity of the sound that it is receiving. A loud sound causes the ear to protect itself by cutting down on its ability to receive sound. If a faint sound follows immediately on a loud sound, the ear is not adjusted to hear it. Because of this phenomenon, faint murmurs that follow loud sounds are heard with difficulty, or not at all. The same is true of faint sounds that follow loud murmurs.

Masking of a different type occurs when a complex sound — one consisting of several tones of different frequencies — undergoes an increase or decrease of intensity. At any given level of intensity, masking of some of the tones by others is likely to occur. The masking effects will, however, vary with intensity. With changes in intensity, some tones may become masked or unmasked and thus change the quality of the sound. When a murmur is transmitted to a different area of the chest and the intensity diminishes, the quality of the sound may change sufficiently to raise some doubt as to whether the murmur is actually a transmitted murmur.

In addition to pitch, quality and loudness, sounds have *duration*, in that they may be short or long. The spacing of sounds in relationship to other sounds gives rise to *timing*.

Transmission of Sound

Sounds produced in and about the heart are heard only after transmission to the chest wall and then to the ear. Some of the factors involved in the transmission of sound are as follows:

1. As sound leaves the source, the intensity diminishes with the square of the distance from the source. On the basis of this factor, sounds should usually be loudest in that part of the chest closest to the point at which the sound is produced; however, other factors often disturb this relationship.

2. As sound is transmitted to the chest wall, it is influenced by reflections that take place at changes in media, i.e., from heart to surrounding muscles, to chest wall or lung. When sound passes from one medium to another, part of the sound is reflected and part passes through. Various factors influence the amount of reflection, but difference in density of the tissues at the interphase is most important. If the media are of approximately the same density, most of the sound passes on and only a small part is reflected; if the media are markedly different in density, a large portion of the sound is reflected. Tissues such as blood and muscle are of about the same den-

sity, and the sound passes through them without much reflection. On the other hand, the lungs, with their air spaces, have a lower density, and sound in going from muscle to lung and from lung to the chest wall suffers a great deal of reflection and is not well transmitted. Because there is such a difference in the densities of the chest wall and of air, only the very loudest sounds can be heard unaided outside the chest.

3. When sound passes through a medium, there is a loss of intensity due to acoustical damping within the medium. Some organs and tissues, such as the lungs and subcutaneous fat, exert a more marked damping effect than others. This damping may be very marked, and the energy of the vibrations at the body surface may be a very small fraction (sometimes as small as a millionth) of the energy of the murmur at its origin. Higher frequencies are damped more than lower frequencies; therefore, the sound, in addition to losing intensity, may also undergo a change in quality, since this depends on the relative frequency makeup of that sound. Thus, as one follows the same murmur over the chest, the quality may change. This change and the change in quality due to masking must be remembered in deciding whether there are one or two murmurs on the basis of the quality of the murmur heard in different areas.

4. Vibrations produced in the heart are probably propagated in the body tissues as low-velocity transverse vibrations, rather than as longitudinal compression waves which would travel with the speed of sound in tissues. The velocity of these transverse waves is about 15–20 meters per second—only one hundredth of the velocity of compressional waves. These transverse vibrations travel over the heart, and where the chamber is in contact with the chest wall, the vibrations emerge and spread across the surface of the chest. The areas where the vibrations emerge on the chest wall constitute the *auscultatory areas*, which have long been associated with the various heart sounds and murmurs.

CHAPTER 2

The Stethoscope

Description

FOR TRANSMISSION OF THE SOUNDS from the chest wall to the ear, the binaural stethoscope is the most commonly used, and the observations described in this book have been made with this stethoscope. Various types of stethoscopes are used, and a basic knowledge of the properties of each is essential. Since stethoscopes have a certain individuality, it is wise to become familiar with one type and use it most of the time.

Although numerous modifications of the stethoscope have been made since Laennec devised the original instrument over 150 years ago, there is still no general agreement on what the characteristics of a stethoscope should be in order to best transmit chest sounds to the ear. Unfortunately, the choice of a stethoscope usually depends upon which instrument is most convenient to carry or is advertised the most. Attempts to compare stethoscopes experimentally have resulted in no general consensus. The experimental procedures are frequently quite artificial and the conclusions drawn cannot be accepted because of obvious flaws in the procedures. Conclusions drawn on a theoretical basis alone are inadequate if not experimentally confirmed. When data obtained by an experimental method (often with obvious flaws) are at variance with accumulated experience of a host of expert auscultationists over the years, it would seem safe to question the data. What will be said here about the characteristics of a good stethoscope represents the experience and experimental work of the authors.

5

EAR PIECES. — For the transmission of sound through a stethoscope, the system should be airtight; any leak markedly attenuates the sounds and permits external sounds to enter the system. The defect is thus more serious in a noisy room than in a quiet room. It is important that the ear pieces be of the right size and shape and that they fit the ear well; the axis of the ear piece should be parallel to the long axis of the external auditory canal. Enough tension must be present in the spring to hold the ear pieces tightly in place. Poor fitting of ear pieces is probably the most common defect in stethoscopes.

TUBES. — On a theoretical and experimental basis, the more firm the tubing, the better the conduction of sound; thus, a metal tubing, although obviously unusable, would be best. However, plastic tubing, especially with a 1/16-inch wall is only slightly less effective. Conduction by rubber tubing will vary with the softness of the tubing and the thickness of the wall. When the wall is fairly thick and the rubber is rather stiff, the conduction may be as good as that with plastic tubing. Frequencies under 500 cycles per second are transmitted almost equally well by metal, plastic and rubber; it is only the higher frequencies that are affected, and then not too significantly.

It has been thought that the volume of the air in the stethoscope should be kept at a minimum; thus, keeping the tubing short and using a 1/8-inch tube bore have been considered important. This would appear to be a mistaken concept since conduction down a tube depends on the resistance in the tube and not on air volume. The resistance in a tube depends, among other factors, on the radius of the tube and the length of the tube. Within limits, the greater the internal diameter, the better the conduction. Thus with tubes of equal length a tube of 3/16-inch internal diameter conducts sounds much better than one of 1/8-inch diameter, and one of 1/4 inch conducts even better than a 3/16-inch tube. The longer the tube, the greater the loss, but the increase in tubing bore is a more important factor, so that a longer tube of 3/16-inch diameter will conduct sounds better than does a shorter tube of 1/8-inch diameter. Using tubing with a 3/16-inch diameter, no significant difference in the functioning of a stethoscope can be noted between tubing 10 inches in length and tubing 15 inches long.

When discussing tubing length, another possible factor should be considered. Conduction of sound by the stethoscope results in peaks and valleys due to resonant factors in the stethoscope. The frequencies of the peaks and valleys are determined in great part by the length of the stethoscope, and in the case of lower frequencies the peaks actually represent an amplification of the sound. The longer the stethoscope, the lower the frequency of the initial peak and the more frequent the peaks. The importance of this factor has not yet been evaluated and it is possible that longer tubing may be advantageous at times.

To summarize, (1) plastic tubing appears to be best, (2) the tubing should have an internal diameter of a least ³/₁₆ inch, and (3) the length of the stethoscope may not be as critical as was previously considered.

Of great importance is the question of whether to use a double- or single-tube stethoscope. A single-tube stethoscope has certain mechanical advantages: its bulk is less, the noise due to rubbing of the tubes on each other is not present, and there is a smaller surface to pick up outside noise. On the other hand, there is some experimental work to indicate that the single-tube stethoscope is inferior to the double-tube stethoscope in conducting sounds in the 150–300 cycles per second frequency range. This is, of course, a highly significant range. The deficiency in conduction is most evident if the internal diameter of the tubing is ⅛ inch, but it is also present to a lesser degree with larger internal diameters. Because this experimental work confirms our clinical experience, we are inclined to accept the experimental work and, therefore, prefer a double-tube stethoscope. It should be pointed out, however, that there is some difference of opinion on this subject among various workers.

CHEST PIECES. — There are two basic types of chest pieces, the bell type and the diaphragm type. Bell chest pieces are of different sizes and shapes. The larger the diameter of the bell, the more efficiently it picks up low-pitched sounds. However, there is difficulty in placing the larger bells on the chests of thin patients and children. The 1-inch diameter has been most commonly accepted as being of sufficient size and still small enough for good placement. The Leatham stethoscope (Fig 2–1, B), because it provides a bell of larger diameter, when it can be used, has a definite advantage for listening to low-pitched sounds. The internal configuration of the bell should

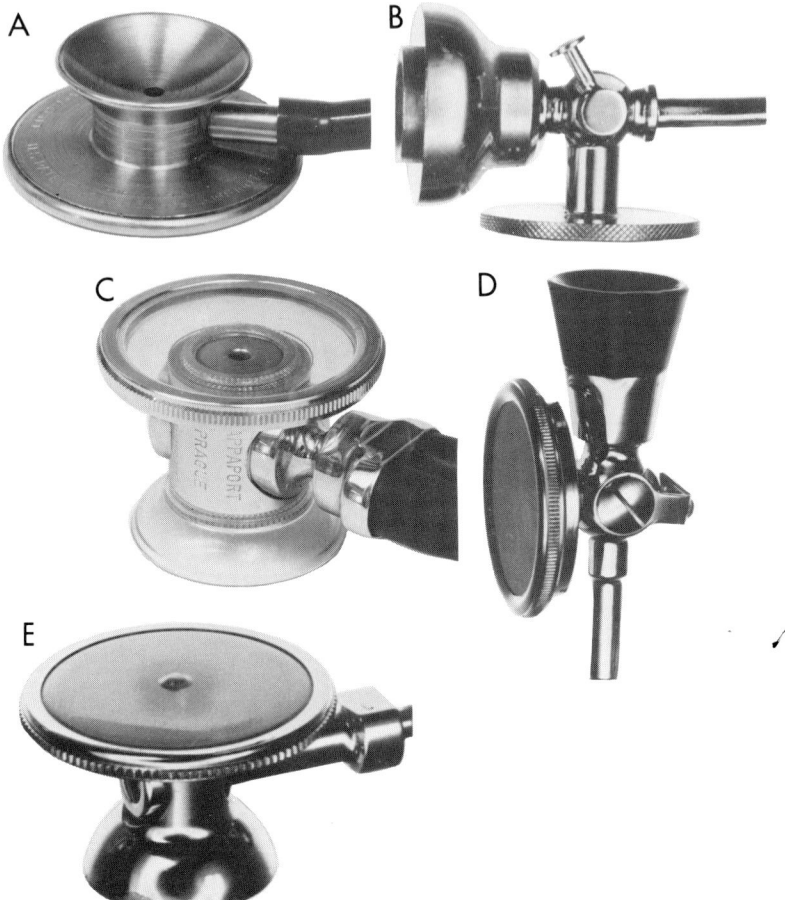

Fig 2–1.—Stethoscope chest pieces (see text). **A,** Littman. **B,** Leatham. **C,** Sprague-Rappaport. **D,** Sprague-Bowles. **E,** Tycos (Howell type).

be one which keeps the volume as low as possible but does not easily fill with skin and thus decrease the effective diameter. The bell chest piece, if used correctly, is best for low-pitched sounds.

Since many heart sounds are in the low-frequency range and best evaluated using the bell chest piece, it is this device to which we have directed our attention recently. Few commercially available stethoscopes come equipped with an adequate bell. In fact, large-diameter bells with thin edges are rare. We use a large, simple bell made of aluminum, fashioned by hand, and designed for maximum sound-gathering (large diameter) and pickup of low-frequency sounds (thin edge that allows a tight seal with minimum pressure). It is made to fit several commercial models, primarily the inexpensive ones readily available to students and house officers. It has proven effective in adult patients. This bell, attached to a familiar Bowles-type stethoscope, is shown in Figure 2–2.

The diaphragm chest pieces likewise vary in shape and size but a diameter of 1⅜ inches is most commonly used. The diaphragm has a relatively high natural frequency of vibration and therefore transmits well those frequencies at or above its natural vibration frequency but attenuates lower frequencies. When the diaphragm is firmly applied to the chest wall (as it should be), damping of the lower frequencies also occurs as a result of the phenomenon described on page 13. Because of these effects, the diaphragm is valuable for hearing high-pitched murmurs and sounds and it helps overcome the mask-

• **Fig 2–2.**—The large, deep bell chest piece is best for detection of low-pitched, low-amplitude sounds. With firm pressure, its thin edge and large size make an efficient "diaphragm" of the skin.

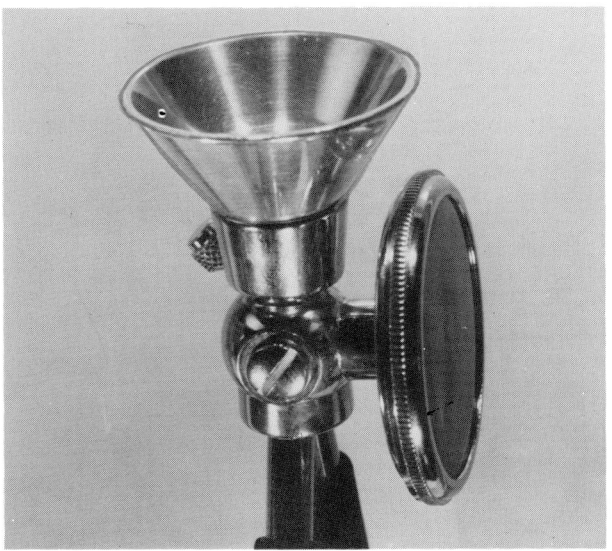

ing effects of low-pitched, loud sounds or faint, high-pitched murmurs which may follow them. A loss in intensity due to the rigidity of the diaphragm is partially compensated for by the increased size of the diaphragm as compared to the bell. The characteristics of a diaphragm chest piece depend on the rigidity of the diaphragm. The stiffer the diaphragm, the higher its natural frequency of vibrations, and the more effectively it will cut off lower frequencies. It does, however, at the same time cut down markedly on the overall sound intensity. The diaphragm can be so soft that it is almost as effective as the bell for low-pitched vibrations but it will not, as a result, be as effective for listening to high-frequency sounds. On the other hand, the diaphragm may be so stiff that it cuts the overall intensity of sound so markedly that it is practically useless. The ideal diaphragm should have a rigidity that cuts off the low frequencies but still transmits high frequencies adequately.

It is questionable whether the newer, more expensive stethoscopes now available have any advantage over, or are in fact as good as, a well-fitted Sprague-Bowles stethoscope (see Fig 2–1).

Amplifying Stethoscopes

These stethoscopes are of value to physicians whose hearing is deficient, but they should not be used as a substitute for a quiet room. Most murmurs of significance can be heard without any amplification. Amplifying stethoscopes with filters are of value for training oneself and for teaching. In any system with amplification, the sound may be different from that ordinarily heard with the binaural stethoscope. The examiner must understand his instrument and be able to recognize the artifacts that are inherent in the instrument and those that result from technical and mechanical difficulties.

Phonocardiography

The production of more adequate instruments for recording heart sounds and murmurs, and a better understanding of the physical principles involved, have opened up a new field of investigative work. With these instruments several advantages are evident: (1) the full spectrum of frequencies can be recorded and a permanent record can be obtained; (2) amplification permits a better study of faint sounds; (3) recording other cardiac events at the same time permits the timing of sounds and murmurs with accuracy; and (4) by the use of filters, vibrations of selected frequency ranges can be recorded. Such recording permits a study of the frequency makeup of murmurs.

Phonocardiography had its origin in auscultation but has become a sophisticated field which feeds auscultation. It has expanded into a science of its own with applications that are not related to bedside auscultation. Some have additional clinical value; many have mainly research value. Phonocardiography is an excellent means of increasing one's knowledge of auscultation. It supplements, but does not replace, auscultation.

A record of heart sounds is only as good as the person who takes it. To have the technician put a microphone in a stated heart area and take a record is essentially worthless. The recordings vary with (1) small changes in location; (2) amplification; (3) background noise in the machine, room and patient; (4) vagaries of the recording instrument and the skill with which the instrument is used; (5) the type of chest piece; and (6) structural factors in the patient.

Spectral phonocardiography differs from conventional phonocardiography principally in that the frequency spectrum of the sounds and murmurs is more evident. This permits a better definition of quality. *Intracardiac phonocardiography* has opened up a new field for investigation. Thus far, the results, for those interested in bedside auscultation, have been very gratifying in that they confirm much that was accepted or suspected. It presents diagnostic possibilities not otherwise available.

Use of the Stethoscope

QUIET BACKGROUND. — Much of what is wrong with everyday auscultation results from its being hurriedly done in a noisy room. For satisfactory auscultation, the room *must* be quiet. One often has the experience of hearing a faint murmur one day and not the next. A common cause is the variation of the level of background noise. When one physician is listening, other members of a group must be quiet. Auscultation in a room that has been soundproofed or partially soundproofed is often a revelation even to one who is familiar with the disturbing effect of external noise. The patient should be comfortable and warm to avoid muscular noises. Frequently, respiration of the patient must be suspended and nasal oxygen temporarily discontinued while one is listening.

POSITION OF THE PATIENT. — For a thorough examination, auscultation must be done with the patient in a sitting, lying, and left lateral recumbent position. An adequate examination can possibly be done in the recumbent position alone, but listening to the heart with the patient only in a sitting position is absolutely inadequate. Typical diastolic murmurs of good intensity when the patient is lying down may not be heard at all when the patient is sitting. In the recumbent position, the patient's arms must not be held over the head, since this will elevate the rib cage and decrease the intensity of the heart sound. Positions most commonly of value for different murmurs will be discussed later.

For most physicians, especially those who are right-handed, listening from the right side of the patient seems more natural and puts the stethoscope in a better position. Sometimes moving one's head up and down will reveal a position in which sounds seem to be heard better.

Occasionally it is advantageous to listen with the patient in the prone position; this may be true in patients with deep chests or those who may have a friction sound. This position is awkward when the patient is in bed or on the examining table and supporting himself by his elbows. It is much more satisfactory to have the patient stand up and lean over in the position shown in Figure 2-3. Muscle noise is at a minimum in this position, and the patient and examiner are much more comfortable. An important additional advantage of this position is that the patient can be made to exercise by touching his toes several times before he assumes the position.

APPLICATION OF THE CHEST PIECE TO THE CHEST WALL. — Although every physician uses a stethoscope, very few have been taught or have learned by themselves that in the use of the bell chest piece there is marked variation in what is heard, depending upon whether the bell is applied very lightly or heavily to the chest wall. When the bell is applied very lightly,

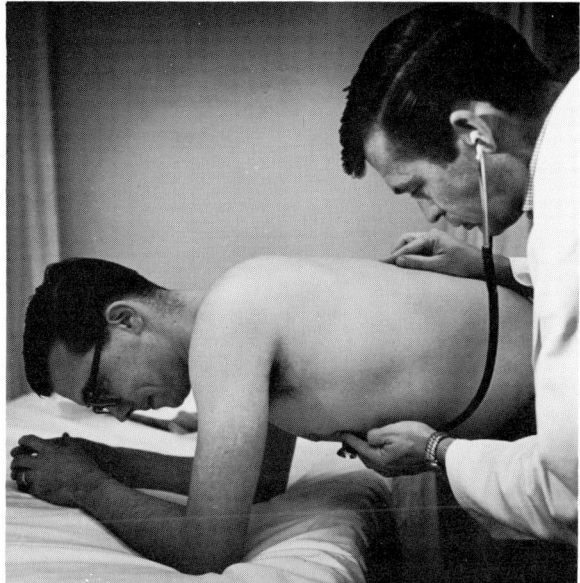

Fig 2–3.—The standing-flexion position. This position is of value when the heart sounds are faint due to a deep chest or emphysema and when a friction rub is being sought.

low-pitched sounds are well heard. Such sounds are atrial sounds, third heart sounds, the middiastolic murmur of mitral stenosis, and often the first heart sound. With heavy application of the bell, the loudness of these sounds is markedly diminished in most individuals (Fig 2–4), especially if the amount of subcutaneous tissue is abundant. The difference in loudness of middiastolic murmurs, third heart sounds, and atrial sounds is of a degree that affects the ability to hear, or not to hear, these sounds. Third heart sounds are infrequently heard, partly because the pressure of the bell on the skin is too great.

This phenomenon has been explained (Rappaport and Sprague, 1941) as follows: When the bell is applied to the skin, the enclosed skin forms a diaphragm. With increased pressure, the skin diaphragm is made more taut and its natural period of oscillation increases. This improves the response to higher pitches, but at the same time there is a general lower-

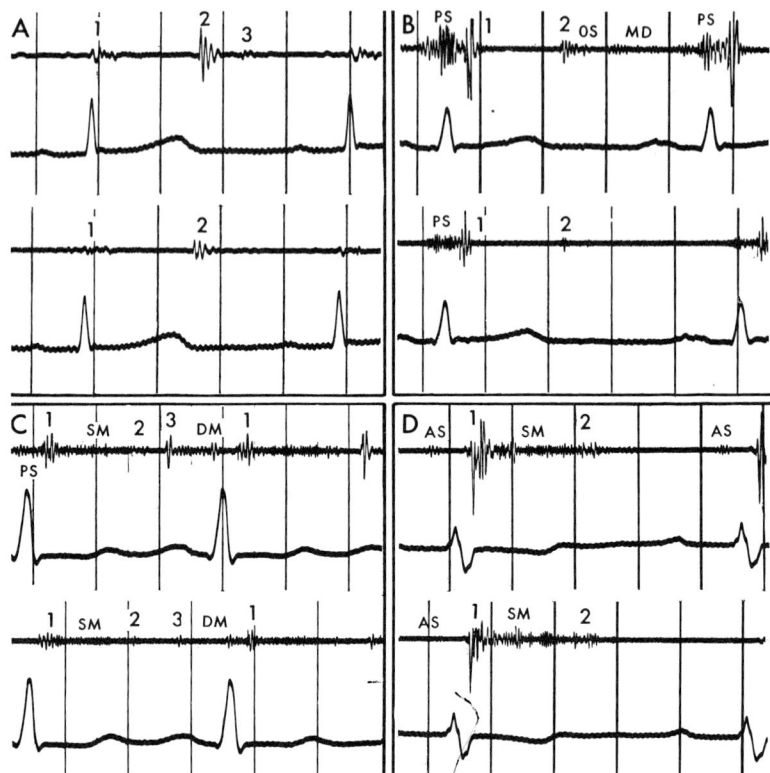

Fig 2–4. — Effect on heart sounds and murmurs of pressure on bell chest piece. In each case, the upper tracing was taken with the bell chest piece held lightly, and the lower tracing with the bell chest piece applied with pressure.

A, normal child. With light pressure, all three heart sounds are clearly heard. With pressure, the first sound becomes very faint, the second sound is less intense but well heard, and the third sound is not heard.

B, patient with mitral stenosis. The upper tracing shows a loud presystolic murmur *(PS)* and a loud first heart sound. The second sound is followed by a faint opening snap *(OS)* and a middiastolic murmur *(MD)*. The rate is slow, and the middiastolic murmur begins to fade before atrial contraction produces a loud presystolic murmur. With pressure on the bell chest piece *(lower tracing)*, the presystolic murmur, which in this case is a rather rough murmur, continues to be well heard, although it is less intense. The first and second heart sounds are diminished in intensity. No middiastolic murmur is heard. In nearly all patients with mitral stenosis, a middiastolic murmur is ing of the sensitivity of the skin diaphragm. As a result, the lower-frequency components of the heart sounds are attenuated, whereas the higher frequencies are still well heard.

This important maneuver of being able to diminish the intensity of low-pitched sounds by pressure on the bell has several implications and applications:

1. To hear faint, low-pitched sounds, the examiner *must* apply the bell lightly to the chest wall.

2. By noting what happens to a sound or murmur when the bell is first applied lightly, and then with pressure, the examiner can judge, to a certain degree, the pitch of a sound or murmur.

3. The high-pitched systolic murmur of mitral regurgitation is less likely to be affected by pressure than are medium-pitched, innocent systolic murmurs.

4. With pressure, the faint, high-pitched, systolic murmur of mitral regurgitation is less affected than is the first heart sound, and the masking effect of the first heart sound is thus diminished. The same is true of the high-pitched, early diastolic murmur of aortic regurgitation and an accentuated second heart sound.

5. In some very noisy hearts with both systolic and diastolic murmurs, it is difficult, because of the amount of sound in systole, to be sure if there is a low-pitched diastolic murmur; with pressure, the total sound is diminished and the low-pitched

---

present, but because of its low pitch, it may not be heard if the stethoscope is applied with too much pressure. The presystolic murmur, which is more rough, continues to be heard.

C, patient with marked mitral regurgitation. Upper tracing shows a systolic murmur *(SM)* persisting throughout systole, a rather faint second sound, and a well-heard third heart sound. Because of the rapid rate, the rumbling diastolic murmur *(DM)* is essentially presystolic. In the lower tracing, the systolic murmur, as recorded, seems somewhat less intense, but this is merely because of a decrease in a few of the lower-pitched vibrations, and actually the systolic murmur to the ear is very little changed. The third heart sound and diastolic murmur are markedly diminished.

D, patient with an atrial septal defect. *Upper tracing:* A clear atrial sound *(AS)* is present. The first sound is followed by a systolic murmur *(SM)* and a split second sound. *Lower tracing:* With pressure, the atrial sound can no longer be heard, although the phonocardiogram shows a few small vibrations.

murmur in diastole may disappear. By holding the bell alternately lightly and heavily and by concentrating on diastole, the examiner can detect the diastolic rumble.

As the size of the bell is increased to over 1 inch in diameter, pressure is less effective in tensing the skin. A larger bell, therefore, has the advantage of picking up low-pitched sounds, even if the examiner is careless in the amount of pressure he applies; this, together with the greater collection area, makes a large bell valuable for low-pitched sounds. On the

Fig 2–5. — Application of the bell to the chest wall. **A,** correct manner. The bell should be applied with as little pressure as is necessary to make an air seal. **B,** incorrect manner. Too much pressure has been applied and low frequency sounds will be damped and not heard.

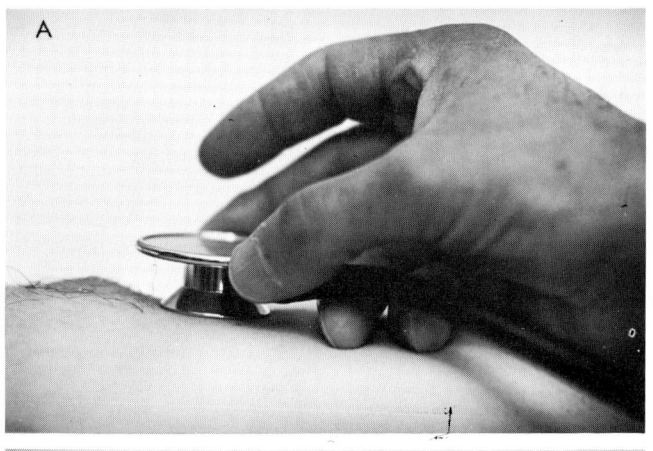

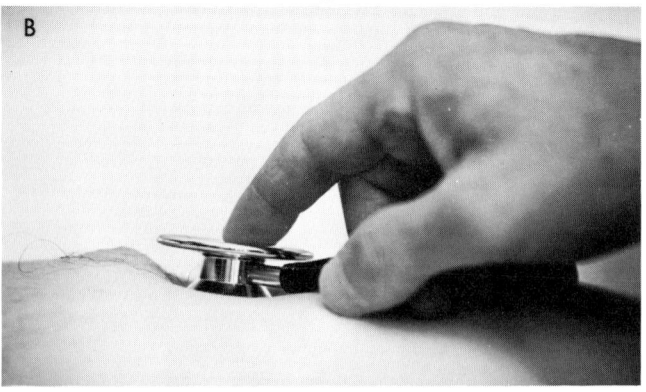

other hand, the larger bell is less effective for determining the effect of pressure on sounds and murmurs.

To apply the bell lightly means application with just enough pressure to make an air seal. This can be done only if the stethoscope endpiece is held as shown in Figure 2–5, A. The endpieces of the newer stethoscopes are not built to be held easily in this position, and this represents a definite defect. The tendency is to press the bell down as shown in Figure 2–5, B.

In contrast to the bell, the diaphragm should be applied with firm pressure.

LOCATION ON THE CHEST WALL.—Too often, auscultation consists of applying the stethoscope merely to the apex. Most murmurs are called *apical* because the apex is the only area where the stethoscope is placed. Whereas auscultation at the apex, the fourth left intercostal space, and the second right and left intercostal spaces may be sufficient when nothing unusual is heard, tracing the point of maximum intensity and transmission of a murmur may require listening in numerous areas over the chest and into the neck, back, lung bases, and even elbows.

The apical area of the heart is usually formed by the left ventricle and it is here that sounds produced at the mitral valve and in the left ventricle are best heard. The area just to the left of the lower end of the sternum is over the right ventricle, and here the sounds produced at the tricuspid valve and in the right ventricle are best heard. Sounds produced at the aortic valve and aorta are usually heard best in the second intercostal space to the right of the sternum, and those at the pulmonary valve and pulmonary artery are usually best heard in the second intercostal space just to the left of the sternum (see Fig 7–1, p. 97).

LISTENING TO THE HEART.—It is true that the physician proficient in auscultation may often quickly recognize a lesion, just as he recognizes a "dog by its bark." Most physicians are not trained to the point at which they can do this, and in many hearts, because of multiple modifying factors, the "bark" may be well disguised and not easily recognized. It may be necessary to listen long and repeatedly to understand and analyze what is heard.

The untrained person must learn to analyze separately the various sounds and phases of the heart cycle. Man has the capacity to direct his attention to the sound he wants to hear. He can listen to the person talking in front of him or ignore what is being said and listen to distant sounds. This ability to direct attention is the keynote to successful auscultation. One listens to the first heart sound, then to the second heart sound, and then specifically to systole and to diastole. Sounds other than those being listened to are ignored. This method permits the ear to hear all that should be heard and partially to overcome masking. We have often had the experience, after listening intently for a middiastolic murmur for several minutes in various positions, of being asked whether there was a systolic murmur and being unable to answer because we had not been listening to systole. One of the greatest aids in learning to direct attention is the graphic method of recording described below.

A sense of rhythm helps in auscultation, and the examiner often subconsciously beats out a cadence while listening. If a third heart sound is being listened for and the examiner beats out "lub-dub-puh" in his mind while listening to the heart, he more easily directs his attention to the point of the cycle where the "puh" should be heard.

CHAPTER 3

Graphic Recording of Auscultation

H. N. SEGALL in 1933 described a graphic method for recording auscultatory findings which has many advantages over
written descriptions. (1) The examiner is forced to listen carefully and separate what is heard into its components — a procedure that, as has been previously emphasized, is the founda-
tion of good auscultation. (2) What is heard can be graphically
shown in a fraction of time taken for writing the same data.
(3) The graphic description is usually much more complete
than a written description, because one cannot ignore or forget
to describe some of the findings. "A systolic murmur was
heard at the apex" may suffice for a written description, but
graphically the intensity and pitch of the murmur must be
shown and its relation to the first and second sounds indicated. (4) A glance serves to show what has been heard, and a
comparison with previous auscultations can be made easily.
The graphic method, with minor modifications from Segall's
original description, has been used throughout this book.

The heart sounds are represented by rectangular blocks,
with the height of the block indicating loudness and the width
indicating duration of the sound. By diagraming the first and
second sounds in one cycle and the first sound of the next cycle, the length of systole and diastole may be shown. Thus, the
sounds at the apex might be indicated as in Figure 3–1, A. A
third heart sound is shown in Figure 3–1, B. The pitch of a
sound is not shown, but if it is unusual it may be indicated by a
word or phrase. A slightly split first heart sound is shown in

19

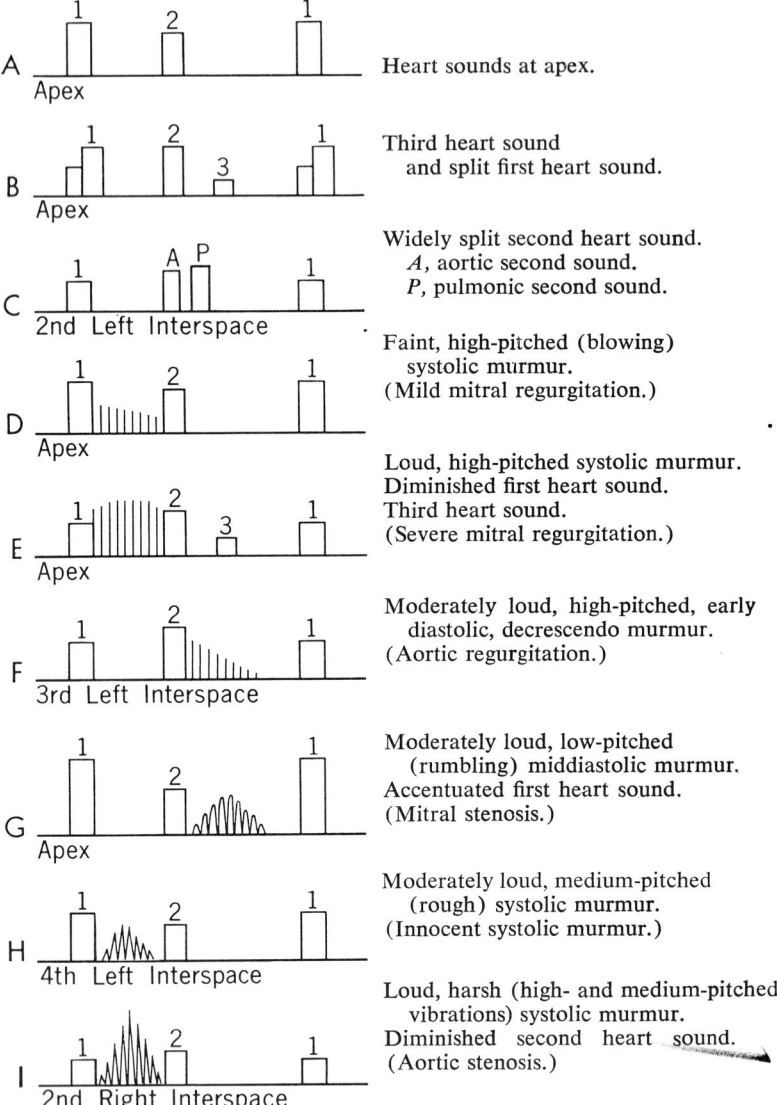

A — Heart sounds at apex.

B — Third heart sound
and split first heart sound.

C — Widely split second heart sound.
A, aortic second sound.
P, pulmonic second sound.

D — Faint, high-pitched (blowing)
systolic murmur.
(Mild mitral regurgitation.)

E — Loud, high-pitched systolic murmur.
Diminished first heart sound.
Third heart sound.
(Severe mitral regurgitation.)

F — Moderately loud, high-pitched, early
diastolic, decrescendo murmur.
(Aortic regurgitation.)

G — Moderately loud, low-pitched
(rumbling) middiastolic murmur.
Accentuated first heart sound.
(Mitral stenosis.)

H — Moderately loud, medium-pitched
(rough) systolic murmur.
(Innocent systolic murmur.)

I — Loud, harsh (high- and medium-pitched
vibrations) systolic murmur.
Diminished second heart sound.
(Aortic stenosis.)

Fig 3–1.—Symbols used in graphic recording of auscultation.

Figure 3–1, B. A more widely split second heart sound is shown in Figure 3–1, C.

A high-pitched, blowing murmur is represented by closely placed vertical lines. Timing and duration are shown in relation to the heart sounds. The height of the lines indicates the loudness. A faint, high-pitched systolic murmur and a loud, high-pitched systolic murmur are indicated in Figure 3– 1, D and E, respectively. A high-pitched, early diastolic murmur is shown in Figure 3– 1, F. A low-pitched, rumbling murmur is indicated by rounded humps. A low-pitched middiastolic murmur is shown in Figure 3– 1, G. Medium-pitched, rough murmurs are indicated by spikes; thus, a moderately loud, medium-pitched systolic murmur is indicated as in Figure 3– 1, H. Harsh murmurs are also indicated by spikes (Fig 3– 1, I). Medium-pitched murmurs rarely become loud without becoming harsh. The intensity then indicates whether the murmur is rough (medium pitched) or harsh (combination of high and medium frequencies).

The location on the chest at which the observations are made is recorded on a diagram of the chest with the heart outline and thoracic cage shown (Fig 3–2, A). The horizontal lines on the right and left are connected by lines to the area on the chest where the stethoscope is placed. For a guide in determining the size of the blocks used to indicate sounds, the standard for sounds at the apex is shown in the fine outline. The intensity of the first heart sound as shown at the apex is considered to be moderately loud or $^3/_6$ on the scale described on page 89. A moderately loud murmur would be drawn to the same height. The expected intensity of the sounds in the second right interspace is also shown, and in this line the second sound is shown as moderately loud or of $^3/_6$ intensity. Since the positions of the first and second sounds are fixed on all the lines, diastole will be of different length for different heart rates. The comparative lengths of diastole at rates of 120, 90, 75 and 60 are indicated by the four marks near the end of each line. When a first sound is placed in the correct rate position, systole and diastole have the expected duration for the observed rate; thus, at a rate of 120, systole and diastole are of approximately equal length, whereas at a rate of 75, diastole is about one and a half times as long as systole.

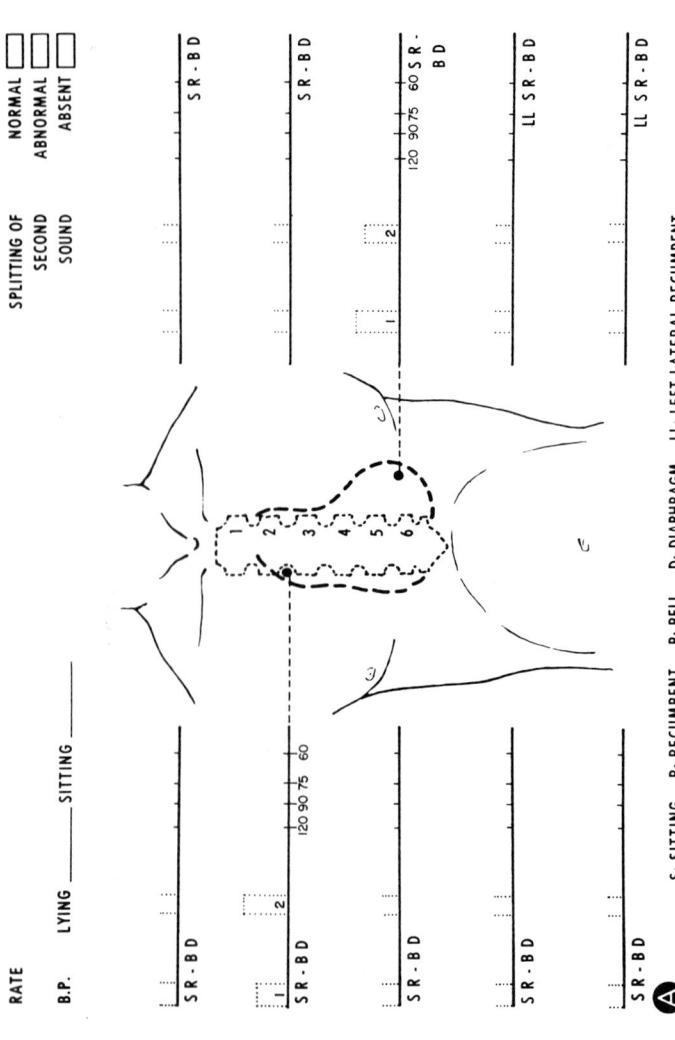

RATE

B.P. LYING _____ SITTING _____

SPLITTING OF SECOND SOUND

NORMAL ▢
ABNORMAL ▢
ABSENT ▢

120 90 75 60

120 90 75 60

S R - B D
S R - B D
S R - B D
S R - B D
S R - B D

S R - B D
S R - B D
S R - B D
LL S R - B D
LL S R - B D

S: SITTING   R: RECUMBENT   B: BELL   D: DIAPHRAGM   LL: LEFT LATERAL RECUMBENT

Fig 3–2.—A, diagram of the chest used for recording the results of auscultation. The standard for the heart sounds at the apex is shown in fine outline on the horizontal line connected to the apex. The expected intensity of the sounds in the second right interspace is also shown. The first heart sound at the apex and the second heart sound in the second right interspace are considered as being of $^3/_6$ intensity. Since the positions of the first and second heart sounds are fixed on all the lines, diastole will be of different lengths for different heart rates. Comparative lengths of diastole at the rates of 120, 90, 75 and 60 are indicated by four marks near the end of each line. The first heart sound of the second cycle should be placed so that it starts at the correct rate. *(Continued.)*

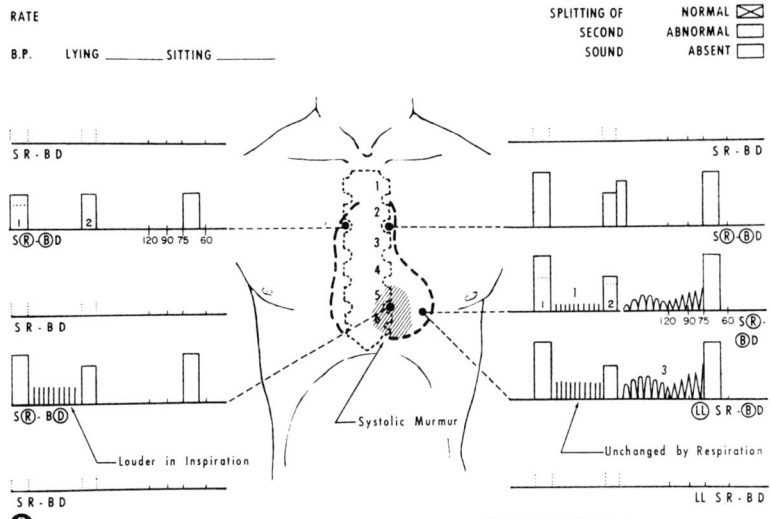

RATE

SPLITTING OF NORMAL ⊠
SECOND ABNORMAL ☐
SOUND ABSENT ☐

B.P.   LYING _____ SITTING _____

S: SITTING   R: RECUMBENT   B: BELL   D: DIAPHRAGM   LL: LEFT LATERAL RECUMBENT

Fig 3–2 (cont.)–B, the use of the chart for the graphic representation of auscultatory findings. The symbols used are described in the text and in Figure 3–1. The dots indicate the location on the chest wall where the stethoscope is placed. The heart rate is 75 as indicated by the fact that the first sound of the second cycle starts at the 75 mark.

The findings at the apex are illustrated for two positions; recumbent *(R)* and the left lateral recumbent *(LL)*. The bell *(B)* was used for listening in both positions. The first heart sound is accentuated as indicated by the fact that it is taller than the faintly outlined first heart sound at the apex. A faint, high-pitched, systolic murmur is present. The number "1" indicates the intensity grade of the murmur (p. 89); the intensity grade is not essential but is occasionally helpful. The intensity can be recognized in this case by comparison with the faintly outlined first sound at the apex which is of ³/₆ intensity. Since this murmur was not changed by respiration (in contrast to another systolic murmur), the phrase "unchanged by respiration" is added on the chart. A moderately loud, low-pitched, rumbling, middiastolic murmur with a presystolic accentuation is present. The number 3 above the murmur is the intensity grade. The same observation regarding intensity is made by comparing this murmur with the faintly outlined first heart sound. The presystolic portion of the murmur is of higher pitch than the middiastolic portion (peaked tops instead of rounded tops). The murmur is louder in the left lateral position than in the recumbent position. The illustrated auscultatory findings are those of a tight mitral stenosis with a slight mitral regurgitation.

Also shown in the diagram is the presence of a faint, high-pitched, systolic murmur localized to a small area at the lower end of the sternum *(shaded area)* and showing an increased loudness on inspiration. This is the murmur of tricuspid regurgitation.

The heart sounds in the second right and second left intercostal spaces are shown. Splitting of the second sound is normal.

The chest piece used in auscultation is indicated by circling the B (bell) or D (diaphragm), and the position of the patient is shown by circling the S (sitting), R (recumbent), or LL (left lateral recumbent).

If the aortic and pulmonic components of the second sound are evident in the second left intercostal space on inspiration, they are both shown. To indicate that they are single or closely split in expiration, *Normal Splitting* is checked. If only one sound is heard on inspiration and expiration, it is diagramed and *Absent Splitting* is checked. If splitting is abnormal, both inspiration and expiration should be diagramed.

The loudness of the murmurs can be judged by comparison with the finely outlined first sound at the apex and second sound in the second right interspace, both of which are considered to be ³⁄₆ (Fig 3–2, A). To make comparisons more exact, one may, at times, place along with the murmurs the loudness number. In Figure 3–2, B, an accentuated first sound, a very faint (grade 1) high-pitched systolic murmur, and a moderately loud (grade 3) low-pitched diastolic murmur (middiastolic and presystolic) are represented at the apex. The bell chest piece was used and the findings at the apex are shown with the patient in both the recumbent and left lateral recumbent positions.

The point of maximum intensity of a murmur may be indicated by an *X* on the diagram, and the area in which a murmur is heard may be shaded.

If the examiner knows, for example, that the first sound must be shown, he listens to see if it is normal, accentuated or diminished, or split. The same is true for other sounds. If a murmur is present and shown in correct relation to the sounds, there can be no question as to whether it is systolic or diastolic. Time and again, a student will listen to a systolic murmur and interpret it as diastolic, or vice versa. If he is asked to listen to the first sound and record it, and then to the second sound and record it, the murmur is almost always correctly placed.

The tendency to careless listening and even more careless recording is avoided by this method. This method need not be used by all physicians on all patients, but it would be well for cardiologists to use it most of the time, and for most physicians to use it some of the time.

ALTERNATIVE METHOD FOR GRAPHIC RECORDING. — Other

methods for graphic recording of auscultation have been used. A commonly used method is one that mimics the phonocardiogram. The sounds, however, instead of being represented by vibrations, are represented by lines. Thus, the sounds at the apex might be represented as shown in Figure 3–3, A. Although relative intensity can be indicated, absolute intensity requires some additional sign or notation. If the time interval between slightly separated sounds can be estimated, it may be indicated (Fig 3–3, B).

Many physicians who used this system have become so accustomed to looking at phonocardiograms in which pitch and quality of murmurs are not clearly evident that they make no distinction between pitch and quality in their designation of the murmurs, and place the main emphasis on their form and duration. Thus, the harsh murmur of aortic stenosis and the blowing murmur of aortic regurgitation are indicated in the same manner as shown in Figure 3–3, C. This neglect of re-

Fig 3–3.—Alternative method for graphic representation of auscultation (see text).

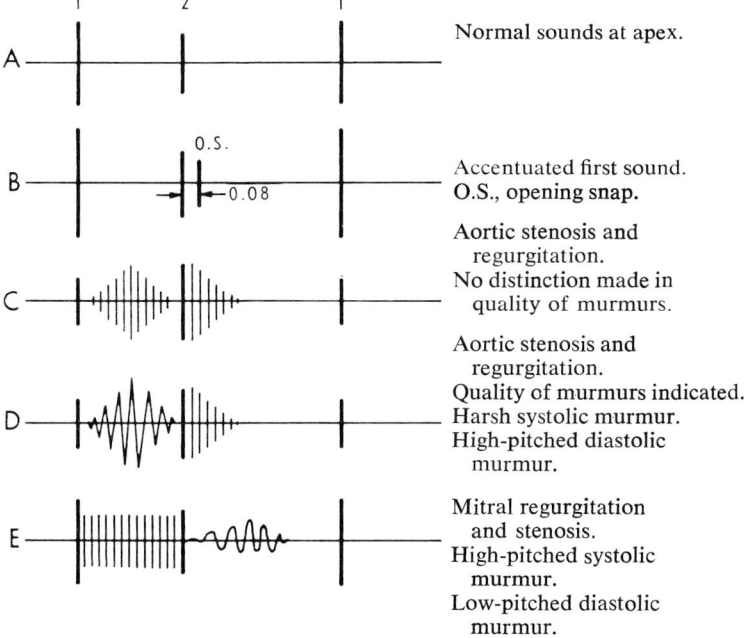

cording pitch and quality is unfortunate and should be avoided (p. 90). If the previously described designations for pitch and quality (p. 20) are used, this method can be quite effective. The murmur of aortic stenosis and regurgitation would be shown as in Figure 3–3, D, and the murmur of mitral regurgitation and stenosis would be indicated as in Figure 3–3, E. This method is not as easy to use on a chart with an outline of the heart as is the method used in this book.

CHAPTER 4

Heart Sounds

Timing of Heart Sounds

IF THE TIME RELATIONSHIP, pitch and intensity are characteristic, the first and second heart sounds are usually recognized with no difficulty; however, at rapid rates systole and diastole become almost equal in length (systole equals diastole at a rate of about 120), and the pitch and intensity of heart sounds may be widely altered. Occasionally, when a tachycardia causes confusion, the heart may be temporarily slowed by having the patient hold a deep breath or by pressure on the carotid sinus.

The first sound occurs at the onset of the apical impulse and the carotid pulsation. The sounds should *not* be timed by the radial pulse, which is just late enough to be confusing. The apical impulse is probably better than the carotid pulsation in most people. If the stethoscope or hand is placed at the apex, the first heart sound will be synchronous with the outward thrust.

Gradually moving the stethoscope from an area where the sounds are clear and timing definite to areas where timing is not clear will sometimes be of value.

The graphic recording of the heart sounds, together with an electrocardiogram, jugular pulse tracing, or apexcardiogram, is sometimes necessary for timing.

The introduction of echocardiography has provided an additional tool for timing heart sounds as well as for understanding the mechanisms of sound production in the heart (Fig 4 – 1).

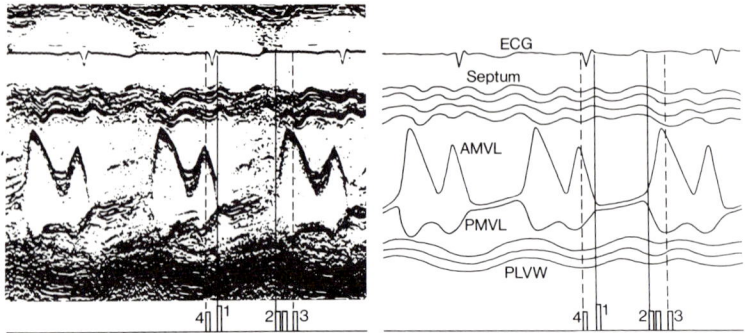

Fig 4–1.—Echocardiogram of a normal mitral valve. The first heart sound is commensurate with the coming together of the anterior and posterior mitral valve leaflets. The second heart sound occurs immediately prior to the separation of these leaflets. In diastole, the leaflets separate widely and then drift together as the initial rapid flow across the valve diminishes. With atrial contraction, the leaflets separate a second time due to increased flow across the valve, then oppose again immediately before the onset of systole. Note that a third heart sound, when it occurs, coincides with the maximal separation of the mitral leaflets, which is the time of peak blood flow into the left ventricle. A fourth heart sound, when it occurs, coincides with the second phase of leaflet separation associated with atrial contraction. This sound, like the third, occurs at a period of increased blood flow into the left ventricle and becomes audible when ventricular compliance is reduced. *AMVL,* anterior mitral valve leaflet; *PMVL,* posterior mitral valve leaflet; *PLVW,* posterior left ventricular wall.

First Heart Sound

DESCRIPTION

The first heart sound consists of several components with varied frequencies, and it cannot, therefore, be accurately classified as having a definite fundamental vibration; there is, rather, a group of vibrations. Those that seem most important in giving the auditory impression are in the 70–110 cycles per second range. As a group, these vibrations are only slightly lower in pitch than those of the second sound, but the second sound has more components among the higher frequencies. If, therefore, the bell chest piece is applied firmly to cut down on low-pitched vibrations (p. 12), the intensity of the first heart sound is decreased more than that of the second sound.

The hemodynamic events producing the major vibrations of the first heart sound have generally been referred to as *closure* of the mitral and tricuspid valves; the leaflets are probably already apposed prior to the first heart sound, thus *closure* is not strictly applicable. It seems likely that the origin of this sound is the abrupt tensing of the leaflets, chordae tendineae and papillary muscles (primarily the leaflets) occurring during the preejection period. There is some evidence that right-sided cardiac events play only a minor role in production of the first heart sound, but this is a current subject of much debate.

Phonocardiographic analysis of the first heart sound commonly shows four recognizable components. The first and fourth components are of low intensity and frequency and are not usually audible (Fig 4–2). The second and third components constitute the audible sound. The first, low-pitched, inaudible component is believed to result from development of tension in the ventricular musculature and the early motion of blood toward the mitral and tricuspid valves before they close. Often some residual vibrations of atrial origin occur at the very beginning of the first sound. The fourth component seems to be due to semilunar valve opening plus some contribution from vibrations of the great vessels (aorta and contained blood) at the onset of ejection. This component, by delay in onset and increased intensity, becomes the ejection click in semilunar valve stenosis.

The audible second and third components may produce a single sound, but often they can be recognized as separate sounds, although they are close together *(closely split)*. This normal splitting, when present, shows a characteristic pattern which can be recognized by listening first at the apex and gradually moving toward the sternum. At the apex, or somewhat lateral to the apex, the sound is usually single. Somewhere between the apex and the sternum, two components of about equal intensity may be recognized. Near the sternum, the split consists of a less intense first component, followed by a louder, somewhat sharper, second component. Near the sternum, the first component often has a crescendo character; and occasionally the impression of a presystolic murmur is erroneously obtained, especially if there is some tachycardia. Splitting is more evident in expiration.

Since hemodynamic studies indicate that the mitral valve closure occurs slightly before tricuspid closure, and since the first of the two audible components is loudest at the apex and

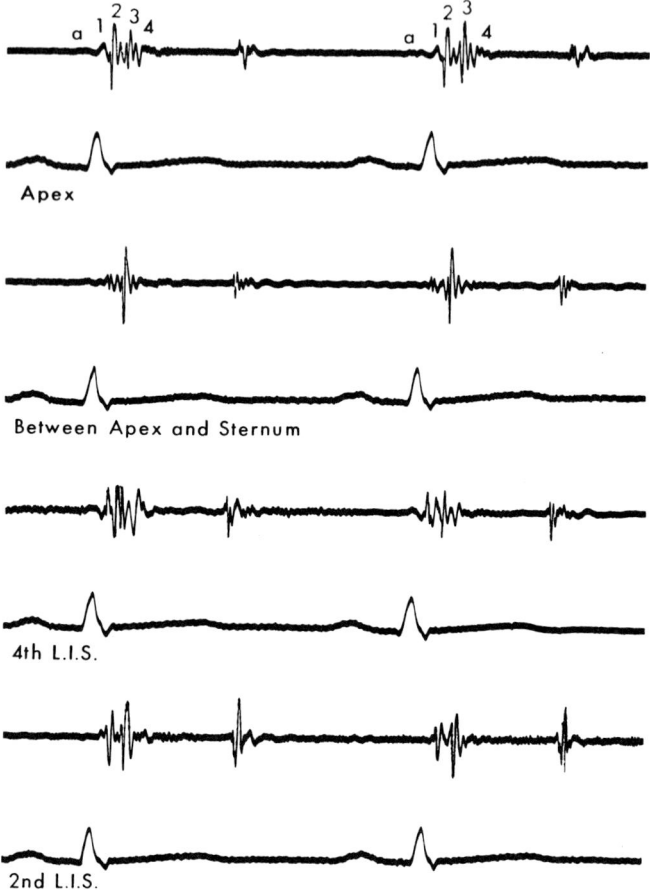

Apex

Between Apex and Sternum

4th L.I.S.

2nd L.I.S.

Fig 4–2. —Variation in the first heart sound in different locations. In the tracing at the apex, the four components of a first heart sound that can be recognized on a phonocardiogram are indicated. The first and fourth components are not usually heard. A fourth sound *(a)* is often evident on the phonocardiogram but not usually heard in normal persons. The variation in the components in different beats is produced by respiration.

The second and third components can often be distinguished on auscultation, especially when they are as clearly separated as in this patient. The first sound then consists of two components; usually the first component (actually the second component as noted above) is loudest at the apex and the second component is loudest along the left border of the sternum (see text). Even when the two components are as clearly separated in most areas as they are in this patient, a blending occurs in some areas (4th L.I.S.) that suggests that the first heart sound consists of more than a combination of two clear-cut components such as is seen in the case of the second heart sound.

the second along the left border of the sternum, it has been postulated that the first component of the sound is produced by the mitral valve and the second component by the tricuspid (see Fig 5–1, p. 54). This has not been accepted by all investigators in the field, but it forms a good working basis for explaining changes observed in various conditions.

The importance of factors other than the vibration of the mitral and tricuspid valve apparatus in the production of the first heart sound is still a matter of controversy. Even if the audible portion of the first sound is initiated by vibration of these structures, other phenomena may contribute. At the onset of ventricular contraction, as the blood moving toward the atria is suddenly arrested by the tautening of the atrioventricular valves, a general vibration is set up in the blood, ventricular musculature, papillary muscles, chordae tendineae, and valves. Each structure may contribute to the sound, although it is quite probable that most of the sound originates in the valves and chordae tendineae. It is also probable that the sudden acceleration of the blood at the end of isometric contraction, which results in the opening of the semilunar valves and the distention of the arteries above the valves, can at times produce audible vibrations which form a part of the first sound. Even when the first sound appears single to the ear, it is undoubtedly composed of several components that sound single, because the components are too close together to be recognized individually, or because there is masking of some components by others. Phonocardiograms often show what appears to be two components at the apex, while the ear will hear only one sound.

The first heart sound is usually loudest at the apex. In this region it is generally louder than the second heart sound, but the two sounds may be of about equal loudness, and the second sound may, at times, be louder than the first, especially if the bell chest piece is applied too firmly. Not infrequently, the first heart sound is louder in the fourth left interspace than it is elsewhere in the precordium. At the base of the heart, the second heart sound is usually louder than the first, and an accentuated first sound in this area should arouse suspicion of the presence of pathology. The first heart sound is usually louder in the second left interspace than in the second right interspace.

Changes in loudness of the first sound and the presence and degree of splitting are noted on auscultation. Variations in pitch are often associated with changes in loudness. When the sound is loud, the pitch is higher then usual, and the sound is "sharp"; low-pitched sounds are "dull" or "muffled." The quality of the first sound is less significant than the loudness or pitch, although occasionally the sound may have an unusual quality, e.g., the resonating and tonelike first sound sometimes heard in mitral stenosis.

The first sound in the sternal region may have a "scraping" quality which is much more evident in the sitting position and on expiration. A sound called the *xiphosternal crunch* has been described. While this term seems to have been used for almost any sound occurring in the region of the xiphoid, it is true that when the patient is in the sitting position, the quality of a split first heart sound in the xiphoid region may occasionally be described as "crunching."

CHANGES IN LOUDNESS

The factors that influence the loudness of the first sound may be *extracardiac* or *cardiac*. The extracardiac factors usually affect both the first and the second heart sounds. Cardiac factors involve primarily the first sound.

Extracardiac Factors Influencing the Intensity of the First Heart Sound

1. THICKNESS OF THE CHEST WALL. — The farther the sound has to travel through the chest wall, the fainter the sound will be because of distance, damping and reflection. In a heavy-chested person, the sounds will be less intense than in a thin-chested person or in children. Fatty tissue is inelastic and a poor transmitter of sound and, therefore, the sound will be faint in obese persons and women with large breasts. Sounds will be less evident in a patient with a deep chest, i.e., a person with a large anteroposterior chest diameter. In these patients, the sounds are better heard in the sitting than in the recumbent position.

2. EMPHYSEMA. — Emphysematous lungs can effectively insulate the heart so that the heart sounds will be faint or inau-

dible. The standing-flexion position (see Fig 2–3, p. 13) is of value in these patients and in those with thick chest walls. Sounds may be best heard over the xiphoid and epigastrium in patients with severe emphysema and occasionally may only be heard in these areas.

3. PERICARDIAL FLUID.—This may diminish heart sounds both by increasing the distance from the heart to the chest wall and by introducing new reflections. Many patients with myxedema have pericardial fluid that may account, in part, for a decreased intensity of the heart sounds. However, since sound is better transmitted by fluid than by lung tissue, heart sounds are occasionally quite normal even in the presence of significant pericardial effusion.

CARDIAC FACTORS INFLUENCING THE INTENSITY OF THE FIRST HEART SOUND

1. POSITION OF THE ATRIOVENTRICULAR VALVES AT THE TIME OF VENTRICULAR CONTRACTION.—Variations in intensity of the first sound have been closely correlated with the position of the atrioventricular valves at the moment of ventricular contraction. If the valves are widely open when the tension in the ventricle is increased, they snap abruptly with production of a loud sound. If the valves have fallen back to the position of closure and are thus partially taut, the amount of sound produced at the time of ventricular contraction is greatly diminished. The amount of sound produced by excursion of the valves from intermediate positions will vary accordingly (Fig 4–3).

The position of the valves during diastole is influenced by the flow of the blood from the atria to the ventricles and by atrial contraction. Immediately after the opening of the valves, there is a period of rapid blood flow during which the valves are wide open. As the flow slows after this sudden filling, the valves are partially taut. The valves then open again but not as widely, since the flow is slower. With atrial contraction and increase in the velocity of flow, there is an approximation of the mitral leaflets; this is due to the Bernoulli effect. To the extent that the intensity of the first sound varies with the position of the leaflets at the onset of ventricular contraction, it would in turn depend upon the time in diastole at which ventricular contraction occurs.

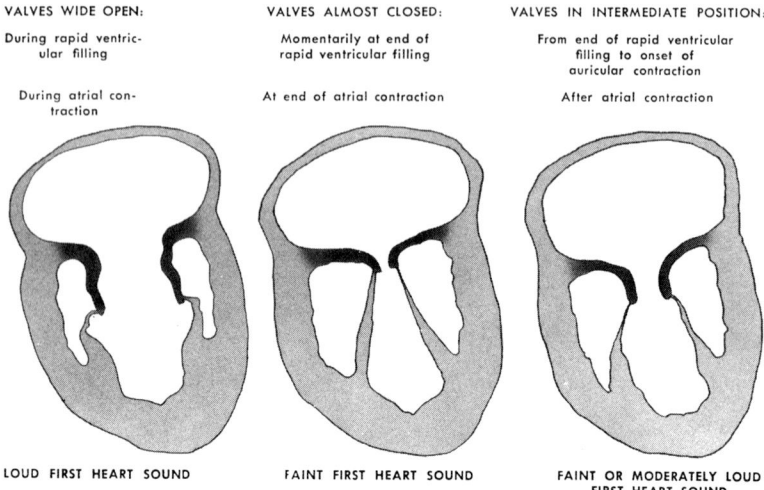

VALVES WIDE OPEN:

During rapid ventric-
ular filling

During atrial con-
traction

VALVES ALMOST CLOSED:

Momentarily at end of
rapid ventricular filling

At end of atrial contraction

VALVES IN INTERMEDIATE POSITION:

From end of rapid ventricular
filling to onset of
auricular contraction

After atrial contraction

LOUD FIRST HEART SOUND

FAINT FIRST HEART SOUND

FAINT OR MODERATELY LOUD
FIRST HEART SOUND

Fig 4–3. — Relation of positions of atrioventricular valves at the time of ventricular contractions to the intensity of the first heart sound.

a. Complete heart block. — The pathognomonic variation in the intensity of the first heart sound in complete heart block has been shown to depend upon the varying relationship of atrial systole to ventricular systole (Fig 4–4). In patients with this condition, the first heart sound is most accentuated when the P-wave precedes the QRS-wave by 0.08–0.12 second and the valves are wide open. The loudness of the first sound decreases as the P-R interval lengthens, and with P-R intervals of over 0.20 second the sound may be markedly diminished. By this time, the valves are partially closed. In some patients, there may be a secondary zone of accentuation of the first sound when the P-R interval increases over 0.25 second. Since a bradycardia with a constant P-R interval (sinus bradycardia or 2-to-1 block) will not show this variation in the first sound, this sign is a valuable diagnostic aid.

b. Variation in the P-R interval. — In acute rheumatic fever, there is often a prolongation of atrioventricular conduction. Accompanying this change in the P-R interval is a change in the loudness of the first heart sound. When the P-R interval is 0.12 second, the first sound is sharp and louder than the second sound. At 0.14 second, the first sound is moderately sharp and louder than the second sound; at 0.16 second, the first and

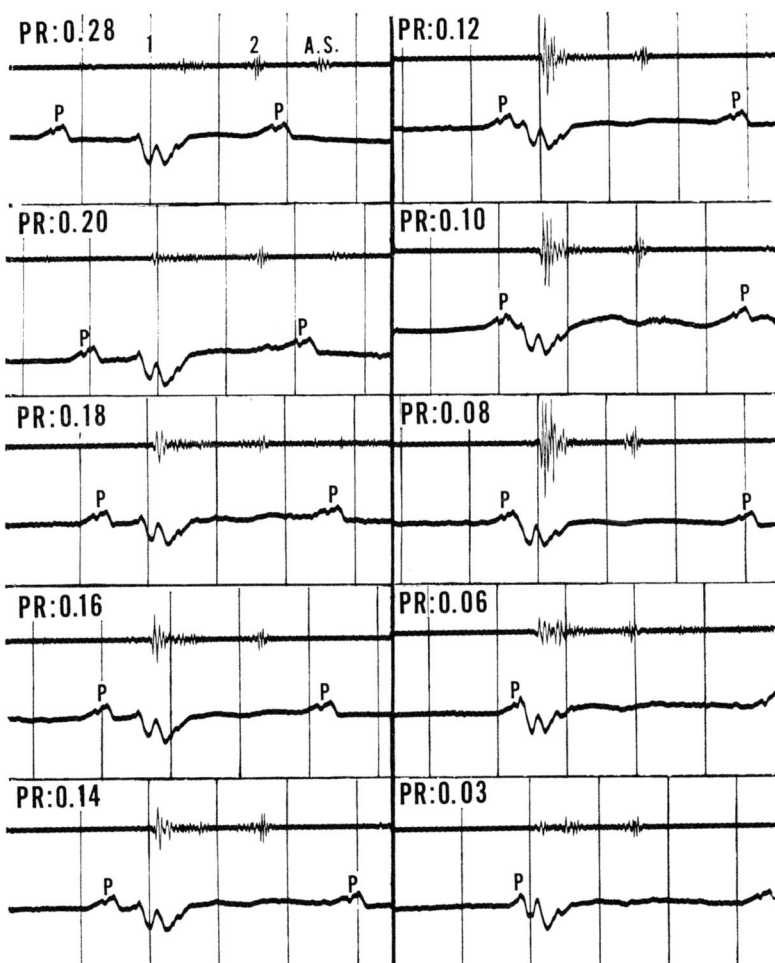

Fig 4–4.—Variation in intensity of first heart sound in complete heart block. When P-wave precedes the QRS complex (W-shaped in this patient) by 0.20 second or more *(upper left)*, the first sound is very faint. The first sound is somewhat louder when the P-R interval is 0.18 second. When the P-R interval is 0.16 and 0.14 second, the first sound is moderately loud. At 0.12 second and 0.10 second, the first heart sound is loud, and at 0.08 second it is very loud. It drops off sharply at 0.06 second and becomes very faint at 0.03 second.

In the upper left strip (PR:0.28), note that the atrial contraction *(A.S.)* produces a very audible sound when it occurs in early diastole and is superimposed upon the phase of rapid ventricular filling. At other times, the atrial sound was sometimes evident but faint.

The time interval between the vertical lines in most of the phonocardiograms shown in the text is 0.2 second.

second sounds are of about equal intensity; at 0.18 second, the second sound is louder than the first sound, and the first sound is definitely diminished in intensity; at 0.20 second, the first sound is faint. Since this correlation between P-R interval and intensity of the first sound is quite good, one has a simple clue as to the presence of prolongation of atrioventricular conduction. Although myocardial weakness can produce a faint first sound, the decreased loudness of the first sound in acute rheumatic fever is most often accompanied by lengthening of the P-R interval. Even in the absence of rheumatic fever, a definitely diminished first heart sound, as compared with the second heart sound at the apex, should make one suspect the presence of a P-R interval at the upper limit of normal or prolonged.

c. *Ventricular tachycardia.* — In some instances of ventricular tachycardia in which the atria are beating at an independent and slower rate than the ventricles, the ventricular beats following very shortly after atrial beats have an accentuated first sound. An accentuated first sound thus occurs at fairly regular intervals. The explanation is similar to what has been previously noted. The variation in the first sound does not occur in the presence of atrial fibrillation or if there is retrograde conduction to the atria. This sign may be of value in distinguishing ventricular tachycardia from other types of tachycardia (p. 161).

d. *Atrial fibrillation.* — In atrial fibrillation, the first sound varies in loudness with the length of the preceding diastole in a manner that would be expected from the description given. Phonocardiographic studies show that the first sound is loudest when it occurs up to about 0.21 second after the preceding second sound when the valves are wide open during rapid ventricular filling. The sound is markedly diminished during the next tenth of a second, as the valves fall toward each other at the end of the rapid filling. A secondary zone of moderate accentuation usually follows. The variation in loudness may be evident to the listener and is of some diagnostic value.

e. *Mitral stenosis and atrial fibrillation.* — An interesting relationship between the intensity of the first heart sound and the length of the preceding diastole is found in some patients with mitral stenosis and atrial fibrillation. The first heart sound is loudest when it occurs early in diastole and gradually diminishes in intensity as diastole lengthens. This has been explained as follows: Because of the stenosis, the ventricle fills slowly. Early in diastole, therefore, the ventricles do not have much blood, and since the pressure in the atria is high, the valve is pushed toward the ventricle. As the ventricles gradually fill, the pressure on the two sides equalizes and the valve gradually rises toward the atrium. This would account for a loud sound early in diastole that gradually decreases as diastole lengthens. Patients who show this variation in the first sound have moderately tight rather than very tight mitral stenosis, often with some regurgitation. With very tight mitral stenosis, the first sound does not show variation in intensity with length of diastole.

2. PATHOLOGIC CHANGES IN THE VALVES. — When, as a result of rheumatic fever, the mitral valve is markedly fibrosed, calcified and bound down so that there can be little motion, the intensity of the first sound is usually diminished.

In the presence of mitral stenosis, the first sound is loud and high pitched if the valve cusps retain their mobility. Several factors may play a part in producing this accentuated sound: (1) because of the stenosis, pressure in the left atrium is increased, filling of the ventricle is slow, and the valve remains deep in the ventricle until ventricular systole occurs; (2) the anterior cusp of the valve may be thickened and shortened, and this tends to produce a higher-pitched sound; (3) the valve ring may be thickened and thus give more support to the valves, and the thickened chordae tendineae may stop the motion of the valve more abruptly than does the normal chordae tendineae; (4) since the pressure in the left atrium is elevated, ventricular pressure must rise to a higher level before the valves close. The closing pressure is increased and the valve is closed more abruptly.

3. EFFECT OF RAPIDITY OF LEFT VENTRICULAR CONTRACTION. — It has become clear that the rate of ventricular contraction is probably the most important single factor influencing the intensity of the first heart sound. A more abrupt tensing of the valve causes the production of higher frequencies, which makes the sound louder to the ear. In addition, experiments have shown a direct relationship between the rate of rise of tension and the intensity of the first sound. A rapid ventricular contraction is not necessarily related to the height of systolic

pressure attained or to the amount of blood ejected (stroke volume). A more abrupt rise in ventricular pressure is a prime factor in the increased first sound heard in exercise, thyrotoxicosis and fever; after drugs such as epinephrine; and in the various hyperkinetic states. It is probably an important factor in mitral stenosis. In this condition, the rate of rise of pressure in the left ventricle is normal or increased, which, combined with the low valvular position and structural alteration, produces the characteristically loud first sound.

Even with prolonged P-R interval or complete heart block. the rate of contraction probably plays a primary role. Atrial contraction contributes a final augmenting stretch to the ventricular myocardium immediately preceding the onset of ventricular contraction. When atrial contraction occurs 0.08 – 0.12 seconds before ventricular contraction, this augmentation is maximal and the first sound is loudest; at longer P-R intervals, the augmentation is progressively less and the first sound becomes softer.

A slow rate of rise of ventricular pressure is a prime factor in the diminished first sound found in myocardial infarction, cardiomyopathy, myxedema, terminal states, and most cases of shock. In all of these instances, other factors may also play a part.

4. MASKING. — Loud systolic murmurs may mask a first heart sound. With training, one may learn to separate the sound from the murmur even though the first impression is that the murmur has replaced the sound. The alternate use of heavy and light pressure with the bell may make a first sound obvious. Often a phonocardiogram will show a first sound when none can be definitely heard with the stethoscope.

ABNORMAL SPLITTING OF THE FIRST HEART SOUND

On the assumption that the two audible components of the first sound are produced by mitral and tricuspid closure in that order (see Fig 5–1, p. 54), one would expect bundle branch block to produce abnormal splitting of the first sound. In *right bundle branch block* this is often, but not always, evident on auscultation. Wide splitting is best heard to the lower end of the sternum or in the apicosternal region. In *left bundle branch block,* abnormal splitting of the first heart sound is rarely evident; the sound is commonly faint or "dull." The abnormal sequence of contraction and the slight delay in its onset may be important factors; there is some evidence that paradoxical movement of the interventricular septum may further influence left ventricular contractility.

In *ventricular premature contractions* and *ventricular tachycardia,* there is asynchronous contraction of the ventricles and splitting of the first sound is usually evident (p. 160). (See Fig 10 – 1, p. 163.)

Splitting of the heart sounds is usually more evident with the use of the diaphragm than with the bell, because the higher-pitched vibrations are more clearly separated than the low-pitched vibrations, which may be prolonged and thus blend.

If the audible portion of the first sound consists only of sound produced by closure of the mitral and tricuspid valves, there are very few conditions other than those mentioned above where an abnormally split first sound should be present. If, however, semilunar and vascular components occasionally or regularly form an audible portion of the first sound, then accentuation of these components in certain pathologic conditions could produce split first sounds. When the ejection components blend with the first sound, as they do at times, no splitting is evident. With pathologic accentuation and often delay of the ejection components, *ejection sounds* may be recognized. In this sense, the presence of an ejection sound does constitute a split first sound. Ejection sounds are discussed on page 62.

The presence of a fourth sound, a short presystolic murmur, or a short early systolic murmur might give the impression of a split first sound.

Second Heart Sound

DESCRIPTION

The second heart sound is produced by vibrations initiated by the closure of the aortic and pulmonary semilunar valves and by the sudden cessation of backflow of the blood. These vibrations occur in the semilunar valves, in the blood, and in the adjacent portions of the aorta and pulmonary artery. The sound produced by the closure of the aortic semilunar valve is usually heard over the entire precordium; that produced by the closure of the pulmonary valve is normally heard in a much smaller area, centering around the second left interspace (Fig 4–5). In expiration, the aortic and pulmonary semilunar valves close almost synchronously and produce a single sound or a closely split sound. With inspiration, there is an asynchrony in the closure, the aortic valve closure occurring before the pulmonic valve closure (see Fig 5–1, p. 54). This may be due to the delay in closure of the pulmonic valve, an earlier closure of the aortic valve, or both factors. Delay in the pulmonic closure is the most important factor and accounts for most of the separation. An earlier aortic valve closure is a significant but much less important event. With inspiration, intrathoracic pressure is decreased and the pressure gradient between the right atrium and extrathoracic veins is increased. An increased flow into the right atrium results in increased filling of the right ventricle, and the increased stroke volume of the right ventricle prolongs its systole and delays the closure of the pulmonic valve. At the same time, inspiration increases the venous capacity of the lungs and left atrium, with a resultant decreased flow into the left ventricle; consequently, the left ventricular ejection time is slightly shorter and the aortic second sound is heard earlier.

Inspiratory splitting of the second sound varies in degree and is commonly most marked in the heart beat at the peak or immediately after the peak of inspiration. It will be evident only in the area where the pulmonic as well as the aortic second sound can be heard. Splitting is best determined with the diaphragm chest piece and is usually evident during ordinary respiration. If respiration is shallow, the patient should be asked to breathe somewhat more deeply, but abnormally deep respiration may be noisy and confusing. Often it is helpful to have the patient take a moderately deep breath and hold it for several seconds (held inspiration), and then let it out and hold it for several seconds (held expiration). It is important to listen to the first few beats in each phase of respiration, because in held expiration, the second sound, which is at first single, often becomes split, although not usually to the degree noted on inspiration. With held inspiration, the second sound, first split, becomes single. If audible expiratory splitting is

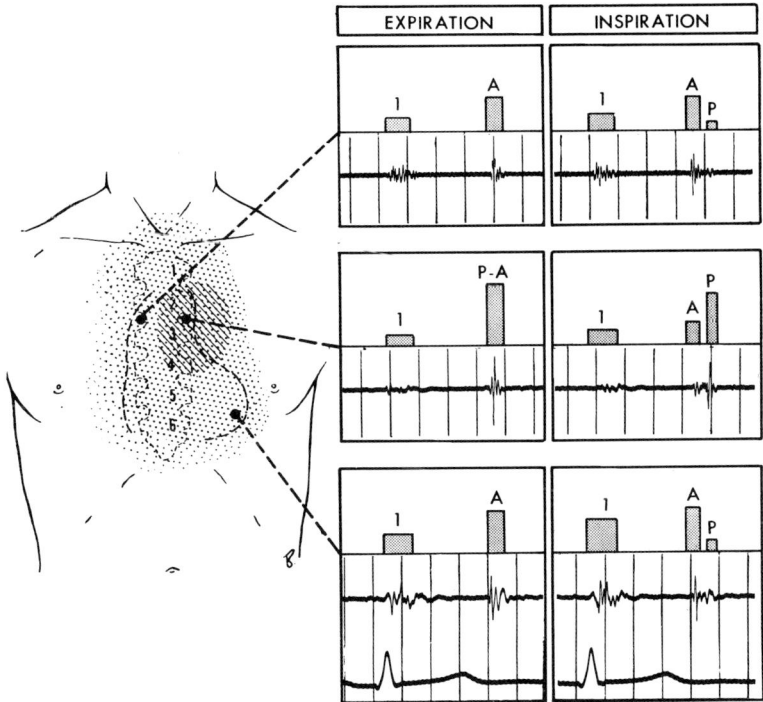

Fig 4–5.—Second heart sound; composition in different areas of precordium and effect of respiration. The *stippling* indicates the area where the aortic second sound is heard; the *shaded* portion is the area in which the pulmonic second sound is normally heard. As is noted, the second sound in the second right intercostal space and at the apex is essentially of aortic origin. In the second left intercostal space the second heart sound is composed of both aortic and pulmonic second sounds. In different persons, the relative intensities of the two components in this area will vary, and often the aortic component is louder than the pulmonic component even in this area. In expiration, the aortic and pulmonic components in most normal persons are superimposed and produce a single sound. In inspiration, right ventricular systole is prolonged and the pulmonic second sound is delayed. In the area, therefore, in which the pulmonic second sound is evident, a splitting of the second sound will occur. In the case illustrated, the pulmonic component of the second sound can be seen on the phonocardiogram during expiration in both aortic and apical regions. It was not evident, however, to the ear.

heard with the patient recumbent, auscultation should be done in the upright position. The normal response is fusion of the two sounds such that expiratory splitting is no longer heard. This is probably due to accentuation of the effect of respiration on venous return in the upright position, which tends to increase the degree of movement of the pulmonic sound.

Recognition of splitting is, like everything else, a matter of training and direction of attention; once the examiner becomes conscious of the occurrence of splitting, it opens a new field of auscultatory enjoyment.

Total right ventricular systole is the most important determinant of the degree of splitting, since ejection must terminate and the right ventricle must relax before closure of the valve. Thus, with prolonged right ventricular systole, splitting may be wide whereas an abbreviated period will tend to cause narrow splitting. Elevated pulmonary diastolic pressure will close the valve with greater force, producing a loud sound. Some have postulated that the elevated pulmonary arterial pressure prolongs right ventricular systole and thus delays pulmonic closure. Indeed, wide splitting of the second sound, unexplained by hemodynamic measurements, has been reported in idiopathic dilatation of the pulmonary artery and is suggested in some studies of pulmonary hypertension. Explanations other than duration of right ventricular systole have thus been postulated. These include (1) backflow of blood due to elevated pulmonary arterial pressure, which may delay closure of the valve and increase splitting; and (2) loss of elasticity of the pulmonary artery, notably when dilated or with chronic pulmonary hypertension, resulting in delayed rebound of the vascular wall, again producing wide splitting. These postulates seem improbable, but it is clear that factors as yet unexplained are operative, especially in certain pathologic states. The most reliable working hypothesis, however, remains the correlation of right ventricular systolic duration with degrees of splitting and pulmonary arterial diastolic pressure with loudness. Since left ventricular ejection period is more constant, aortic closure has less influence on splitting. Exceptions include delayed closure in left bundle branch block, severe aortic stenosis and hypertensive heart disease with failure, and early closure when left ventricular stroke output is markedly diminished.

Phonocardiograms indicate that the pulmonic component of the second sound may be present in the aortic area (see Fig 4–5); however, here it is faint, masked by a preceding louder aortic component, and not normally heard. The aortic second sound is often louder than the pulmonic second sound in the *pulmonic area.* Both the aortic and the pulmonic second sounds may occasionally be louder in the third left intercostal space than in any other area. Although the phonocardiogram may show a faint pulmonic sound at the apex, the second sound at the apex is almost entirely aortic in origin. An easily identified pulmonic closure sound in this area suggests pulmonary hypertension. Occasionally, in an apparently normal individual, the pulmonic second sound may be evident in inspiration over most of the precordium.

Since the second heart sound is usually single or very slightly split on expiration and clearly split on inspiration, the expression "normally split" is used to indicate this finding.

The wider distribution of the sound produced by closure of the aortic semilunar valve probably results from the much higher closing pressure in the aorta and the deeper location of the aorta. The sound produced by the closure of the pulmonary valves is less intense because of the lower closing pressure. But since the pulmonary artery is close to the chest wall, the sound is well heard, although in a small area. During the first three to four decades of life, the second sound in the second left intercostal space is usually louder than the sound in the second right intercostal space. In older people, the situation is reversed. This change in relative intensities may result from the increase in the systemic pressure, the change in the relative position of the aorta and pulmonary artery, and the changes in the structure of the aorta and aortic valve that occur with age.

The second sound is normally louder at the base than at the apex. At the base, the second heart sound is louder than the first heart sound. At the apex, the second heart sound is not usually as loud as the first heart sound, but may be of equal intensity and not infrequently is louder than the first sound.

Variations to be noted in the second sound are *changes in loudness* and *changes in degree of splitting.* Changes in quality of the second sound occur and sometimes are significant but, generally, are less important than changes in loudness.

CHANGES IN LOUDNESS

An increased or decreased intensity of the aortic second sound results in a change of intensity of the second sound in the second right intercostal space and apex. In persons in whom the heart sounds are faint at the base because of emphysema or a heavy chest wall, the character of the second heart sound at the apex gives a clue to changes in the aortic second sound; for example, the second sound at the apex may be increased in hypertension. An increase in the pulmonic second sound results in a loud pulmonic second sound in the second left intercostal space. Since the sound is also more widely heard, splitting of the second sound may be evident in a wide area, including the second right intercostal space, down the left border of the sternum, and often at the apex.

The factors that produce changes in loudness of the second sound may be divided into *extracardiac* and *cardiac*. The *extracardiac factors* are similar to those that influence the first heart sound (p. 32), and the two heart sounds are usually affected at the same time. Fibrosis of one or the other of the upper lobes of the lungs may increase the second heart sound in the area without especially affecting the first heart sound.

The *cardiac factors* affecting the loudness of the second sound are: (1) the pressure in the aorta or pulmonary artery; (2) pathologic changes in the valves; (3) changes in the structure of the valve ring and great vessels and (4) masking.

1. ARTERIAL PRESSURE. — The greater the closing pressure in the vessel, the louder is the sound produced by closure of the valve. Exercise, excitement and essential hypertension increase the pressure in the aorta and may increase the aortic second sound (see Fig 4–8, I). Any of the many conditions associated with pulmonary hypertension — congenital heart disease, mitral stenosis, congestive heart failure, and idiopathic pulmonary hypertension — will produce an increased pulmonic second sound (see Fig 4–8, D).

The faster the pressure falls during the latter part of systole, the more abrupt is the closure of the valve. The result may be a greater proportion of high-pitched vibrations and a louder sound. The increased aortic second sound in some patients with aortic regurgitation may, in part, be produced by this mechanism.

A fall in systemic blood pressure due to hypotension, circulatory failure or shock will result in a diminished aortic second sound. With infundibular and valvular pulmonary stenosis, the pulmonic second sound will be diminished or absent, due in part to the low closing pressure.

In congestive failure in older patients, the relative loudness of the aortic and pulmonic second sounds may show changes that are of diagnostic value. When the failure in these patients is compensated, the aortic second sound is louder than the pulmonic second sound. When failure occurs, the pulmonary artery pressure increases and the pulmonic second sound increases. At the same time, the systemic pressure may decrease and the aortic second sound decrease. Thus, the pulmonic second sound will be louder than the aortic sound. As the patient improves with treatment, the pulmonary artery pressure decreases and the systemic pressure increases. The aortic second sound first becomes equal to the pulmonic second sound and then becomes louder.

2. PATHOLOGIC CHANGES IN THE VALVES. — If the valve remains flexible, mild thickening of the valve, such as occurs with rheumatic fever and possibly arteriosclerosis, may increase the second sound. If the valves are markedly thickened and calcified and the motion is limited, the second sound is diminished or absent, as in calcific aortic stenosis.

3. CHANGES IN THE STRUCTURE OF THE VALVE RING AND GREAT VESSELS. — Arteriosclerotic or syphilitic changes in the vessel may increase sound production. Dilation of a vessel may change the quality of a sound, and in aortic aneurysm the second sound may have a peculiarly resonant quality. With dilation of the pulmonary artery, the pulmonic second sound may be increased in the absence of increased pressure. Arteriosclerosis of the aorta may increase the aortic second sound, especially if there is some dilation. Temporary mild hypertension, such as occurs in persons who are blood pressure hyperreactors, is less likely to be associated with an accentuated second sound than is a persistent hypertension of the same degree with aortic changes.

4. MASKING. — A loud systolic murmur may mask a normal or somewhat diminished second sound in mitral regurgitation (aortic second), pulmonic stenosis (aortic second), aortic stenosis (pulmonic second), and patent ductus arteriosus (aortic and pulmonic second).

ABNORMAL SPLITTING OF THE SECOND HEART SOUND

In infants, the degree of inspiratory splitting is less than it is in older children, and it is often difficult to recognize splitting because of the rapid heart rate and respiration. In children, some degree of inspiratory splitting can almost always be recognized. In many adults, especially if the second sound is not too well heard because of a heavy chest wall or emphysema, splitting may not be evident. Inspiratory splitting becomes less with age, due mainly to less delay in the pulmonic second sound. In older persons, the pulmonic second sound may be faint and only the aortic second sound will be heard in the second left interspace. No reason may be evident for the absence of recognizable splitting in some normal persons. Often, even when a clear splitting is not evident, a definite change in the quality of the second sound occurs with respiration. A slight degree of splitting may normally be present in expiration. Before deciding that there is an abnormal degree of splitting in expiration, it is wise to try held expiration.

Immediately following a Valsalva maneuver, wide splitting (up to 0.08 – 0.10 second) of the second sound occurs. This splitting gradually narrows with succeeding beats, so that in six to eight beats a single second sound is nearly always present. This wide splitting immediately after the maneuver is explained by the sudden increase in venous return to the right ventricle. This increases filling of the right ventricle, prolongs right ventricular ejection time, and delays the pulmonic second sound. As the right ventricle passes on the extra blood to the left ventricle, right ventricular ejection time shortens and left ventricular ejection time lengthens. The splitting, therefore, decreases and the aortic and pulmonic second sounds merge into a single sound. This occurrence of a single sound after several seconds is of diagnostic significance (p. 182).

Abnormalities of splitting recognizable on auscultation consist of: (1) absence of splitting on inspiration so that only one sound is heard during both inspiration and expiration; (2) an abnormal degree of splitting on expiration; (3) an abnormal degree of splitting on expiration with no increase in the splitting on inspiration (fixed splitting); and (4) a reversal of the effect of respiration on splitting (paradoxical splitting).

Splitting is *absent* in some congenital and acquired heart conditions, owing to the following causes. (1) Only one valve may be producing sound. In many patients with the tetralogy of Fallot, only the aortic sound can be heard (see Figs 4 – 8, G and 11 – 7, p. 190). The second sound may have a pure and tonelike quality. With a truncus arteriosus only one valve is present to produce sound. (2) One of the sounds may be masked by a loud murmur; this masking may occur in aortic or pulmonic stenosis (see Fig 11–6, p. 187). (3) One sound may be so accentuated and booming that it masks the other sound. This situation may occur with pulmonary or systemic hypertension (see Fig 4–8, D and I). By listening in an area where the sound is not so intense, one may sometimes recognize splitting, e.g., listening in the fourth left intercostal space in pulmonary hypertension. (4) The position of the great vessels may be abnormal, altering the usual transmission of sounds from the semilunar valves; for example, in transposition of the great vessels the pulmonary valve is posteriorly situated and only the aortic closure sound may be audible.

Splitting is *abnormal* in the following conditions:

1. RIGHT BUNDLE BRANCH BLOCK. — In this condition, excitation of the right side of the heart is delayed, and, as a result, the pulmonary valve closure is delayed. Splitting of the second sound is present in expiration and is further increased and marked in inspiration (Figs 4–6 and 4–8, B). The diagnosis of right bundle branch block can often be made or suspected on this finding alone. The degree of expiratory splitting will vary with the degree of bundle branch block. Most patients with electrocardiograms showing partial right bundle branch block and having QRS complexes of less than 0.10 second do not have abnormal splitting.

2. LEFT BUNDLE BRANCH BLOCK. — Excitation of the left

Fig 4–6.—Increased splitting of second sound in right bundle branch block. The splitting is evident on expiration and becomes more marked on inspiration. The aortic second sound *(A)* precedes the pulmonic second sound *(P)*. There is a faint systolic murmur in this patient, but most of the vibrations, other than the heart sounds, are due to respiration and muscle noises.

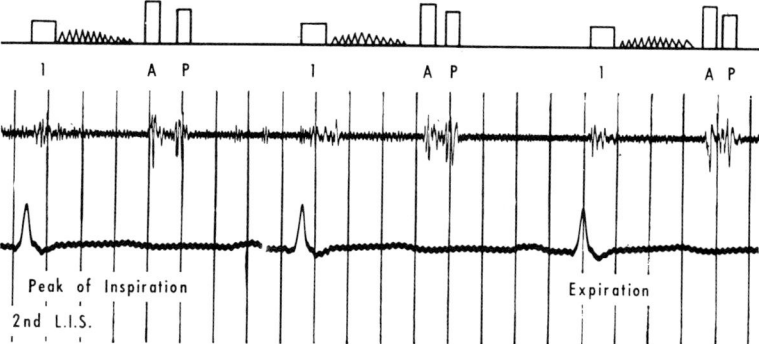

side of the heart and aortic closure are delayed. In expiration, therefore, the aortic component of the second sound will occur after the pulmonic component, and a splitting of the second sound is evident. With inspiration the pulmonic second sound is delayed and falls at the same time as the aortic sound (Figs 4–7 and 4–8, G). There is thus a splitting in expiration and a single sound in inspiration—a reversal of the usual state and hence the name *paradoxical splitting*. The paradoxical splitting of the second sound in left bundle branch block is not as easily determined as is the abnormal splitting in right bundle branch block—possibly because it is more common in age groups where splitting may normally not be very evident.

3. INCREASED RIGHT VENTRICULAR EMPTYING TIME.—This may result from an increased stroke volume of the right ventricle (diastolic overload) or an increased systolic load on the right ventricle (systolic overload).

In atrial septal defects the right ventricle receives an increased amount of blood during diastole, but it pumps the blood out against a normal pressure—hence the term *diastolic overload*. Because of the shunt, the right ventricle pumps more blood with each beat than does the left ventricle. This prolongs right ventricular systole, delays the pulmonic second sound, and gives an abnormal degree of splitting during expi-

Fig 4–7.—"Paradoxical splitting" of second sound in congenital aortic stenosis. Because of the aortic stenosis, the left ventricular systole is prolonged and the aortic second sound is delayed. In expiration, therefore, when the right ventricular systole is short, the pulmonic second sound occurs early and there is splitting. In inspiration, right ventricular systole is prolonged and the pulmonic second sound now falls at about the same time as the aortic sound, giving a single or almost single sound.

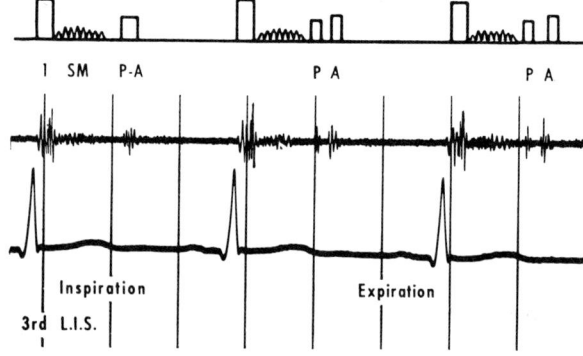

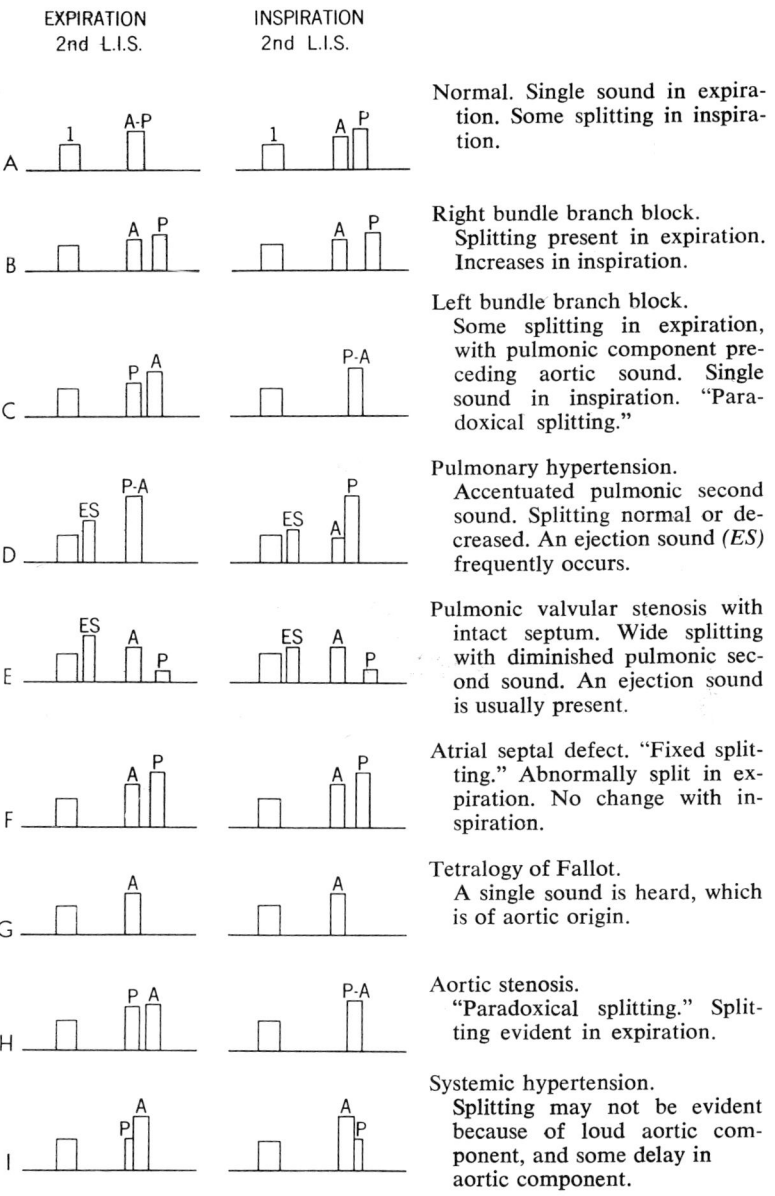

EXPIRATION
2nd L.I.S.

INSPIRATION
2nd L.I.S.

A. Normal. Single sound in expiration. Some splitting in inspiration.

B. Right bundle branch block. Splitting present in expiration. Increases in inspiration.

C. Left bundle branch block. Some splitting in expiration, with pulmonic component preceding aortic sound. Single sound in inspiration. "Paradoxical splitting."

D. Pulmonary hypertension. Accentuated pulmonic second sound. Splitting normal or decreased. An ejection sound (ES) frequently occurs.

E. Pulmonic valvular stenosis with intact septum. Wide splitting with diminished pulmonic second sound. An ejection sound is usually present.

F. Atrial septal defect. "Fixed splitting." Abnormally split in expiration. No change with inspiration.

G. Tetralogy of Fallot. A single sound is heard, which is of aortic origin.

H. Aortic stenosis. "Paradoxical splitting." Splitting evident in expiration.

I. Systemic hypertension. Splitting may not be evident because of loud aortic component, and some delay in aortic component.

Fig 4–8.—Changes in the second sound. *A*, aortic second sound. *P*, pulmonic second sound. *ES*, early ejection sound.

ration (Fig 4–8, F; see Fig 11–5, p. 181). With most atrial septal defects, the splitting is not significantly increased by inspiration; *fixed splitting* is present. Inspiratory splitting depends upon a differential effect of inspiration on the filling of the right and left atria (p. 40); with both atria connected by the defect, there is a common reservoir, and this differential effect does not occur. It is also possible that in some patients the flow into the right atrium, because of the shunt, may be so great that inspiration does not further significantly increase the filling of the right atrium. Significant inspiratory increase in splitting does, however, occur at times; occasionally, even normal splitting (single or closely split sound in expiration) may occur in patients with proved atrial septal defects.

② Pulmonary valvular and infundibular stenosis represents a *systolic overload*, which prolongs right ventricular ejection time and produces a delay in the pulmonic second sound and abnormal splitting on expiration. Since the pulmonic sound is often diminished in intensity, the splitting may not always be evident. The splitting may also be masked by a prolonged systolic murmur (see Fig 11–6, p. 187). Increase in splitting is most evident if the stenosis is not too severe. ③ In pulmonary hypertension, the expected delay in pulmonic second sound due to systolic overload may not occur; an earlier closure of the pulmonic valve, because of the high diastolic pressure, may be one factor and, as already indicated, right ventricular systole may be shortened due to an inability to maintain a normal stroke output. ④ Dilation of the pulmonary artery without pulmonary hypertension will, at times, be associated with an abnormally split second sound in expiration which will increase somewhat with inspiration.

4. INCREASED LEFT VENTRICULAR EMPTYING TIME.—This condition occurs with a systolic overload (aortic stenosis and systemic hypertension) or a diastolic overload (patent ductus arteriosus). In patients with mild aortic stenosis, normal splitting of the second sound occurs. If the stenosis is moderately severe, no splitting on inspiration may be evident. Severe aortic stenosis will delay the aortic second sound enough so that the pulmonic second sound precedes the aortic second sound, and *paradoxical splitting* occurs (Figs 4–7 and 4–8, H). If a loud systolic murmur masks the pulmonic second sound, or if the aortic second sound is faint, splitting may not be heard.

In systemic hypertension the aortic second sound may be delayed and no splitting evident (Fig 4–8, I). Since hypertension commonly occurs in an age group in which splitting may not be evident for other reasons, the significance of this finding is not great. If there is associated left ventricular failure, paradoxical splitting may occur.

If the myocardium of the left ventricle is weakened by ischemia, inflammation or fibrosis, a normal load may represent a systolic overload and result in prolongation of left ventricular systole. Thus, paradoxical splitting may occasionally occur in the acute stages of myocardial infarction, in myocardiopathies, and in any condition producing a weakened myocardium.

In patent ductus arteriosus, there is a diastolic overload on the left ventricle which is putting out more blood than is the right ventricle. This delays the aortic second sound and may, on occasion, give a paradoxical splitting. Unfortunately, from an auscultatory standpoint, the lesions which are severe enough to produce these changes also produce so much murmur that recognition of the components of the second sound is often difficult.

When the second heart sound is normally split, it is usually obvious. Certain sounds may mimic splitting of the second sound and when the latter is abnormal, these sounds must be differentiated. The most important ones are: (1) a third heart sound, (2) opening snap of the mitral or tricuspid valve, (3) late systolic click and (4) pericardial knock. These are discussed in subsequent sections.

Third Heart Sound

The normal third heart sound occurs shortly after the second heart sound (0.13 to 0.18 second) (see Fig 2–4, p. 14). Because of its low intensity and low pitch (lower than either of the other heart sounds), it is not commonly heard, although it can often be recorded. The frequency with which it is heard depends upon how often it is looked for in the correct manner. (1) It is best heard in children and patients with thin chest walls. (2) The room must be quiet and the patient recumbent or in the left lateral position; the sound may disappear if the patient sits up. (3) The examiner must apply the bell chest piece very lightly to the chest wall and must concentrate on early diastole. (4) The third sound is usually best heard at the point of the apex impulse or just medial to the apex impulse. (5) It is best heard usually during expiration; the third sound may disappear if the breath is held after deep inspiration. (6) The sound is increased by exercise, pressure on the abdomen, or lifting of the legs. (7) For some reason, the sound is best heard at the very start of auscultation. Some type of accommodation occurs with continued listening, which makes the sound less evident.

If attention is paid to the factors mentioned above, a normal third heart sound may be heard in many children and in some adults. Further discussion of the third heart sound will be found on page 75.

CHAPTER 5

Abnormal and Extra Heart Sounds

THE FIRST AND SECOND HEART SOUNDS are associated with abrupt changes in direction and velocity of blood flow. Other cardiac events which do not usually produce sound because the changes are not so marked can, under unusual or abnormal conditions, produce vibrations of a pitch and intensity that can be heard (Fig 5–1). In this chapter, those sounds will be considered which are associated with (1) atrial contraction; (2) opening of the semilunar valves and distention of the large vessels; (3) opening of the atrioventricular valves and (4) rapid filling of the ventricles in early diastole. Systolic clicks will also be described.

The term *gallop rhythm* has been widely used when an extra sound is added to the first and second heart sounds. If the three sounds are unevenly spaced and of unequal intensity, they give the impression of a gallop, especially at faster heart rates. This term is actually no longer of value; it should be dropped together with its various classifications for the following reasons:

1. Most of the time the three sounds do not have a gallop cadence and, therefore, *gallop* as a descriptive term is of little value.

2. Since the extra sound of a gallop rhythm may be of varied timing and origin, the statement that a patient has a gallop rhythm has little meaning until the extra sound is identified. On the other hand, the statement that a patient has a fourth sound needs no further explanation, and nothing is added by saying that he has a gallop rhythm. Classification of gallop

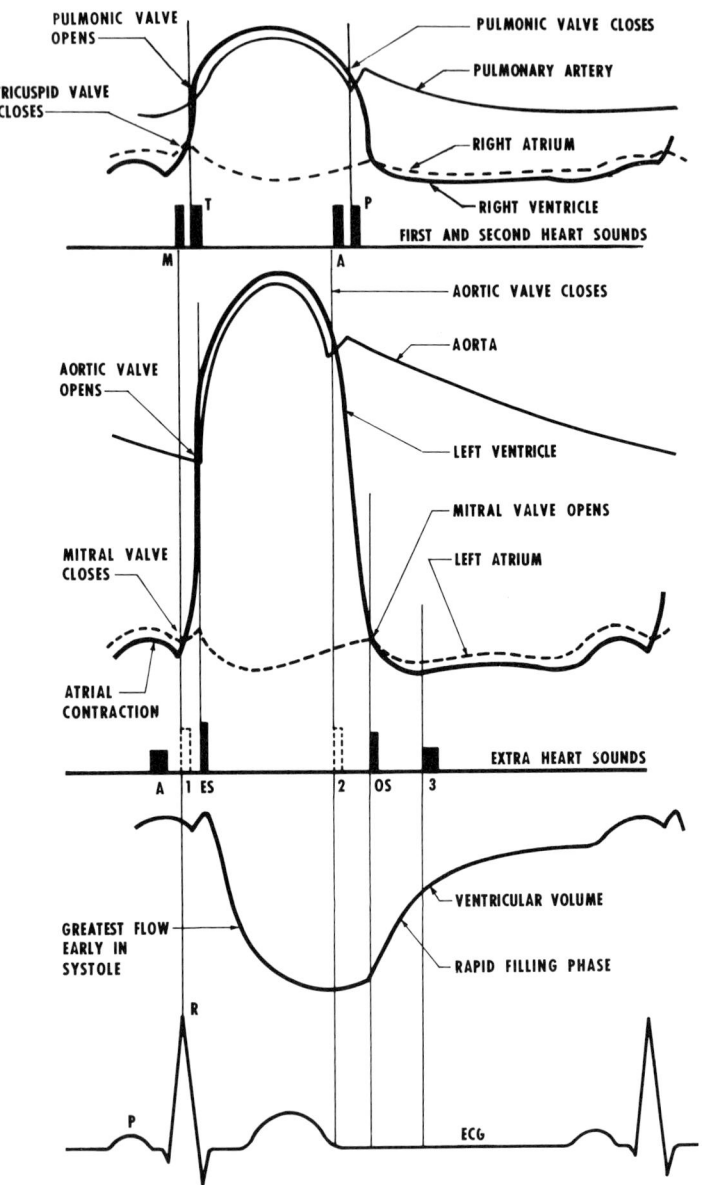

Fig 5–1.—Time relationships of various cardiac events to the occurrence of the first and second heart sounds and extra heart sounds. From the top downward are represented the pressure changes in the right side of the heart, the timing of the first and the second heart sounds, pressure changes

rhythms is based on identification of the extra sound. When, however, the extra sound is identified, classification is superfluous.

3. If the term gallop is used to indicate that the extra sound is abnormal rather than normal, a clinical interpretation is engrafted on an auscultatory finding. Whether an extra sound is normal or abnormal depends on the clinical setting in which it occurs. A child with no normal third heart sound may develop a third heart sound with acute rheumatic fever, but this abnormal third heart sound may not be as loud as a normal third heart sound heard in another child. The least confusion results if the extra heart sound is identified and then the decision of normality or abnormality is made in the clinical context.

4. Finally, the term gallop does not even designate whether the extra sound is in systole or diastole.

The same criticisms hold for the term *triple rhythm*. It adds

---

in the left side of the heart, the timing of extra heart sounds, the ventricular volume curve, and the electrocardiogram.

The first heart sound is produced by tensing of the leaflets of the mitral *(M)* and tricuspid *(T)* valves. Left ventricular contraction proceeds at a greater rate and causes the mitral valve to close slightly before the tricuspid. This produces normal splitting of the first heart sound which can be frequently recognized. The onset of the first sound is usually at the peak of the R-wave of the electrocardiogram.

The second heart sound is produced by closure of the aortic *(A)* and pulmonic *(P)* valves. In inspiration, the aortic valves close before the pulmonic valves and the aortic second sound is, therefore, earlier than the pulmonic second sound and there is splitting of the second sound. In expiration aortic and pulmonic closure may occur simultaneously with production of a single second sound. The second sound usually occurs at the end of the T-wave of the electrocardiogram. It is the start of isometric relaxation.

The fourth sound *(A)* is usually heard about 0.08 to 0.10 second after the beginning of the P-wave on the electrocardiogram. Its distance from the first sound will vary with the P-R interval and with the condition producing the fourth sound.

An aortic ejection sound *(ES)* occurs at the end of left ventricular isometric contraction when the ventricular pressure exceeds the aortic pressure and the aortic valves open. A pulmonic ejection sound occurs just as the pulmonic valves open. The ejection sounds may, at times, form a part of the first heart sound.

The opening snap *(OS)* of the mitral and tricuspid valves occurs when the ventricular pressure falls below that in the atrium. This sound is not heard unless there is some pathologic change in the mitral or tricuspid valves. The beginning of rapid filling phase of the ventricle starts with the opening snap.

The third heart sound occurs near the end of the rapid filling phase of the ventricle.

nothing to a simple statement of the presence of an abnormal sound of a specific type.

It is too much to expect that the word gallop will leave our auscultatory vocabulary, but perhaps if the word is always used with a descriptive adjective and no effort is made to classify "gallop rhythms," the same end can be accomplished. Thus we can speak of an atrial sound or an atrial gallop and an abnormal third heart sound or a ventricular gallop.

Fourth Sound

With as descriptive a term as *atrial sound*, it may be reasonable to use this term rather than *fourth heart sound* for a sound which, when present, is the initial sound in the cardiac cycle. It is true, however, that *fourth sound* is the term most commonly used; in addition, vibrations that produce it arise largely within the ventricle and it is this chamber that information derived from the atrial sound concerns. The term fourth sound will therefore be used here, being synonymous with *atrial sound; atrial gallop* and *presystolic gallop* are terms sometimes used but are probably best discarded.

Phonocardiograms often show some vibrations at the beginning of the first heart sound (see Fig 4–2, p. 30). These have been attributed to atrial contraction, since they occur before the onset of the QRS complex of the electrocardiogram. Occasionally, in normal persons, a fourth sound may be audible immediately before the first heart sound (Fig 5–2). In pathologic conditions, a fourth sound is frequently heard and may be quite loud, indeed louder than the first heart sound. Just as an increased awareness of the occurrence and significance of splitting of the second heart sound added new depth to auscultation, so also will an increased awareness of the occurrence and significance of fourth sounds add depth in the future.

The fourth sound is low pitched (in the 40–60 cycles per second range), although when loud it is somewhat higher pitched. It is usually not as loud as the first sound but may, at times, be louder. Because it is low pitched, it must be listened for with the bell of the stethoscope, and the larger the bell the more likely it is to be heard. The bell must be applied very lightly to the chest, and the room must be quiet. The sound is

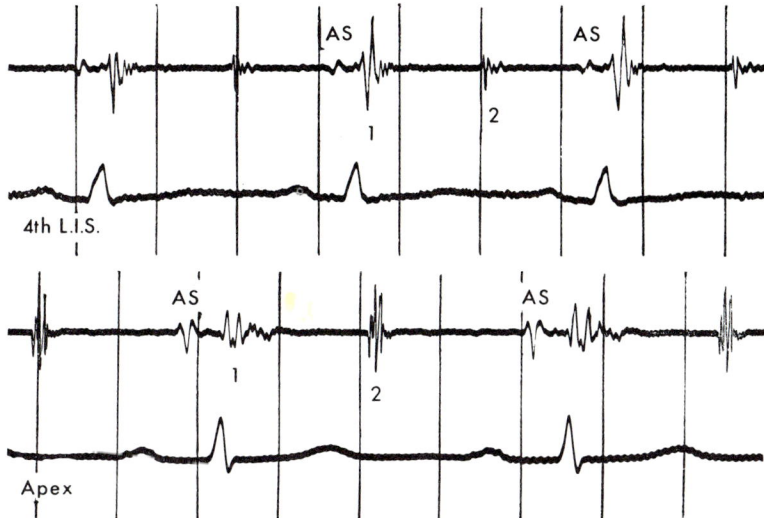

Fig 5–2. — Fourth sounds. *Upper tracing*: A fourth sound *(AS)* was heard along the left border of the sternum in a 28-year-old woman with a normal cardiovascular system. Because of the location in which it was maximum and the increase in intensity with inspiration, it was felt that the sound had its origin in the right side of the heart. Fourth sounds produced in the right side of the heart are occasionally heard in patients with atrial septal defects (see Fig 2–4, D, p. 14) and with pure pulmonary stenosis. *Lower tracing*: A fourth sound *(AS)* in a 48-year-old man with systemic hypertension and some left ventricular hypertrophy.

best heard when the patient is in the recumbent position. It may be more evident shortly after mild exercise, such as several sit-ups. Sitting up and standing tend to diminish or eliminate a fourth sound; however, if the sound is loud, it may persist. Venous tourniquets decrease a fourth sound. During a Valsalva maneuver, the fourth sound is diminished, but it increases immediately afterward.

In the absence of prolongation of the P-R interval, the interval between the fourth sound and the first heart sound varies with the severity of the condition producing the fourth sound. If the condition improves, the interval shortens until the fourth sound may no longer be obvious.

A fourth sound may be produced by either left or right atrial contraction. A *left-sided fourth sound* is usually best heard at the apex over the left ventricle. It is loudest on expiration (Fig 5–3, A), coinciding with maximal venous return to the left

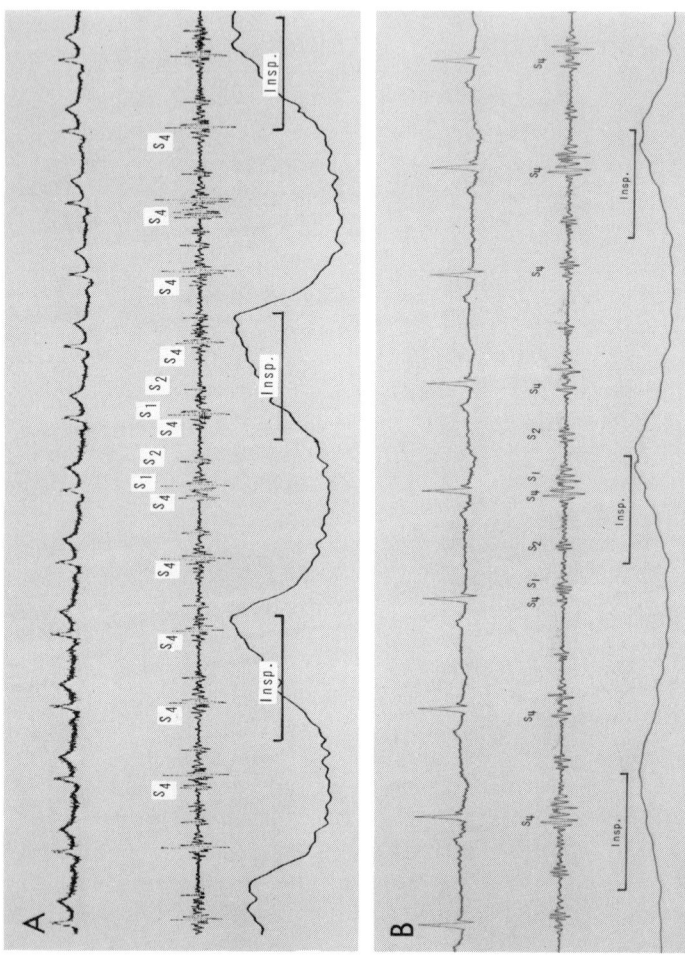

Fig 5–3. – **A,** A left-sided fourth sound. Patient had an acute myocardial infarction. Note the marked increase in intensity of the S_4 during the expiratory phase of respiration. *Insp.,* inspiration. **B,** A right-sided fourth sound. This patient had severe chronic pulmonary disease. Note the increase in intensity of the S_4 during inspiration.

heart, and this characteristic is of great value in recognizing the sound when it is faint. If the bell is applied very lightly at the apex, with the patient in the left lateral recumbent position, a fourth sound will wax and wane with respiration; while it is loudest on expiration, it may often be heard *only* on expiration. The variation in intensity is less obvious with louder fourth sounds. Occasionally, a distinct apical bulge, coincident with atrial contraction, may be felt and seen before the more forceful apical impulse.

When the fourth sound is prominent and widely separated from the first sound, it may give the impression of a short murmur (referred to as the *atrial systolic murmur*) and be confused with the presystolic murmur of mitral stenosis.

Since the "normal splitting" of the first heart sound is usually not evident at the apex (p. 29), a clearly split sound at the apex should lead one to consider the presence of a fourth sound or a systolic ejection sound (p. 62). A faint or moderately loud first sound and a louder ejection sound may be mistaken for a fourth sound followed by a first sound. A systolic ejection sound occurs after, instead of before, the apical impulse. It is higher pitched than a fourth sound and usually is not affected by sitting up. Because of its low pitch, a faint fourth sound will not be heard with a diaphragm; ejection sounds, on the other hand, are usually heard with the diaphragm.

A right-sided fourth sound is best heard along the left border of the sternum and, as opposed to the left-sided fourth sound and the split first sound, is increased by inspiration (Fig 5–3, B). This helps distinguish it from the normally split first heart sound often heard in this area, since the splitting is more evident on expiration.

Atrial contraction at the end of diastole forces more blood into the ventricles, abruptly increasing ventricular volume and pressure. This sudden distention of the ventricles is sharply curtailed and produces the vibrations which are recognized as the fourth sound and the apical bulge. From a practical standpoint, it is really immaterial whether the sound is produced by the stretching and rebound of the ventricular muscle, stretching and tensing of the chordae tendineae and papillary muscles, or partial closure of the atrioventricular valve; all of these factors may play a part. There is evidence that partial atrioventricular valve closure occurs during atrial contraction in very close proximity to the fourth sound and before the first sound, and is probably the main cause of the fourth sound. Two primary factors seem operative: (1) the low-volume, high-velocity jet produced by atrial contraction tends to reduce the pressure between the thin flexible leaflets, bringing them into apposition toward the end of atrial contraction, and (2) since the chordae tendineae from each papillary muscle are inserted into both cusps, stretching of the papillary muscles and chordae tendineae tends to partially close the valve.

Since atrial contraction does not usually produce an audible sound, the increased sound production in pathologic conditions must result from an increased resistance of the ventricle to distention and, probably, a more forceful atrial contraction. The reduced compliance (increased resistance to distention) may be due to muscular hypertrophy, myocardial ischemia, diffuse or localized fibrosis, inflammation, or some other type of myocardial involvement. An excessive amount of residual blood may, at times, be a factor. As a result of the decreased compliance, a higher ventricular enddiastolic pressure is needed and the force of atrial contraction is increased; eventually, atrial hypertrophy may occur. Right-sided fourth sounds occur in atrial septal defects, and their occurrence may be related to the excessive amount of blood in both the right ventricle and the right atrium at the time of atrial contraction.

OCCURRENCE. — To hear a fourth sound it is necessary to *listen specifically for it*. If this is done, one is soon amazed at the frequency with which this sound is heard and feels keenly disappointed if it is not heard in patients with hypertension or coronary artery disease, especially with some cardiac enlargement. Left- and right-sided fourth sounds are sometimes heard in apparently normal persons; their significance in these persons is not clear (see Fig 5–2).

A left-sided fourth sound is most commonly heard in *systemic hypertension* (see Figs 5–2 and 5–3, A) and may possibly be the earliest evidence of ventricular hypertrophy. Lowering the blood pressure with drugs reduces the intensity of the sound.

In coronary artery disease, a fourth sound can usually be heard during an ischemic episode and is extremely common following acute myocardial infarction, diminishing or disappearing as the infarction heals. A fourth sound persists if there is some cardiac enlargement; occasionally it persists in the absence of enlargement. A fourth sound would seem to be of more serious import in coronary artery disease than in hypertension. A prominent atrial wave in the apexcardiogram has been associated with the presence of coronary artery disease and angina. When the atrial wave is prominent, a fourth sound is almost always present (Fig 5–4). A fourth sound is often present in this condition when the apexcardiogram is normal, and the sound would appear to be a more sensitive indicator of the presence of pathology.

Fourth sounds and third heart sounds are especially common in *myocardiopathies* (see Fig 14–1, p. 217), and the presence of these sounds should always alert one to this diagnosis.

In *aortic stenosis* of moderate or severe degree, a left-sided fourth sound is heard and its presence indicates a left ventricular-aortic pressure gradient of significant degree. A right-sided fourth sound may be heard in *pulmonary stenosis* with intact septum and in *pulmonary hypertension;* here, again, it indicates significant pathology.

Fourth sounds may be present for years; their presence does

Fig 5–4. —Apexcardiogram *(middle curve)* and phonocardiogram *(upper curve)* on a patient with an old myocardial infarction. The patient had no symptoms other than angina on more than average exertion and his heart size was slightly over normal. Note the prominent atrial wave *(AW)* apexcardiogram and the fourth sound *(AS)* on the phonocardiogram. Fourth sounds can be heard in many patients of this type in whom the atrial wave is not abnormally prominent. The mitral valve opens at the O-point *(O).*

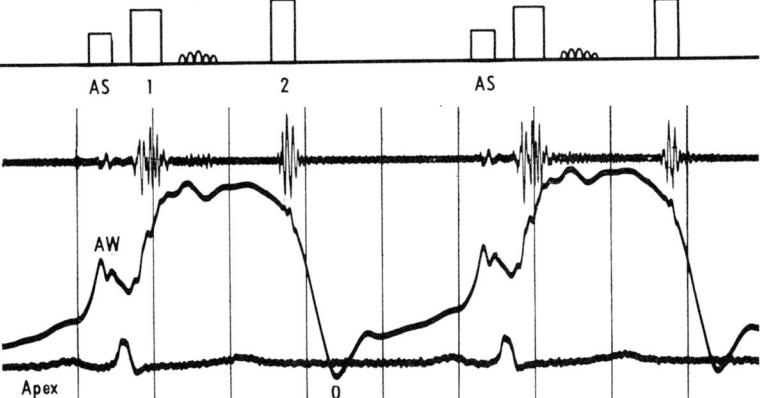

not mean that *cardiac failure* is present or even remotely imminent, although they may indicate the presence of ventricular hypertrophy, fibrosis or myocardial disease. With ventricular failure, however, especially with hypertrophy or myocardial ischemia, a fourth sound is exceedingly common. Needless to say, fourth sounds do not occur in the presence of atrial fibrillation.

With *delayed atrioventricular conduction,* a fourth sound may often be heard in the absence of any other evidence of cardiac pathology. The first sound is faint because of the prolonged P-R interval, and the fourth sound may be louder than the first heart sound. When conduction is prolonged, the fourth sound may, at more rapid rates, be early or middiastolic rather than presystolic. In *complete heart block*, a sound produced by atrial contraction can usually be heard and is most evident in early diastole when the atrial contraction is superimposed on the phase of rapid ventricular filling (see Fig. 4–4, p. 35).

Ejection Sounds

Depending on the auscultatory impression, these sounds have been called *ejection sounds* or *ejection clicks.* They have often been more specifically identified as *early systolic sounds (clicks)* or *early systolic ejection sounds (clicks).* Shortening the term to *ejection sound* does not appear to produce any confusion.

As previously noted (p. 29), the first sound usually has vibrations which, because of timing, have been considered by some investigators to be related to the sudden opening of the semilunar valves and distention of the great vessels at the onset of ejection (see Fig 5–1). Others believe that neither of the above events contributes to the audible first sound and that the audible components are produced entirely by the mitral and tricuspid valves. It seems reasonable that opening of the semilunar valves does produce vibrations that under normal conditions are of low intensity and are fused with the late vibrations that comprise the first sound, and therefore are "inaudible." Certain pathologic states produce hemodynamic changes which combine to increase the intensity of these vibrations and delay their onset. These are referred to as *ejec-*

tion sounds or *ejection clicks*. Examples of these pathologic states include: (1) the presence of a stenotic, but mobile, semi-lunar valve; (2) the ejection of a greater than usual amount of blood by the left or right ventricle, or both ventricles; and (3) a more forceful ventricular ejection due to the presence of hypertension in the aorta or pulmonary artery. Under these circumstances, isometric contraction is prolonged and the semilunar valves open under greater pressure. An aorta or pulmonary artery that is somewhat dilated because of the increased pressure may be more likely to vibrate in the audible range with additional dilatation. Another example of a pathologic state is (4) the presence of marked dilatation of the pulmonary artery or aorta that sometimes occurs without elevated pressures.

The increased sound may be the result of the sudden arrest of the upward movement of a dome-shaped, stenotic semilunar valve, the more sudden and forceful dilation of the aorta or pulmonary artery, or the impinging of a jet on the vessel wall. It is possible for one or all of these factors to be involved in any particular case.

The auscultatory sensation may take a number of forms: (1) the first sound may be prolonged and may not be recognized as being split; (2) the first sound may be moderately split, with both components giving a fairly similar sound sensation; (3) a moderately to widely split sound may occur, with the second component being higher pitched and clicking in quality.

The auscultatory sensation produced by ejection sounds, in addition to the variations noted above, depends on whether the listener uses the bell or diaphragm chest piece. The ejection sound is sharper and more click-like with the use of the diaphragm, and what may sound like a prolonged first sound with the bell will be clearly split with the diaphragm. This is due to the presence of low-frequency sounds which are longer lasting and blend the two sounds. The higher-frequency vibrations are more clearly separated.

Ejection sounds may be produced on the right side (pulmonary ejection sounds) or on the left side (aortic ejection sounds) of the heart.

PULMONARY. — These sounds are usually of maximum intensity in the second or third left interspace, but may be heard down along the left border of the sternum. They are not usually heard at the apex. Most often they are sharp and clicking in quality and markedly affected by respiration (Fig 5–5), being louder on expiration and much fainter or actually disappearing on inspiration. When the first sound appears loud and snapping in the second left interspace, especially when it is louder in this area than at the apex, the presence of an ejection sound produced at the pulmonary valve and artery should be suspected. The first sound may not be evident in the pulmonic area, but by listening between the apex and the second left interspace, both the first sound and ejection click may sometimes be heard.

Occurrence. — Pulmonary ejection sounds occur in most instances of pulmonary valve stenosis (p. 188) (see Fig. 5–14, C), except in some of the very mild and, occasionally, in some

Fig 5–5. — Pulmonary ejection sound in pulmonary hypertension with dilation of pulmonary artery. This sound *(ES)* is best heard in the second and third left intercostal spaces and is loudest in expiration. It has a clicking quality. The auscultatory impression is very similar to that of a split first sound with a loud second component. The sound is not heard at the apex *(lower tracing)*. A high-pitched diastolic murmur *(DM)* is present *(upper tracing)* and is produced by pulmonary regurgitation. As is generally true, a high-pitched murmur is much more evident to the ear than on a tracing.

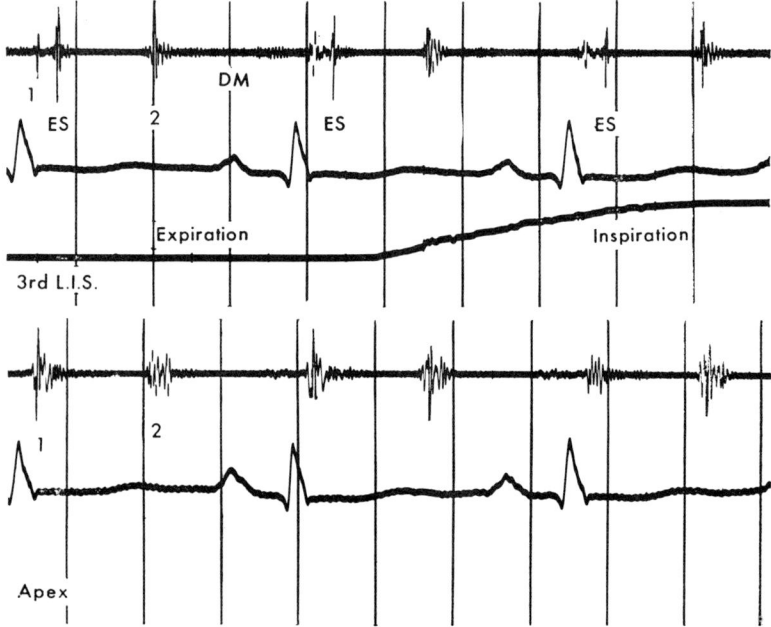

of the very severe cases. An ejection sound may be masked by the systolic murmur in the second left interspace but may be evident in the third left interspace.

A pulmonary ejection sound may occur in pulmonary hypertension, whether primary or secondary. It tends to be less click-like than in pulmonary stenosis and less affected by respiration; it is often heard farther down the sternum.

A pulmonary ejection sound may, at times, be heard in conditions associated with increased right ventricular output, such as atrial septal defect or ventricular septal defect. It may be present with a dilated pulmonary artery with no shunt and

Fig 5–6.—Aortic ejection sound in a patient with mild congenital aortic stenosis. This sound *(ES)* was well heard at the apex and at the second right intercostal space. Its intensity was not appreciably affected by respiration. The first sound was faint, especially in the aortic area. A rough systolic murmur *(SM)* of maximum intensity at the second right intercostal space was present. The murmur was faint at the apex.

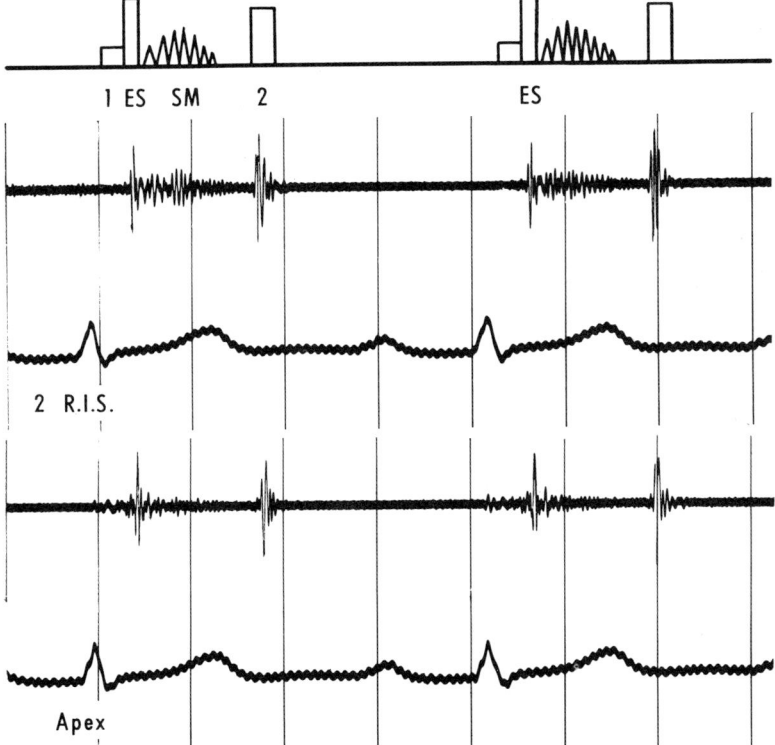

no pulmonary hypertension. Some patients with "idiopathic" dilatation of the main pulmonary artery actually exhibit very mild valvular pulmonic stenosis and an ejection sound.

AORTIC. — These sounds are usually best heard at the apex, but are also heard along the left border of the sternum and in the aortic area (Fig 5–6). An aortic ejection sound should be considered if the first sound is definitely split at the apex or somewhat lateral to the apex. This is especially true if the second component is higher pitched and somewhat click-like. Unlike the pulmonary ejection sound, the aortic ejection sound is not affected by respiration.

Occurrence. — An aortic ejection sound is present in almost all instances of *congenital aortic stenosis* and tends to be click-like in quality. *Rheumatic aortic stenosis* may occasionally have an ejection sound at the apex.

An aortic ejection sound associated with an ejection murmur places the level of obstruction at the valve, ejection sounds being rarely heard in supravalvular, discrete subvalvular or muscular subaortic stenosis.

Systemic hypertension may be associated with an ejection sound, but this does not appear to be especially common; a fourth sound at the apex is much more common.

Fig 5–7. — An aortic ejection sound in a patient with marked aortic regurgitation. The sound was not sharp and clicking in quality but sounded like the usual first sound. Quality of a sound is not recognizable on the ordinary phonocardiogram, but comparison with Figure 5–6 illustrates the difference in duration of the sound which is related somewhat to the quality. The diastolic murmur of aortic regurgitation is not usually especially evident at the apex but was in this patient because of its intensity.

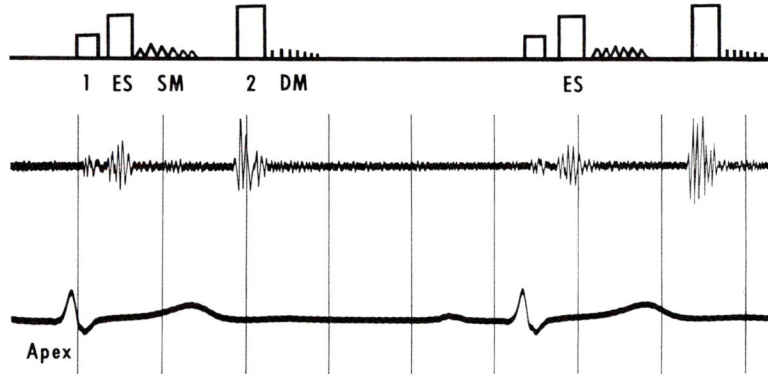

Aortic regurgitation of significant degree is commonly associated with an ejection sound that can be heard at the apex. It is not especially click-like in character and sounds like a split first sound (Fig. 5–7). The same type of ejection sound may occasionally be heard with a large patent ductus arteriosus or with coarctation of the aorta. In the latter, a congenitally bicuspid aortic valve should be suspected. An ejection sound may, on rare occasion, be heard in a normal individual with an overactive heart.

Systolic Clicks

Systolic clicks are sharp clicking sounds which generally occur later in systole than ejection sounds, although they may occur during any part of systole (Fig 5–8). They are usually single but may be multiple and are usually best heard between the lower end of the sternum and the apex. These sounds have previously been referred to as *systolic gallops* and have been regarded as benign. They have also been heard in connection with pericarditis, and thickened, roughened areas of the pericardium have been demonstrated in such pa-

Fig 5–8.—Systolic click. This patient had an atrial septal defect, and the midsystolic click *(SC)* was heard only on one occasion. The patient had been seen several other times and no systolic click was heard. The click was most evident on expiration. It was not heard in the pulmonic or aortic region, but was confined to the area between the apex and the left border of the sternum.

Note the split second sound which is characteristic of atrial septal defect. In this condition, the split second sound is often evident at the apex, despite the absence of an accentuated pulmonic sound. A middiastolic murmur *(DM)* is frequently heard in the apicosternal region in patients with atrial septal defects.

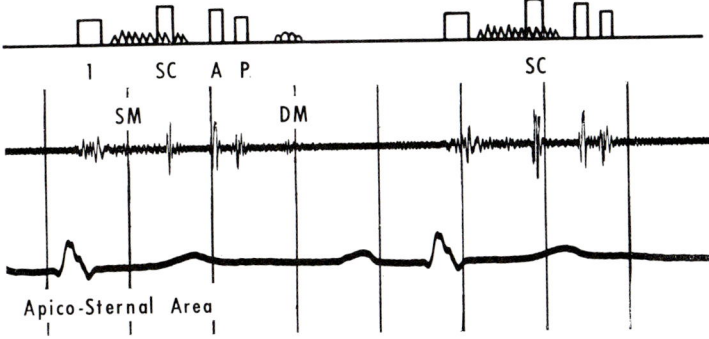

tients. Recent experience demonstrates that in most instances
they are due to a degree of mitral valve prolapse with or without mitral regurgitation.

The most important systolic click is that associated with the
so-called *click-murmur syndrome* (Fig 5–9). In this entity, a

Fig 5–9.—Midsystolic click with late systolic crescendo murmur. The
upper tracing was taken when the patient was 43 years old and about a
month after a murmur was found for the first time. This patient had had
frequent examinations and no murmur had ever been heard before. He had
no complaints at this time and the heart was normal in size. The systolic
click was heard at the apex and along the left border of the sternum. The
murmur started with the click and was crescendo in character. It was loudest
at the apex but was heard quite well in the apicosternal region.

The lower tracing was taken three years later, at which time the patient
had congestive failure, and his heart was enlarged. At this time he had a
loud holosystolic murmur and a middiastolic sound which, because of the
rapid rate, was probably a summation sound, although at slower rates it
may have been primarily a third heart sound.

This patient was operated upon and found to have ruptured chordae
tendineae. Following a plastic repair, the murmur has become faint and the
heart size has returned to normal.

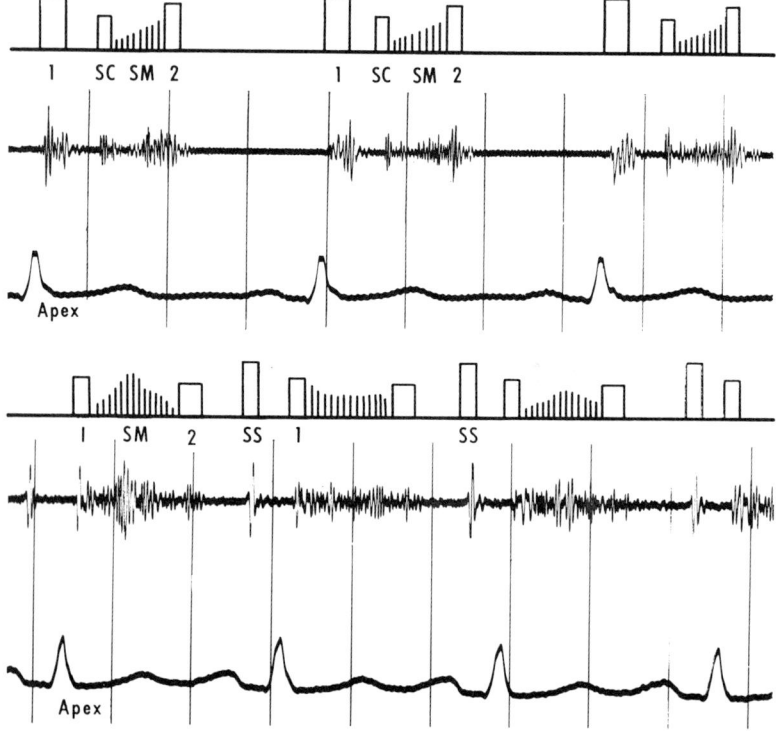

late systolic murmur begins with a midsystolic click and continues to the second sound. The pathologic mechanism has been shown to be prolapse of a leaflet of the mitral valve (usually the posterior leaflet) late in systole; this allows regurgitation, which begins with the prolapse and builds up to the second sound. The click is due to sudden tensing of the prolapsed leaflet or chordae tendineae, or both, just prior to onset of the regurgitant flow. This click is much more widely heard than innocent systolic clicks, and it often has the intensity pattern on the precordium of an opening snap of the mitral valve (p. 71). Other evidence of cardiac involvement, including left atrial enlargement, may be present although the findings are often stable for months or years. The characteristic click and late systolic crescendo murmur are best heard in the supine position; in the erect position the click tends to move toward the first sound and the murmur tends to occupy more of systole, occasionally becoming holosystolic with the click hard to detect. The click-murmur syndrome has been associated with "idiopathic" mitral prolapse, sometimes due to myxomatous degeneration, redundancy of a leaflet ("floppy valve"), and papillary muscle dysfunction due to ischemic heart disease. Both atrial and ventricular dysrhythmias occur and sudden death has been reported. These entities are treated in greater detail in subsequent sections.

Opening Snap of the Mitral Valve

A stenotic mitral valve that has retained some degree of flexibility may produce a sound when it opens. This sound usually occurs 0.08–0.10 second after the second sound, and has been called the *opening snap of the mitral valve* (see Fig 5–1.) Phonocardiograms occasionally show small vibrations at this point in normal persons, but usually no audible sound is present. In such cases of mitral stenosis, the valve resembles a hammock with a hole in the middle (see Figs 12–4 and 12–5, pp. 198 and 199). During systole, the hammock bulges into the atrium. At the end of systole, as the pressure in the left ventricle drops below that in the left atrium, the hammock is snapped back and bulges into the left ventricle. The higher the pressure in the left atrium, the more forcible is the movement of the valve and the louder the sound. Other factors in-

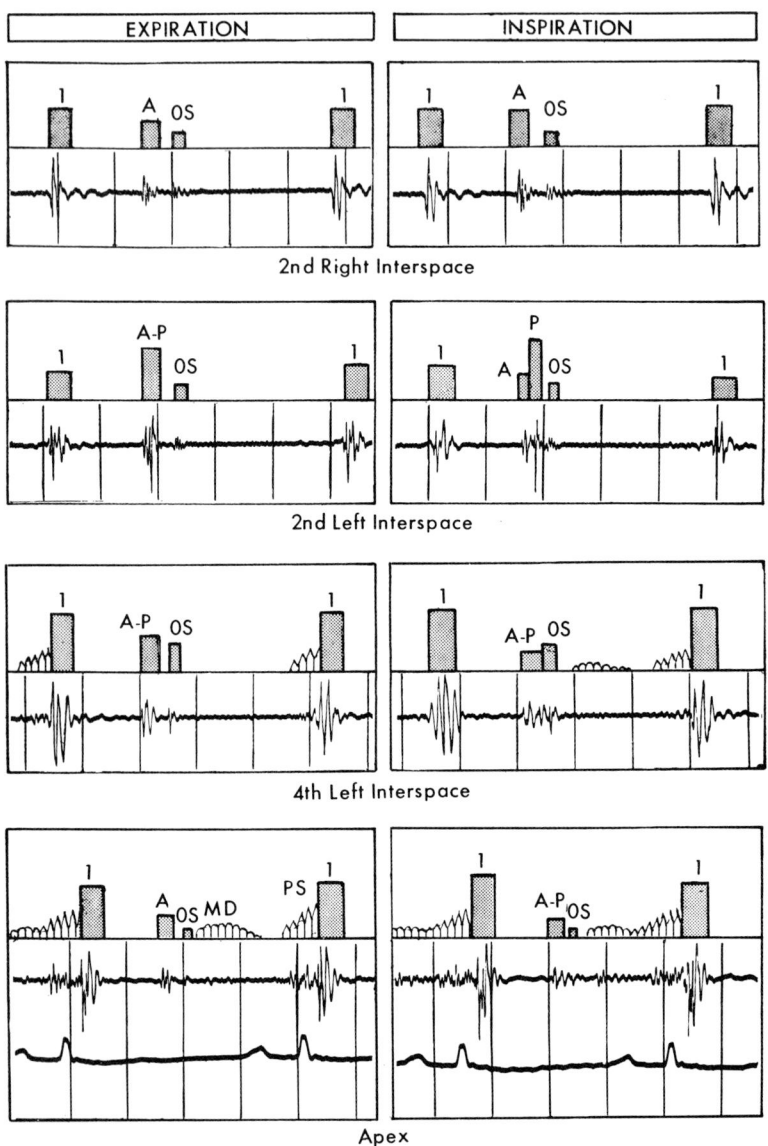

Fig 5–10. —Opening snap of mitral valve. The opening snap of the mitral valve *(OS)* is usually loudest in the fourth left intercostal space. In this area it has a clicking quality. It is most evident in expiration but is usually recognized in inspiration. In the second left interspace, the opening snap is usually heard in expiration. However, in inspiration in this area the pulmonic second sound *(P)* moves into the space between the aortic second sound

volved in the increased sound production would be similar to those resulting in an increased first sound in mitral stenosis (p. 37).

The sound is medium pitched and of a snapping or clicking quality. It may be louder in some areas than the second heart sound, which it often resembles. It is always associated with a good, and usually accentuated, first heart sound. The opening snap may be heard over the entire precordium but is best heard along the left border of the sternum at about the fourth intercostal space (Fig 5–10). In this area, the sharp, snapping character is marked, and the sound can be easily recognized. At the apex, the opening snap is less intense and may be masked by the middiastolic murmur unless attention is directed toward it. In the pulmonic area, the opening snap must be separated from a split second sound. Separation can usually be accomplished by recognition of both the split second sound and the opening snap, on the basis of differential changes that occur on respiration; these are described in detail below. In the aortic area, the opening snap is often well heard, but it has less of a snapping quality. It is probably the most commonly heard extra sound in this area. When it is clearly evident in the aortic area, the opening snap can usually be heard in the suprasternal notch.

The opening snap of the mitral valve usually indicates a flexible valve, but, in persons over 40 years of age, the valve may be thickened or leathery and unsuitable for *finger fracture commissurotomy* (p. 206). Since it is often an early sign of mitral stenosis, the opening snap is not, in itself, an indication for operation. The snap is not heard, with few exceptions, when the valve is markedly fibrosed and calcified and cannot move. It persists after the onset of atrial fibrillation and, in

---

(A) and the opening snap, and it is often difficult to hear the opening snap after the pulmonic sound, especially if the pulmonic second sound is accentuated. With careful listening, all three sounds can occasionally be distinguished. The opening snap is usually well heard in the second right intercostal space and is the most common extra sound heard in that area. Since the pulmonic second sound is not evident in this area, the sound is equally well heard in inspiration and in expiration. The opening snap is present at the apex, but usually is not as loud as in the fourth left intercostal space. Often the accentuated first sound and the middiastolic *(MD)* and presystolic murmurs *(PS)* mask the opening snap.

most instances, after mitral commissurotomy, even though the clinical results may be excellent.

Since the time interval between the beginning of the second sound and the opening snap of the mitral valve represents the time from the closing of the semilunar valves until the pressure in the left ventricle falls below that in the left atrium, the higher the left atrial pressure, the shorter will be the time interval between the second sound and the opening snap (see Figs 5–1 and 8–1, p. 128). This interval can, with training, be estimated on auscultation with a fair degree of accuracy, and may be of some value in estimating the severity of the stenosis. If the left atrial pressure decreases as a result of mitral commissurotomy, the interval between the second sound and the opening snap should increase. Unfortunately, the correlation between the degree of stenosis and the interval between the second sound and the opening snap is not always good.

The opening snap can be distinguished from a split second sound on the following bases:

1. A split second sound is loudest in the pulmonic area; the opening snap is loudest to the left of the sternum in about the fourth intercostal space. When the pulmonic component is accentuated, a split second heart sound may be heard along the left border of the sternum. It is in these patients that the split second sound is most likely to be mistaken for an opening snap. Differentiation depends on the respiratory variation in the second sound. The fixed splitting of the second sound in patients with atrial septal defects is not infrequently mistaken for an opening snap. In these patients, the pulmonic component is loudest in the second left interspace, and careful listening in this area fails to show the respiratory variation described below.

2. With careful listening in the pulmonic area during respiration, both the split second sound and the opening snap can be recognized. On expiration, the splitting of the second sound is minimal or absent, and the opening snap is evident at a definite interval after the second sound. On inspiration, the splitting of the second sound is increased and becomes evident (see Figs 5–10 and 5–11). The opening snap maintains a constant interval to the aortic, or first, component of the second sound; and when the second sound is split, the pulmonic

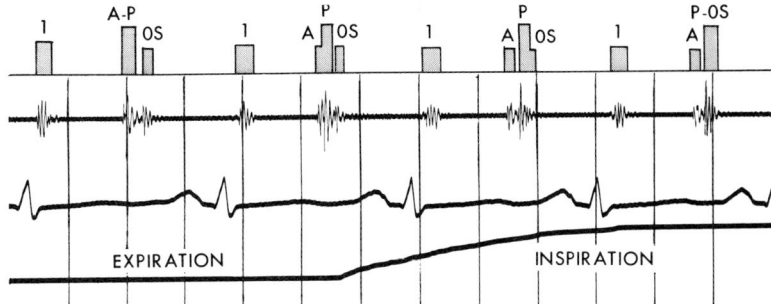

Fig 5–11.—Opening snap of mitral valve. In this patient, the opening snap *(OS)* is quite close to the aortic *(A)* and pulmonic *(P)* second sound on expiration, and the splitting that occurs on inspiration is enough to place the pulmonic second sound on top of the opening snap. The two sounds heard on expiration are, therefore, (1) the combined aortic and pulmonic second sounds and (2) the opening snap. On inspiration, the two sounds are (1) the aortic second sound and (2) the combined pulmonic second sound and opening snap.

component moves into the interval between the aortic second sound and the opening snap. Since the pulmonic second sound is often somewhat accentuated, the opening snap, which now immediately follows it, is heard with difficulty. When the pulmonic second sound is not loud, all three sounds may often be recognized on inspiration. On expiration, a very obvious snap that follows a single second sound is heard. When the opening snap closely follows the second sound, the pulmonic second sound, during inspiration, may actually be superimposed on the opening snap (Fig 5–11).

When the pulmonic second sound and opening snap are quite loud, the aortic second sound may be masked; this means that the pulmonic second sound and opening snap are the only sounds heard in this area. From the preceding description, it is readily appreciated that an erroneous impression of paradoxical splitting of the second sound results; this is relatively common and is referred to as *pseudoparadoxical splitting* of the second sound. This combination of sounds may occasionally appear "fixed" and be confused with atrial septal defect.

3. The opening snap of the mitral valve is usually evident in the aortic area, and here it follows the aortic second sound at an interval which is not affected by respiration.

4. Although a split second sound may occur with or without an accentuated first heart sound, the opening snap of the mitral valve occurs only with a good or accentuated first sound.

5. The characteristic murmur of mitral stenosis, of course, tends to confirm the presence of an opening snap.

The opening snap can be distinguished from a normal or abnormally accentuated third heart sound on the following bases:

1. The third heart sound is of much lower pitch and does not have the sharp character of the opening snap in the fourth left intercostal space.

2. The third heart sound, whether normal or abnormal, is more widely separated from the second heart sound (0.12–0.18 sec) than the opening snap.

3. The third heart sound is loudest near the apex and, unless quite loud, is not easily heard elsewhere in the precordium.

An *opening snap of the tricuspid valve* may also occur. It is of maximum intensity at the lower end of the sternum and may be well heard, or even maximum, along the lower right border of the sternum. Since the opening snap of the mitral valve is much more common and is widely heard, caution must be exercised in making the diagnosis of an opening snap of the tricuspid valve. It may be considered when the opening snap is of maximum intensity at the lower end of the sternum or to the right of the sternum, in the presence of other evidence of tricuspid stenosis.

It should be possible to distinguish the tricuspid opening snap phonocardiographically, since with respiration the opening snap should maintain a constant time interval with the pulmonic component of the second sound rather than with the aortic component. A phonocardiographic study of several patients with tricuspid stenosis associated with mitral stenosis indicates that the opening snap of the tricuspid valve usually occurs just before that of the mitral valve, and is difficult to recognize by ear in the presence of an opening snap of the mitral valve. With marked tricuspid stenosis, the normal inspiratory splitting of the second sound is decreased, possibly because filling of the right ventricle is limited by the stenosis.

Third Heart Sound

The third heart sound, when abnormal, has been given many titles. The timing of an abnormal third heart sound appears to be exactly like that of the normal third heart sound, and normality or abnormality depends on the context (age, clinical condition, etc.) in which the sound occurs. We have tried to stay with the term *third heart sound.* When the sound is abnormal, the term *ventricular gallop sound* or *ventricular gallop* may be used with some justification. *Early diastolic ventricular rapid filling sound,* or just *ventricular filling sound,* has been used. The terms *protodiastolic gallop* and *early diastolic gallop* have nothing to recommend them.

A third heart sound is commonly heard in children if sought for in the manner already described (p. 51). It can be recorded even more frequently on the phonocardiogram. It may be present in young adults at times, especially if they have thin chest walls or a hyperkinetic circulatory system, but is heard infrequently in persons over the age of 30 with normal hearts.

PRODUCTION. — There is no unanimity of opinion regarding the mechanism of production of the third heart sound, and the following description is a personal synthesis of some of the suggested mechanisms. The sound occurs at the end, or near the end, of early diastolic rapid filling of the ventricle when active relaxation is over. As the ventricle fills and the mitral annulus moves up and the apex down, the papillary muscles and chordae tendineae are tensed. Because of the manner in which the chordae tendineae are inserted into the valves, tensing of the chordae tendineae partially closes the valves. This partial closure of the valves and the slight increase in resistance to ventricular filling at the end of active relaxation combine to produce a sudden slowing of flow into the ventricle, and the almost-closed ventricle reacts with a shock and vibration to the changed condition. The presence of a palpable shock at the time of the third sound indicates that more than the falling together and tensing of the valves is involved. The entire ventricle — musculature, blood, chordae tendineae and valves — is set into vibration, although it may well be that most of the audible vibrations are produced by the valves and chordae tendineae.

As a person grows older, there is either a decrease in production of sound, a decrease in transmission of sound to the surface, or both, and no third heart sound is usually heard. Under pathologic conditions, the following factors favor sound production: (1) increased atrial pressure at the end of systole and in early diastole; this may result from an increased amount of blood in the atrium, as in mitral regurgitation, or as a result of failure of the ventricular myocardium; and (2) pathologic changes in the myocardium, such as inflammation and fibrosis, which impair the compliance of the ventricular muscle and make the transition from active relaxation to distention more abrupt.

In mitral regurgitation, there is an increased amount of blood under increased pressure in the atrium at the end of ventricular systole; therefore, flow into the ventricle is rapid and under greater pressure. A dilated mitral ring may exaggerate the condition. The ventricle would be expected to fill quickly, and the point at which sudden change in inflow occurs would be sooner. The third sound would, therefore, tend to be earlier in diastole than usual, and this is indeed often the case. If the atrioventricular valve is narrowed, as in mitral stenosis, the production of a third heart sound would be ruled out due to the slow filling of the ventricle.

DESCRIPTION. — Whereas the third sound normally heard in children is best heard at the apex and appears to be produced in the left side of the heart, a third sound may be produced by pathology in either the left side, the right side, or both sides of the heart. In most cases, those produced in the right side of the heart can be separated from those produced in the left.

When the sound is produced in the left side of the heart, it is best heard at the apex over the left ventricle. With increase in intensity, it has a wider distribution. It may be loudest at times in the mesocardiac area, although, when loudest in this area in a patient with left heart failure, the presence of both right and left third heart sounds should be suspected. Loud third heart sounds may be more obvious than the second sound and be mistaken for the second sound, especially in mitral regurgitation.

Right-sided third heart sounds are best heard along the left border of the sternum and in the mesocardiac area. They have the same auscultatory quality as the left-sided third sounds. A right-sided third sound may occasionally be heard in the right supraclavicular fossa when not heard elsewhere, and, in patients with emphysema, it may be most evident in the region of the xiphoid or slightly below the xiphoid.

Left-sided third heart sounds are usually more evident during expiration but when faint, they tend to show a waxing and waning which are difficult to correlate with respiration or any other obvious factor. Right-sided third heart sounds usually increase in intensity with inspiration.

Since the third sound occurs usually from 0.13 to 0.18 second after the second heart sound, it is definitely later than the opening snap of a mitral valve or the second component of a split second sound. It is also of much lower pitch, and the bell endpiece, applied lightly, must be used. A palpable and visible shock or bulge often occurs with a third heart sound and may be more obvious than the sound. At normal heart rates, the sound is in early diastole. As the rate increases, the sound maintains its relation to the second sound and may become middiastolic or actually presystolic. With atrial fibrillation, its position in diastole varies with the length of diastole; the intensity also varies with different beats.

Third heart sounds, when not loud and not due to the presence of pathology, may disappear when the patient sits up or stands up. If loud and due to pathology, they are more likely to persist, although their intensity may decrease. The intensity of the third heart sound is also decreased by tourniquets and during a Valsalva maneuver, although it will be increased after the Valsalva maneuver. Tourniquets do not affect a split second sound or an opening snap. When the third heart sound is due to the presence of pathology, it may disappear as the pathology improves. If it persists despite treatment, the prognosis may be poor.

OCCURRENCE. — The third heart sound is most significant when it occurs in a setting indicating or suggesting the presence of impaired myocardial reserve. A left-sided third heart sound may occur in left ventricular failure from any cause — coronary artery disease, hypertension, aortic valvular disease, etc. (see Fig 5–14, F). The third heart sound is especially common in the myocardiopathies, and its presence should always lead one to consider this diagnosis. Conditions causing right ventricular failure, such as pulmonary hypertension, pulmonary embolus, and some congenital heart diseases, will produce a right-sided third sound. Right ventricular failure secondary to mitral stenosis may result in a right-sided third heart sound. Failure of the left ventricle can eventually produce failure of the right ventricle, and left and right third heart sounds may be present.

In adults with cardiac pathology, fourth sounds are more common than third sounds, and are less serious from a prognostic standpoint. A patient with hypertension may have a fourth sound for many years with no other evidence of heart involvement, or only evidence of some left ventricular hypertrophy. With failure, this patient may develop a third heart sound and, if the heart rate is rapid, a summation sound. With improvement of the failure, the third heart sound leaves and the fourth sound remains.

In *constrictive pericarditis,* an early diastolic sound (pericardial knock) may be heard which is closer to the second sound than is the usual third sound (see Fig 5–14, I). Nevertheless, this sound is a rapid filling sound and probably occurs early because the ability of the ventricle to fill is limited by the constrictive pericarditis. The sound is of higher frequency than the usual third heart sound and is more widely heard. After a successful operation, it may disappear or occur later and have a lower pitch.

Summation Sounds (Summation Gallop)

When atrial contraction is superimposed on the phase of rapid ventricular filling, the two factors that can produce a diastolic sound are merged. If there was a tendency toward subaudible third and fourth sounds, the merging of these two now produces an audible sound. If a fourth and third heart sound were present together, a single louder sound is now heard (Figs 5–12, 5–13 and 5–14, G). If either sound was present without the other, the new sound is now louder. This sound has been called a *summation sound* or *summation gallop.* The auscultatory impression is that of a "gallop" and, in this case, one might justifiably call the auscultatory impression that of a "gallop rhythm."

For a summation sound to be present, there must be: (1)

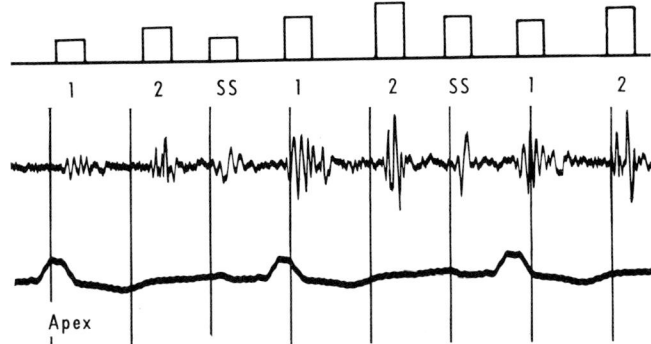

Fig 5–12.—Summation sound in a patient with arteriosclerotic heart disease and failure. The rate is rapid and the summation sound *(SS)* occurs in middiastole.

Fig 5–13.—*Upper tracing:* Quadruple or cogwheel rhythm occurring in a patient with arteriosclerotic heart disease in failure. When the heart rate is slow, a third heart sound *(3)* and a fourth sound *(4)* are evident. There is a prolonged P-R interval.

Lower tracing: Same patient when the heart rate is increased with exercise. There is now a single sound which is a summation sound and is louder than either the third heart sound or the fourth sound was previously.

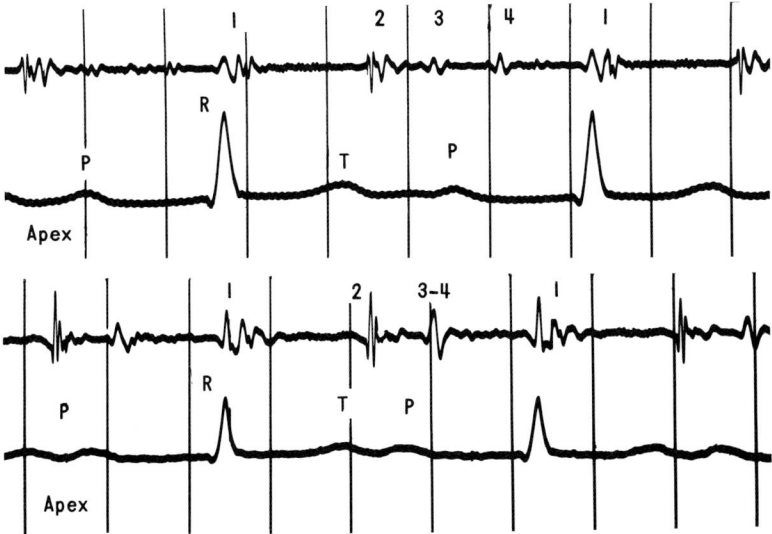

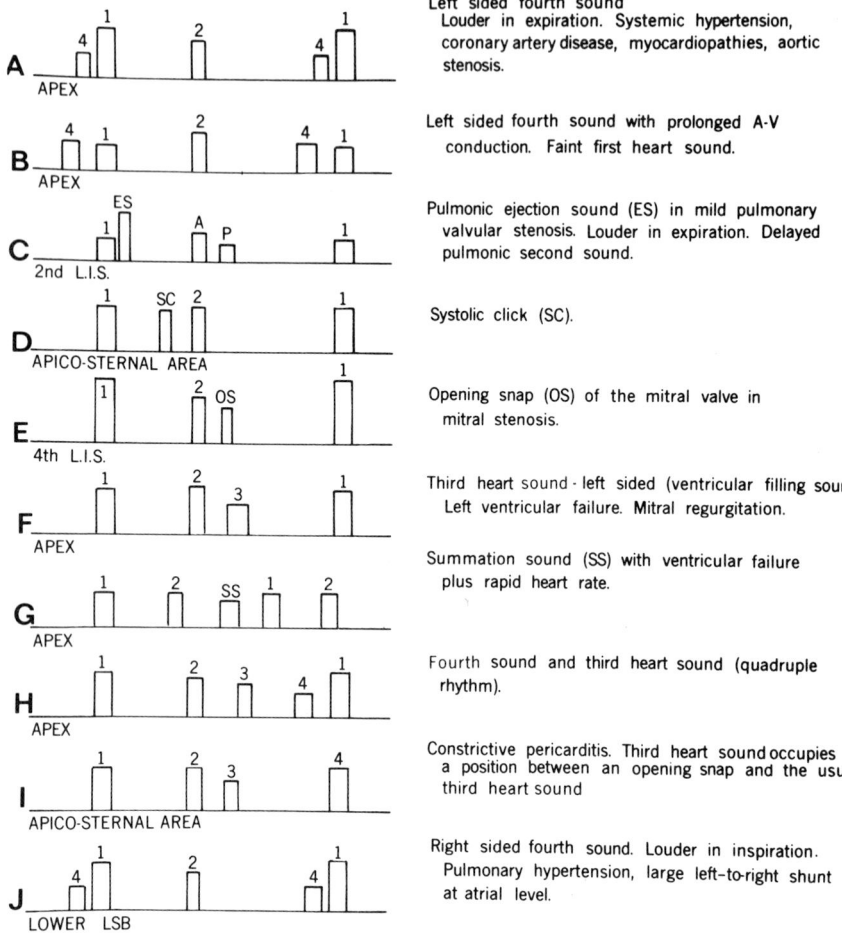

A APEX

Left sided fourth sound
Louder in expiration. Systemic hypertension, coronary artery disease, myocardiopathies, aortic stenosis.

B APEX

Left sided fourth sound with prolonged A-V conduction. Faint first heart sound.

C 2nd L.I.S.

Pulmonic ejection sound (ES) in mild pulmonary valvular stenosis. Louder in expiration. Delayed pulmonic second sound.

D APICO-STERNAL AREA

Systolic click (SC).

E 4th L.I.S.

Opening snap (OS) of the mitral valve in mitral stenosis.

F APEX

Third heart sound - left sided (ventricular filling sound). Left ventricular failure. Mitral regurgitation.

G APEX

Summation sound (SS) with ventricular failure plus rapid heart rate.

H APEX

Fourth sound and third heart sound (quadruple rhythm).

I APICO-STERNAL AREA

Constrictive pericarditis. Third heart sound occupies a position between an opening snap and the usual third heart sound

J LOWER LSB

Right sided fourth sound. Louder in inspiration. Pulmonary hypertension, large left-to-right shunt at atrial level.

Fig 5–14. — Table of extra heart sounds.

superimposition of the atrial contraction on rapid ventricular filling. This requires either a rapid heart rate, a prolonged P-R interval, or a combination of the two. A summation sound will not occur with atrial fibrillation; (2) an underlying tendency to abnormal sound production (pp. 56 and 75).

Summation sounds tend to be louder than third sounds or fourth sounds and are more widely heard. The shock or bulge of the chest wall, sometimes seen with the third heart sound or fourth sounds, is more common with a summation sound. With left ventricular failure, the summation sound is best heard over the left ventricle but is often more widely heard. With right ventricular failure the summation sound is in the apico-sternal area. A pulsus alternans and left bundle branch block are often associated findings. The summation sound is most common in ventricular failure associated with chronic coronary artery disease, hypertension, acute myocardial infarction and myocardiopathies.

Because the presence of a third heart sound is of greater prognostic significance than a fourth sound, it is important to attempt to determine which, if any, sound persists when the heart rate is slowed. If the heart rate is slowed by carotid sinus pressure, breath-holding, or cardiac therapy, the findings will depend on the underlying cardiac status: (1) no extra sounds may be heard; (2) only the fourth sound or the third heart sound may persist; or (3) the fourth and third heart sound may both persist and, if the rate is slow enough, give what has been called a *quadruple* or *cogwheel rhythm* (see Figs 5–13 and 5–14, H). With a mildly slowed rate, there may be only a slight separation of the third and fourth sounds, and the impression of a short diastolic rumble may be obtained, since the two sounds will not be recognized as separate. If atrial fibrillation occurs at either a rapid or slow rate, the atrial component leaves and the third heart sound may or may not be heard.

As a general rule, the fourth sound and third sound tend to occur under similar circumstances, that is, with decreased ventricular compliance. The fourth sound is a more "sensitive" indication of this condition and therefore tends to occur earlier and persist longer than the third sound. This is best understood by realizing that by the end of diastole the great majority of ventricular filling has occurred and that atrial contraction is an attempt to further stretch and "fill" the ventricle.

CHAPTER 6

Murmurs: General Considerations

Production

IT HAS GENERALLY BEEN BELIEVED that most murmurs are produced by turbulent blood flow. The center part of the blood stream flows faster than the periphery; and above a certain velocity, turbulence occurs because of this difference in the speed of flow. It appears unlikely, theoretically and experimentally, that this turbulence can generate enough acoustical energy to produce detectable murmurs (Bruns, 1959). As a river flows past a rock or obstruction, a wake is produced. In our thinking, this type of response has been mistakenly equated with turbulence. Whereas turbulence indicates a randomness, fluid flowing past an obstruction results in a periodic fluctuation, which is a much more efficient producer of sound. Vortices form a wake downstream from the obstruction. A vortex in the circulatory system is a small amount of blood having a whirling or circular motion and tending to form a vacuum in the center; this draws blood toward it. The pressure fluctuations in the wake result from the flow of blood from other areas to fill the space occupied by the vortex just prior to its being shed; they are, thus, the response of the mass of blood comprising the wake to the shedding of the vortices. The frequency of shedding of the vortices determines the pitch of the sound produced. The vibrations and sound are produced in the blood and only secondarily transmitted to and through the heart and vascular structures.

Some of the theoretical and experimental implications

of sound production by vortex formation may be listed as
follows.

1. The intensity of a murmur is markedly dependent on
velocity of blood flow, since it varies as the fourth power of
velocity. The murmur of mitral stenosis may not be heard at
rest, but becomes evident with exercise, tachycardia, and thyrotoxicosis. On the other hand, a quite evident murmur of mitral stenosis may disappear with the decrease in blood flow
which results from decompensation or severe myxedema.
Most murmurs are louder after exercise. In anemia, there is an
increased velocity of blood flow, and murmurs are common.

2. The pitch of a murmur increases with the velocity of
blood. The velocity of blood through an obstruction will depend on the pressure gradient across the obstruction. Murmurs associated with high differences in pressure will be
higher pitched (e.g., left ventricle to left atrium in mitral regurgitation) than those associated with low pressure differences (e.g., left atrium to left ventricle in mitral stenosis). The
frequency also depends on the size of the orifice; higher frequencies are obtained with small orifices, and lower frequencies are obtained with obstructions of moderate size. Since
most obstructive orifices and protuberances into the stream
are rough and of unequal size, instead of obtaining one basic
frequency, there are numerous frequencies, and noise, instead
of a note, is produced.

3. A sudden constriction of a vessel, followed by a return to
the original size, will result in vortex formation and a murmur.
A sudden dilation of a vessel without a previous constriction
will produce vortices; in comparison with the dilation, the
normal vessel is now relatively constricted. Mitral stenosis
and aortic stenosis constitute a constriction that produces a
murmur. Similar murmurs may be heard when the left ventricle is dilated and the mitral valve is of normal size, or when
the aorta is dilated and the aortic valve is of normal size. The
normal mitral and aortic valves are relatively constricted in
relation to the dilated left ventricle and aorta.

4. When blood flows through an orifice and vortices are
formed and shed, the frequency of the sound at the orifice
approximately equals the shedding frequency. A sound of this
frequency is transmitted upstream. Downstream, the vortices
tend to coalesce, and in this region the sound produced has a

lower frequency than at the orifice. Thus, in some patients with aortic stenosis, the murmur heard in the aortic area and aorta tends to be lower pitched and harsher than the higher-pitched murmur heard at the apex of the heart. Other factors may play a part in this phenomenon.

5. Projections into the blood stream represent wake-forming obstructions and are producers of sound. A roughened valve or an arteriosclerotic projection into a vessel can produce sound.

OTHER SUGGESTED MECHANISMS OF MURMUR PRODUCTION. — When a regurgitant stream passes the edge of a valve and causes it to vibrate, a murmur is produced in the same manner that a note is produced in a reed instrument. *Collision murmurs* may originate when the cardiac or vascular wall is struck by a current of blood, e.g., when a stream of blood through a stenosed aortic or pulmonary valve strikes the vessel wall. Normal structures, such as the chordae tendineae, or unusual structures, such as the so-called *ventricular moderator bands*, may be set into vibration and produce rather musical murmurs. It should be noted that these structures may produce a musical murmur merely by acting as vortex-producing obstructions.

It is conceivable that the entire heart, or a major section of the heart or great vessels, may be set into vibration at its natural frequency by the motion of the blood through it. Some such mechanism may play a part in the production of *innocent* systolic murmurs.

Regurgitation and Stenosis

REGURGITATION. — A valve that cannot close, and thus permits the reflux of blood, is said to be *regurgitant*. Regurgitation may occur either because of pathologic changes involving the valve or because of changes in the supporting structures around the valves. The pathologic changes in the valves may vary from minor deformities to marked thickening and shortening of the cusps and chordae tendineae with immobilization of the valves. Changes in the supporting tissues consist of dilation of the valve ring and, in the case of the atrioventricular valves, dilation of the ventricles to the point where the chordae tendineae may not be long enough to permit the valve edges to approximate. Involvement of the valve cusps is called *organic regurgitation*. When the valve cusps are not involved, the terms *functional regurgitation* and *relative regurgitation* have been used. The terms *insufficiency* and *regurgitation* are generally used interchangeably, and, since regurgitation is more widely used, we have used this term in this edition.

STENOSIS.—A decrease in the size of a valve, due to pathologic changes in the valve, produces an *organic stenosis*. The term *relative stenosis* is used when the valve itself is normal but the chamber or vessel beyond the valve is enlarged. Murmurs produced at a normal valve, because of an increased flow through the valve or a relative stenosis, are often called *flow murmurs*—a good descriptive term.

Description of Murmurs

TIMING AND DURATION.—*Systolic murmurs.*—Systolic murmurs have varied timing and duration. If the murmur extends throughout systole (from the first to the second sound), it is called a *holosystolic* or *pansystolic murmur*. Holosystolic would appear preferable on the basis of derivation. If the murmur does not extend throughout systole, it may be primarily early, mid, or late systolic. A systolic murmur may start loud and fade—a *decrescendo murmur;* or start faint and increase in intensity—a *crescendo murmur*. These murmurs may or may not be holosystolic. Some murmurs first increase in intensity to a peak and then decrease—a *crescendo-decrescendo murmur*. These have been called *diamond-shaped murmurs,* and they may or may not be holosystolic.

Systolic murmurs have been divided into *midsystolic ejection murmurs* (usually called *ejection murmurs*), produced by forward flow through the aortic and pulmonary valves, and *holosystolic regurgitant murmurs,* produced by backward flow through the atrioventricular valves, or flow from the left to the right ventricle in ventricular septal defect (Leatham, 1958). The main basis for this division is the difference in the timing of the murmur in relation to the first and second sounds. The dynamic basis for this difference is illustrated in Figure 6–1. The flow through a deformed or stenotic aortic valve does not start until left ventricular pressure begins to exceed aortic pressure at the end of isometric contraction. With aortic steno-

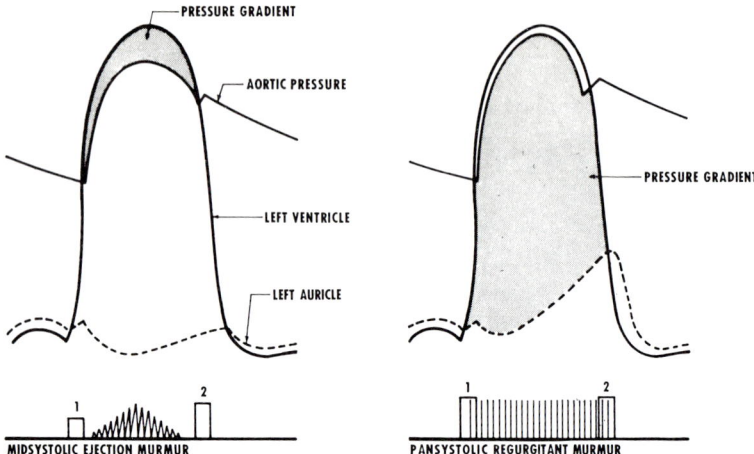

Fig 6–1.—Basis for division of systolic murmurs into midsystolic ejection murmurs and pansystolic (holocystolic) regurgitant murmurs (see text). The midsystolic ejection murmur is produced by forward flow through the aortic or pulmonic valve. It starts at the end of, or after, the first heart sound and stops before the second heart sound. The left ventricular-aortic pressure gradient and consequently, the murmur are maximum in midsystole.

The holosystolic regurgitant murmur starts with the first heart sound and lasts throughout systole, and may actually extend somewhere into the second heart sound. Here the pressure gradient remains high throughout systole.

sis, the gradient between the left ventricle and the aorta increases to midsystole; the velocity of flow and the intensity of the murmur, therefore, increase to midsystole. As the pressure in the left ventricle falls, the gradient decreases and reaches zero at the closure of the aortic valve. The murmur, accordingly, decreases in intensity and stops before the second sound. Since the first sound or an ejection component usually extends to the end of isometric contraction, there may be no significant or auscultatory recognizable interval between the first sound and the onset of murmur, but the murmur starts with low intensity and builds up to a peak. The crescendo-decrescendo shape (diamond shape) can be recognized with training. The cessation of the murmur before the second sound is the most easily recognized characteristic. It must be noted that the murmur stops before the second sound of the side of the heart involved. Thus, the pulmonary ejection murmur of pulmonary stenosis stops before the delayed pulmonic second sound but extends beyond the aortic second sound (see Fig 11–6, p. 187). When the murmur is not due to stenosis but to increased flow through the valves or to valvular deformity, the flow velocity and murmur reach a peak early in systole; with stenosis, the peak is later.

The holosystolic regurgitant murmurs (mitral regurgitation, tricuspid regurgitation, and ventricular septal defect) are produced by flow from a high-pressure chamber (left and right ventricle) into a low-pressure chamber (left and right atrium). This difference in pressure is present at the very onset of systole and actually persists for a short period after the onset of the second sound (see Fig 6–1). These murmurs should thus, theoretically, be holosystolic.

The classification of systolic murmurs into ejection murmurs and holosystolic regurgitant murmurs has been of mixed value. It has served to call attention to the dynamics of murmur production and the importance of differences in timing in the diagnosis of systolic murmurs. On the other hand, there have been some undesirable consequences:

1. In placing great emphasis on the timing and phonocardiographic shape of murmurs, many physicians have lost sight of the important differences in pitch and quality in these murmurs and even, at times, of the importance of the site of maximum intensity. The pitch and quality are more easily recognized by most physicians than are the finer details of timing. It can be shown that if the second sound is faint or absent, most physicians who interpret a murmur as diamond shaped do so by recognizing the quality of the murmur rather than the shape of the murmur; they have associated a certain quality with the diamond shape.

2. Not all regurgitant murmurs are holosystolic, and not all ejection-type murmurs are due to flow through the aortic and pulmonary valves. Faint and moderately loud mitral regurgitant murmurs are not usually recognizably holosystolic to the ear, and many crescendo and decrescendo mumurs of mitral regurgitation require a magnified phonocardiogram to pick up a stray vibration that will classify them as holosystolic. The murmur of ventricular septal defect may have all the characteristics of an ejection murmur.

3. There is a good deal of confusion in the use of the term *ejection murmur*. It was defined originally as a murmur pro-

duced by flow through the aortic and pulmonary valves. Since this murmur is rough or harsh in quality and crescendo-decrescendo in form, the term ejection murmur has been used for any murmur having these two qualities, with no regard to etiology. Murmurs heard over peripheral arteries are described as ejection murmurs, and the literature contains many references to ejection murmurs heard in patients with mitral valve disease, ventricular septal defects, and lesions of unknown etiology. Perhaps the term *ejection-type murmur* might be used for the rough-to-harsh, crescendo-decrescendo murmurs not produced by flow through the aortic and pulmonary valves.

When the length of diastole varies in different beats, as it does in atrial fibrillation or with premature contractions, aortic and pulmonary systolic (ejection) murmurs behave differently from the murmurs of mitral and tricuspid regurgitation. The murmur of aortic stenosis, for example, is much louder after a long diastole than after a short diastole, whereas the murmur of mitral regurgitation, within limits, shows little variation in intensity with the length of diastole (Fig 6–2). The left ventricular-aortic pressure gradient is sensitive to changes in left ventricular filling and aortic pressure. During a long diastole, the aortic pressure falls to a lower level than during a short diastole; at the same time, left ventricular filling is increased. These factors result in a high-pressure gradient and a loud murmur. The reverse is true with a short diastolic pause. In mitral regurgitation, there is always a high-pressure gradient (see Fig 6–1), and changes in left atrial and left ventricular pressure with change in length of diastole do not affect this high-pressure gradient enough to produce significant variations in the intensity of the murmur.

Diastolic murmurs. — Diastolic murmurs may occupy one or another portion of diastole and may be described as *early diastolic* when they start with the second sound, *middiastolic* when there is a short pause after the second sound, and *late diastolic* or *presystolic* when due to atrial contraction. A *continuous murmur* is heard in systole and diastole and has the same quality in both phases.

INTENSITY. — The *point of maximum intensity* of a murmur is usually the most important characteristic of the murmur and must be determined accurately. Murmurs produced in dif-

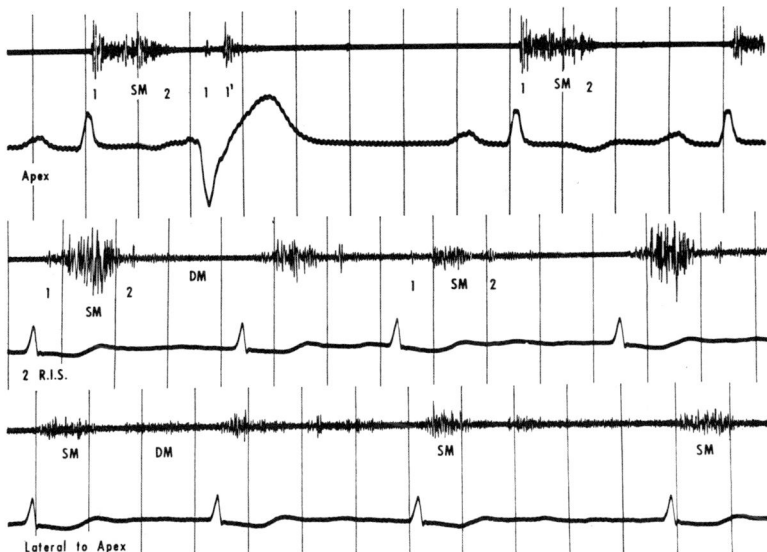

Fig 6-2.—The effect of varying duration of diastole on the intensity of mitral and aortic systolic murmurs. The *upper tracing* was taken on a man with severe mitral regurgitation due to ruptured chordae tendineae. Note that following a ventricular premature contraction there is a long diastolic pause during which the heart can fill to a greater than usual degree, but that the systolic murmur on the subsequent beat is essentially of the same intensity as the systolic murmur on the regular beat at the beginning of the strip. The ventricular premature contraction shows a split first heart sound. There is very little murmur following the ventricular premature contraction because the ventricle at that point had very little blood in it.

The *middle* and *lower tracings* were taken on a woman who had an aortic stenosis with some aortic regurgitation and a mitral regurgitation with some mitral stenosis. The middle tracing was taken in the area in which the aortic systolic murmur was loudest. Note the marked variation in the systolic murmur depending on the length of the preceding diastole—the longer the diastole, the louder is the succeeding murmur. The lower tracing was taken in the area where the murmur of mitral regurgitation was loudest; note that this murmur shows very little variation with the duration of the preceding diastole. This woman had the diastolic murmurs of aortic regurgitation and mitral stenosis, in addition to the systolic murmurs.

ferent portions of the heart are transmitted to different locations on the chest wall.

Freeman and Levine's system (1933) of grading intensity on a basis of 1 to 6 works very well. A system based on 1 to 4 does not give an adequate range. In the 1 to 6 system, the numbers have the following connotations:

1 — Very faint
2 — Faint
3 — Moderately loud
4 — Loud
5 — Very loud
6 — Loudest possible

Grade 1 murmurs can be heard only with concentration in quiet rooms. Grade 6 murmurs usually can be heard without holding the stethoscope on the chest wall. The intensity number should be followed by a 6 to indicate that the scale of 6 has been used; thus, a loud murmur would be indicated by 4/6.

The loudness of a murmur, like the loudness of the heart sounds, will vary with extracardiac factors. This variation must be taken into consideration when correlating the intensity of a murmur with the amount of valvular involvement.

It has been noted that the intensity of a murmur will vary with velocity of blood flow. Since heart rate is often closely correlated with cardiac output and, therefore, velocity of flow, murmurs may be less evident at slow rates than at rapid rates. This fact should be recognized in making a comparison of murmurs on different occasions.

PITCH AND QUALITY. — Murmurs are noises, and their quality depends on their frequency makeup (p. 2). If white noise (sound containing all frequencies) is passed through a band-pass filter so that only those frequencies between certain limits get through, the resulting sounds, depending on the bands chosen, will mimic the murmurs and sounds produced by the heart (Fig 6-3). The sound obtained by passing only a very narrow band in the region of 360-370 cycles per second mimics the sound that is ordinarily called high pitched and blowing and is characteristic of the murmurs of mitral regurgitation and aortic regurgitation when they are not too loud. It is to be noted that the band-pass filter does not cut off the frequencies sharply but rather in a sloping degree, which permits some higher and lower frequencies to pass in lesser intensity.

If the upper limit of the band-pass filter is put at 460 and the lower limit is gradually lowered from 460 so as to pass lower frequencies, the sound produced becomes gradually more harsh. When a band of frequencies from 180 to 460 is being passed, the sound obtained is harsh and has the quality asso-

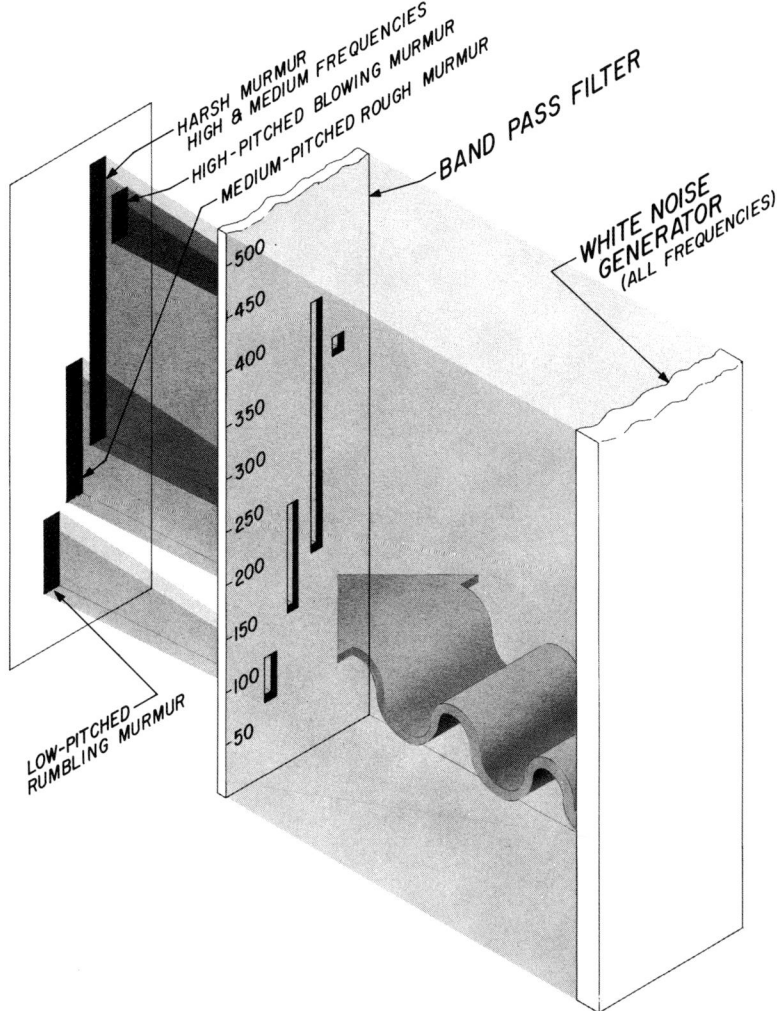

Fig 6–3.—Relation between the pitch and quality of murmurs and the frequency bands which mimic them. A white noise generator produces all the audible sound frequencies in a random manner. This white noise is passed through a band-pass filter which permits only certain frequencies to get through. The frequencies below 120 are considered low frequencies; those from 120 to about 250 are medium frequencies; and those over 300 are high frequencies. The harsh murmur of aortic and pulmonic stenosis is mimicked by a band of frequencies from 180 to 460, and thus consists of medium- and high-frequency vibrations. The high-pitched, blowing murmur of mitral and aortic regurgitation is mimicked by a narrow band of frequencies around 360. A medium-pitched, rough murmur is mimicked by a band of frequencies from 120 to 250, and a low-pitched, rumbling murmur by a band from 70 to 110.

91

cated with the loud murmur of aortic and pulmonic stenosis. A harsh murmur is thus a murmur that has high and medium frequencies. If a medium frequency range of 120 to 250 is passed, the impression is what we prefer to call a *rough murmur* — the type associated with aortic and pulmonic *flow murmurs* of faint to moderate intensity. The rumbling or low-pitched murmurs fall in the 70 – 110 frequency range. The fact that the murmurs are so closely mimicked by the frequency bands does not indicate that these are the only frequencies produced by the heart; it does indicate that the auditory impression made by the murmur depends primarily on the frequencies in the band.

These differences of pitch and quality can be taught and learned, and are extremely important in diagnosis. The mushrooming of phonocardiography has led to a neglect in the teaching of these differences in pitch and quality. The ordinary phonocardiogram gives information about the timing and shape of murmurs but tells little about pitch and quality. It is, therefore, understandable that many physicians who use phonocardiograms place marked emphasis on the shape and finer timing of murmurs and neglect the pitch and quality. I believe that the pitch and quality of a murmur are often more easily recognized and taught than the finer timing of a murmur and are very important to auscultation, if less important to phonocardiography. The ideal approach is to combine recognition of pitch and quality with an understanding of the finer details of timing.

When a murmur consists of such a narrow band of frequencies that the pitch becomes clear, and a fundamental tone, and even some overtones, are present, the murmur sounds musical. Some murmurs of aortic stenosis and mitral regurgitation may be described as musical. The term *musical murmur* is, however, commonly used in connection with unusual sounding murmurs having a very distinct musical quality. Almost any systolic or diastolic organic murmur may, in rare instances, have an unusual quality. Musical sounds may occur with pericarditis and they may be heard in hearts that are otherwise normal. Some of these murmurs may be very loud and audible without a stethoscope. Those produced because of pericardial changes or in the right side of the heart are often much louder on inspiration. *Whooping* and *honking* sounds may occupy part or all of systole. The *cooing* diastolic murmur is usually associated with a retroverted aortic cusp.

EFFECT OF EXERCISE ON MURMURS. — Exercise increases the velocity of blood flow and, in most instances, the loudness of murmurs. Occasionally, at rapid heart rates and with the extraneous noises incident to the exercise, murmurs may become less evident. Exercise is valuable for increasing the intensity of faint murmurs, and often important murmurs may be heard only after exercise. On the other hand, faint murmurs of no significance may be heard in normal persons after exercise. They have the characteristics of innocent systolic murmurs (p. 120) and not of the murmur of mitral regurgitation. Exercise is of no value in distinguishing *innocent* murmurs from *organic* murmurs, since both are usually increased in loudness. For evaluation of the degree of valvular involvement and for comparison of auscultatory findings on different days, observations made with the patient at rest are more valuable than those made after exercise.

Transmission of Murmurs

The following three phases of the transmission of murmurs are worthy of consideration.

1. FACTORS INFLUENCING THE LOCATION OF THE POINT OF MAXIMUM INTENSITY OF A MURMUR. — This point is determined by the location of the valve involved and the chamber in which the vibrations occur. The direction of the flow of blood through the valve is of great importance in locating the murmur because the vibrations are produced downstream. Any surgeon can prove this by noting on which side of a pathologic valve the thrill is felt. The importance of the direction of the stream of blood is illustrated in the case of aortic valve lesions. In aortic stenosis, where the wake is downstream, the murmur is best heard in the second and first right interspaces and up into the neck. In aortic regurgitation, where the wake is upstream, the murmur is best heard along the left border of the sternum.

Another factor influencing the point of maximum intensity is the nature of the tissues between the point of origin of the murmur and the chest wall. In an open chest, it can easily be shown that the murmur of mitral regurgitation is best heard over the left atrium. The left atrium, however, is separated from the chest wall by sound-insulating tissue—the lung. The murmur is, therefore, best heard over the left ventricle at the apex.

2. FACTORS INFLUENCING THE TRANSMISSION OF A MURMUR FROM THE POINT OF MAXIMUM INTENSITY.—The most important factor influencing the transmission of a murmur is the intensity of the murmur. The louder a murmur, the greater is the area over which it will be heard; very loud murmurs will be heard all over the chest and may be transmitted by the bones of the arms to the olecranon process. This, however, does not mean that the bones play an important role in the transmission of most murmurs. Bones transmit sounds much better than soft tissues because of their rigidity. The murmurs, however, are produced in the soft tissues, and a marked difference in the density and structure occurs at the interphase between the soft tissues and the bones. Most of the sound, when it reaches this interphase, will be reflected, and very little sound will enter the bones. If a very loud murmur is present, it may enter the bones in some strength and be widely transmitted by the bones.

3. CHANGES IN QUALITY OF MURMURS ON TRANSMISSION.— The reason why the quality of a murmur may change on transmission has been discussed on pages 3–4. An additional factor influencing the quality of transmitted murmurs might be considered. Most structures, when set into vibration, have a natural vibration frequency. In transmitting sound, these structures exaggerate frequencies similar to their natural frequency. Frequencies lower than the natural frequency are transmitted much better than higher frequencies. The lungs have a natural frequency somewhere between 130 and 180 per minute and they should, therefore, favor transmission of frequencies at and below this range. What the natural vibration frequency of the heart is, and how it affects transmission, are not known.

Relation of Murmurs and Thrills

A thrill is a palpable manifestation of a murmur; the fingers instead of the ears are used to determine the presence of vibration. Since the fingers are much less sensitive and discriminating than the ears, the vibrations have to be more intense before they are felt. The fingers, furthermore, do not make the fine distinction of pitch and quality. A thrill does not tell more about the nature of the underlying lesions than the ear has already learned. The association of a thrill with certain lesions, such as aortic stenosis, in the minds of most physicians, has done more harm than good. Many lesions which, when severe, produce a thrill, should and can be recognized by auscultation long before the onset of the thrill.

Thrills are most commonly felt in association with loud, harsh murmurs. High-pitched murmurs, such as the murmurs of aortic and mitral regurgitation, are not usually associated with thrills. Very low-pitched murmurs might, theoretically, be felt better than they can be heard, since the fingers are sensitive to vibrations that the ear cannot hear (below 20 per second).

CHAPTER 7

Systolic Murmurs

THE QUESTION IS OFTEN ASKED, "How significant is a systolic murmur?" The answer is, "What systolic murmur and at what stage in its development?" The importance of systolic murmurs is often judged by their loudness, and it is true that there may be a correlation between the loudness of a systolic murmur and the presence of underlying pathology. Some innocent murmurs, however, may be loud, especially in children, and some faint organic murmurs may be very significant. Most loud organic murmurs, other than congenital murmurs, must have been faint at one time. Criteria other than loudness are better when one is judging the importance of a systolic murmur. Most systolic murmurs can be correlated with the underlying pathology, and the question then becomes not what is the significance of the murmur, but what is the significance of the pathology.

The Systolic Murmur of Mitral Regurgitation

TIMING AND DURATION.—The murmur of mitral regurgitation is systolic because it is produced by a regurgitation through a valve which should be closed during ventricular systole (Figs 7–1 and 7–2). The murmur is usually holosystolic, especially if it is of moderate or marked intensity. The murmur is not necessarily of the same intensity throughout systole, and most often it is not; it may be crescendo, decrescendo, or even crescendo-decrescendo or diamond shaped. Not all mitral regurgitation murmurs are holosystolic. A late

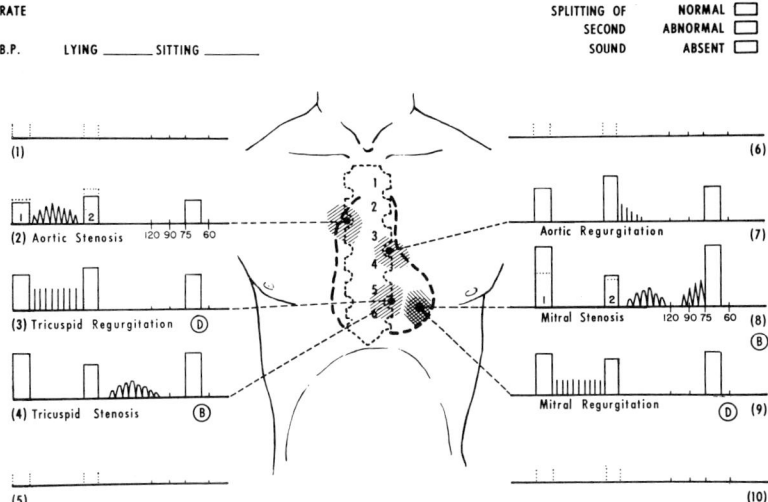

Fig 7-1.—Areas in which murmurs produced at aortic, mitral, and tricuspid valves are heard when they are faint. These are also usually the areas in which these murmurs are of maximum intensity when they are loud. With increase in heart size, the point of maximum intensity of the mitral and tricuspid murmurs may move laterally.

Fig 7-2.—Murmur of mitral regurgitation. The holosystolic character of the murmur is illustrated. The intensity shows some variation but remains very much the same throughout systole. The murmur (SM) starts with the first heart sound and continues up to the second heart sound. Both heart sounds may be masked by the murmur. A third heart sound, which is often heard in severe mitral regurgitation, is present. When the third heart sound is loud, it may be mistaken for a masked second heart sound. Although the murmur is so loud that the first heart sound is not very evident to the ear, the phonocardiogram shows a good first heart sound.

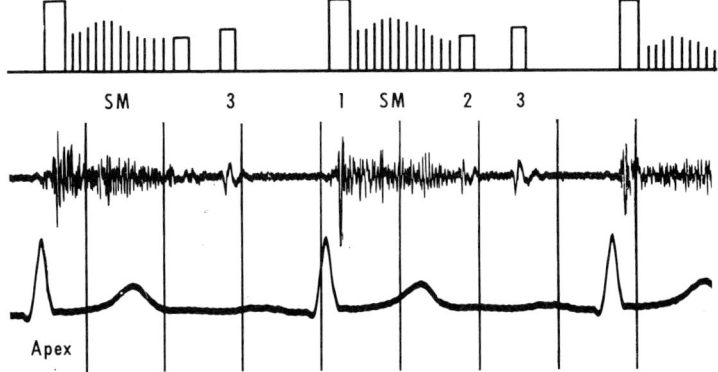

systolic murmur has been clearly identified with mitral regurgitation. When the murmur of mitral regurgitation is of only $^2/_6$ intensity — the type not usually studied or recorded for publication — it does not give the ear the impression of being holosystolic. Many decrescendo or crescendo murmurs of mitral regurgitation in which the murmur sounds either as though it starts after the first sound or stops before the second sound, require, as has been mentioned, a phonocardiogram to pick up a stray vibration after the first sound or before the second sound to interpret them as holosystolic. When these murmurs are made less intense by the use of amyl nitrite, they are no longer holosystolic even on the magnified phonocardiogram.

Several factors are probably involved in the variations in intensity during systole of the murmur of mitral regurgitation: (1) in cases of marked mitral regurgitation where there is a high-pressure V-wave in the atrium, the gradient at the end of systole would be significantly decreased and could account, in part, for a decrescendo murmur; (2) when the chordae tendineae have been shortened by scarring or where the ventricle is dilated so that there is relative shortening of the chordae tendineae, the valves may not approximate early in systole but gradually close as the ventricle expels its blood and decreases in size (Fig 7–3); (3) if one of the papillary muscles is weakened or fibrosed, as is often the case in myocardial infarctions, or if several chordae tendineae are ruptured or lengthened, it is conceivable, and seems to be proved by some angiocardiographic studies, that a valve which was completely closed early in systole would partially prolapse in late systole as the heart emptied itself. In this case, a late systolic murmur would result (Fig 7–4). As will be noted later, a late systolic murmur is not an uncommon finding in acute myocardial infarctions.

POINT OF MAXIMUM INTENSITY AND AREA OF TRANSMISSION. — Maximum intensity is usually at the apex. If the murmur is faint, it is heard only in a small area at the apex (see Fig 7–1). When of moderate intensity, the murmur may be heard medially in diminishing intensity. If the heart is not enlarged, the murmur is poorly transmitted toward the axilla, since the lungs effectively dampen it. If the murmur is loud, and especially if the heart is enlarged so that it is closer to the chest wall laterally, the murmur may be clearly heard in the axilla and even posteriorly in the lung bases. Unless the murmur is

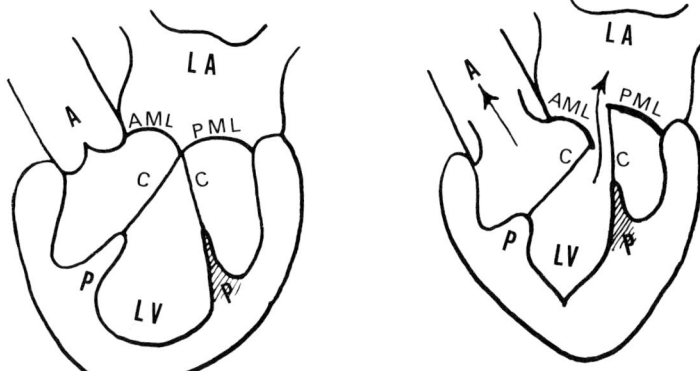

Fig 7–3.—Mitral regurgitation due to papillary muscle dysfunction. At the onset of systole **(left)** the anterior and posterior mitral valve leaflets *(AML* and *PML)* approximate. Later in systole **(right)** the anterior papillary muscle *(P, nonhatched)* contracts while the posterior papillary muscle *(P, hatched)* fails to contract because of ischemia or infarction. Part of the posterior leaflet is allowed to prolapse into the left atrium *(LA)* during systole, producing regurgitation. This process may involve either papillary muscle. *C,* chordae tendineae; *LV,* left ventricle; *A,* aorta.

very loud, it is poorly transmitted above the third intercostal space into the basal area. Very loud murmurs such as occur with ruptured chordae tendineae are widely heard and may, at times, be louder in unusual locations. Occasionally, these murmurs seem to be maximum just within the apex rather than

Fig 7–4.—Late systolic murmur which developed in a patient following an inferior myocardial infarction and is probably due to weakening of the posterior papillary muscle with prolapse of the mitral leaflet into the atrium during late systole (see text).

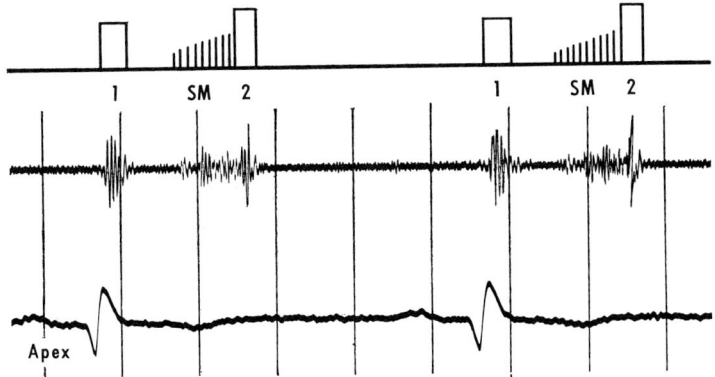

at the apex and, rarely, they may be maximum at the base. With leakage resulting from involvement of the anterior leaflet, the murmur may be loudest at the base. Leakage due to posterior leaflet involvement results in murmurs transmitted more to the axilla and posterior lung base; and transmission of such murmurs to the thoracic spine and upward occasionally results in the murmur being audible in the head. Lung pathology that changes the position of the heart may also change the position of the murmur.

PITCH AND QUALITY.—When the murmur is of faint or moderate intensity, it is characteristically high pitched and has a *blowing* quality. A murmur with this characteristic pitch and quality and of maximum intensity at the apex can be considered as due to mitral regurgitation in the absence of other corroborative findings. As the murmur increases in intensity, it may remain essentially high pitched, but usually becomes more harsh because of the addition of medium-pitched components. This change in pitch and quality, in part, may be due to the greater amount of sound produced and, in part, may be associated with differences in pathology of the valve. The murmur of mitral regurgitation associated with rupture of chordae tendineae is loud and harsh and has a quality similar to that of aortic stenosis.

Since the murmur is high pitched, the *diaphragm chest piece* is best for its detection.

POSITION OF THE PATIENT.—The murmur is usually evident in all positions, but when faint it may be best heard with the patient in the left lateral position immediately after exercise. In some patients, it is best heard when they are sitting up, leaning forward and to the left. For faint murmurs, the room must be quiet, and it may take a minute or two of concentration on systole to hear the murmur. One is often asked, "Why worry about such a faint murmur? Does it have any significance?" The answer is definitely "Yes." The murmur is characteristic and, even if it is faint, it indicates mitral regurgitation. In a child with questionable symptoms of acute rheumatic fever, this is a highly important finding.

EFFECT OF RESPIRATION.—With inspiration, the murmur remains unchanged or diminishes somewhat in loudness. This is probably due to the increased size of the lungs and their increased dampening effect on the heart sounds and murmurs.

CHANGES IN THE HEART SOUNDS. — With a fibrotic, immobile valve the first sound may be diminished. If the valve remains flexible, the first heart sound may be normal and, actually, if some mitral stenosis is present, it may be increased. Loud systolic murmurs may mask the first sound so that even if it is normal it may appear to be faint or absent. If the bell chest piece is held first lightly and then heavily in contact with the chest wall, the change that occurs in loudness of the first sound will make the sound more evident. With loud murmurs, the second sound may also be masked at the apex.

Splitting of the second sound is usually normal but may be increased in severe mitral regurgitation because of rapid emptying of the left ventricle with early closure of the aortic valve. In some patients with marked mitral regurgitation, the pulmonic second sound may be accentuated in the absence of pulmonary hypertension of significant degree, and an erroneous diagnosis of marked pulmonary hypertension may be made. The cause of the accentuation is not clear, but it could be due to an enlarged left atrium forcing a mildly dilated pulmonary artery closer to the chest wall.

An abnormally loud third heart sound is often present with marked degrees of mitral regurgitation (see Fig 7–2). This third sound may be louder than, and be mistaken for, the second heart sound. The presence of a third heart sound in a patient with mitral valve involvement is of diagnostic value, since it indicates that the valvular lesion is predominantly regurgitation and not a stenosis (p. 132). An atrial sound is only occasionally heard.

RELATION OF LOUDNESS OF MURMUR TO DEGREE OF MITRAL REGURGITATION. — It is frequently stated that in some patients no mitral regurgitation is present even though there is a loud murmur, and that a marked mitral regurgitation can occur with practically no murmur. Although these situations do occur, they are, in our opinion, uncommon; a surprisingly good correlation between the intensity of the murmur and the degree of mitral regurgitation (as determined in operation for mitral stenosis) will be found if the following factors are taken into consideration:

1. If all the auscultatory phenomena are decreased because of emphysema, large breasts, or obesity, a faint murmur is

more significant and must be interpreted in relation to the loudness of the other sounds.

2. The murmurs of mitral regurgitation and tricuspid regurgitation must be differentiated (p. 108).

3. A loud first sound will mask a following systolic murmur. The masking may be overcome in part by using the diaphragm or by using the bell with pressure. Attention must be directed to systole.

4. In the presence of loud or moderately loud systolic murmurs in the aortic area, systolic murmurs at the apex must be interpreted cautiously (p. 113).

If these factors are taken into consideration, the correlation between the intensity of the murmur and the degree of regurgitation is good, although some discrepancies will be observed.

Conditions Producing Mitral Regurgitation

Mitral valve closure depends upon the smooth functioning of a number of components, including the mitral leaflets, the mitral annulus, the left atrium, the chordae tendineae, the papillary muscles and the underlying left ventricular wall. Improper functioning of any of these elements of the mitral complex leads to asynchrony of mitral closure and regurgitation. Examples of this include the following.

1. *Rheumatic involvement of the valves.*

2. *Calcification of the mitral annulus fibrosis.* — Due to its attachment to the "fibrous skeleton" at the base of the heart, the mitral annulus has a relatively rigid structure. Dilatation of the ring probably occurs rarely as a cause for mitral regurgitation. In fact, the annulus normally provides a sphincter-like action during systole, decreasing the area that the leaflet must seal. Calcification occurs frequently in the mitral ring and hinders the normal contraction of the ring during systole. This produces a systolic murmur that is usually moderately harsh and holosystolic.

3. *Papillary muscle dysfunction.* — The most common form of mitral regurgitation is that due to dysfunction of the papillary muscle (see Figs 7–3 and 7–4) and ischemic heart disease is the leading cause of this condition. Rarely, with acute myocardial infarction, the tip or belly of the muscle may rup-

ture, producing acute and fulminant mitral regurgitation. More commonly, function of the muscle is transiently impaired during acute ischemic attacks. This can sometimes lead to severe mitral regurgitation and even transiently pulmonary edema.

A number of other conditions interfere with the proper function of one or both papillary muscles, resulting in mitral regurgitation. Such conditions include left ventricular dilatation (Fig 7–5) causing abnormal alignment of the attached papillary muscles and infiltration of the papillary muscles by infection, fibrosis or diseases such as amyloid. Depending on the papillary muscle involved and the severity of the underlying condition, the murmur, which is located at or near the apex, may be holosystolic, crescendo, decrescendo, or confined to early, mid or late systole. The murmur often is transient and audible only during an acute attack of ischemia. At such a time the first heart sound may be increased. Systolic clicks may occur with papillary muscle dysfunction in the presence or absence of a murmur.

(4.) *The click-murmur syndrome.*—Mid to late systolic clicks, single or multiple, occur alone or in conjunction with a

Fig 7–5.—Mitral regurgitation due to a dilated left ventricle. At the onset of systole **(left)** the dilated ventricle *(LV)* with normal papillary muscle *(P)* causes the chordae tendineae *(C)* to be relatively short, not allowing approximation of anterior and posterior mitral valve leaflets *(AML* and *PML)*. As a result there is regurgitation into the left atrium *(LA)*. As the ventricle contracts later in systole **(right)** the leaflets now approximate, and the mitral regurgitation decreases. *A,* aorta.

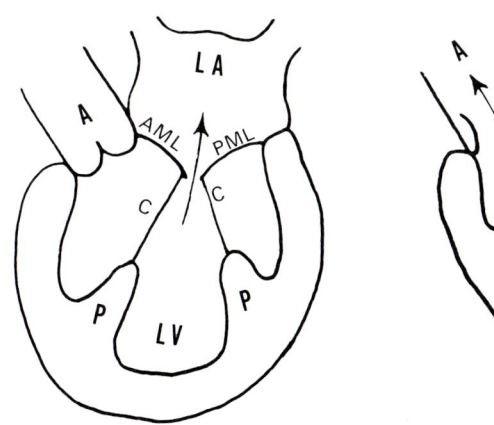
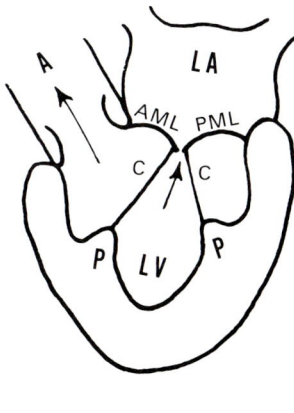

late systolic murmur. Long considered innocent, these findings have clearly been shown to originate from prolapse of a mitral leaflet producing mitral regurgitation usually of mild degree. The murmur occurs at the time of maximal billowing of the valve leaflet into the left atrium. The click appears to arise from sudden tensing of slack chordae tendineae, to a sudden increase in tension in normal chordae or to an abrupt halt in excursion of this billowing leaflet (Fig 7–6). Some possible explanations of the click-murmur syndrome include: (1) some of the chordae are elongated and allow prolapse of a leaflet, usually the posterior one (Fig 7–7); (2) redundant leaflet tissue is present; and (3) the free left ventricular wall under the posteromedial papillary muscle contracts abnormally and fails to provide proper support to the papillary muscle. Any one or a combination of these would result in prolapse of the mitral leaflets, causing mitral regurgitation. The syndrome is occasionally associated with atrial or ventricular arrhythmias, vague symptoms of chest pain, and nonspecific ST-T changes on the electrocardiogram. Sudden death has been reported

Fig 7–6.—Echo of click-murmur syndrome. Echocardiogram of a patient with a midsystolic click and late systolic murmur. Only the anterior mitral valve leaflet *(AMVL)* is well seen. In midsystole, a portion of the leaflet is seen to prolapse posteriorly and remains displaced until the onset of diastole. A murmur appears shortly after the first sound and in this case is crescendo-decrescendo, ending with the second sound. Shortly after the beginning of the prolapse, a click occurs which is believed to result from sudden tautening of the prolapsing leaflet and the associated chordae. See also Figure 7–7.

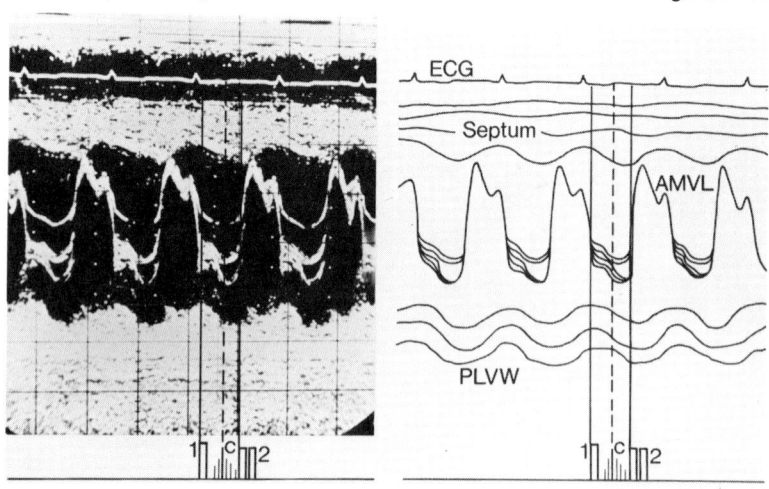

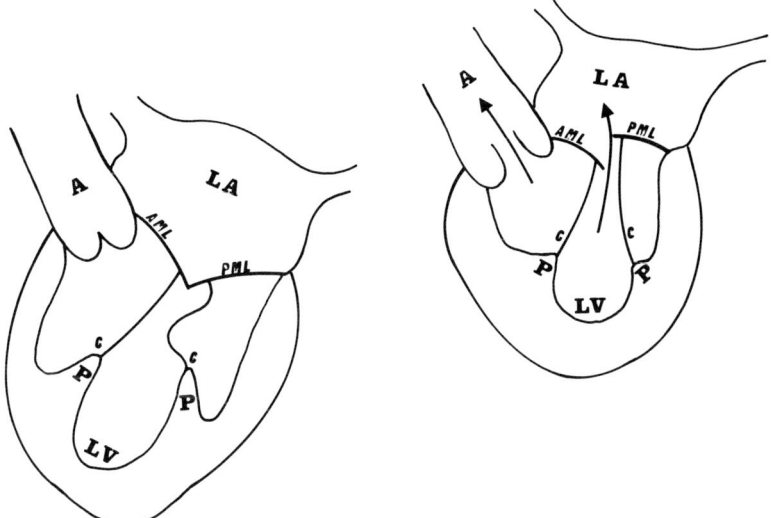

Fig 7–7.—The click-murmur syndrome due to abnormally enlongated chordae *(C)* to the posterior leaflet of the mitral valve *(PML)*. At the onset of systole **(left)** the mitral valve leaflets approximate. As left ventricular ejection proceeds **(right)**, the elongated chordae allow the posterior leaflet to prolapse into the left atrium *(LA)*, producing mitral regurgitation. *AML*, anterior mitral valve leaflet; *P*, papillary muscle; *LV*, left ventricle; *A*, aorta.

and attributed to arrhythmia. Progression of mitral regurgitation also occurs on occasion, and there is a risk of endocarditis with this entity. However, in the vast majority of cases, the syndrome is entirely benign.

The auscultatory findings in the click-murmur syndrome vary with changes in posture. Procedures that decrease the enddiastolic ventricular volume exaggerate the degree of mitral leaflet prolapse. On sitting or standing the click tends to occur earlier in systole, and the late systolic murmur tends to become holosystolic. Under these circumstances a systolic "whoop" may also be heard, sometimes only transiently. Squatting produces the opposite physiologic effect; that is, it increases the venous return to the heart and places the mitral valve under greater tension. This effectively decreases the degree of prolapse and returns the murmur to the late systolic position.

Other maneuvers also influence the findings in the click-murmur syndrome. The Valsalva maneuver decreases venous return and left ventricular volume and thereby increases the loudness of the murmur. This is in contrast to other forms of mitral regurgitation where the murmur becomes less conspicuous during the Valsalva straining phase. Use of a vasopressor to increase systemic resistance accentuates the murmur of some forms of mitral regurgitation (p. 251). Inhalation of amyl nitrite has the opposite effect.

(5) *Chordal rupture.*—Acute severe mitral regurgitation is usually due to rupture of one or several chordae tendineae. The clinical presentation is that of sudden cardiac failure and a loud systolic murmur. The murmur tends to be decrescendo and widely transmitted. A third sound is often heard and, as a point of differentiation from rheumatic mitral regurgitation, a loud fourth heart sound may be present. A presystolic bulge at the apex may accompany the fourth sound. On chest radiograph, the heart size is usually normal without the left atrial enlargement that characterizes chronic mitral regurgitation. Signs of pulmonary edema develop and persist in some cases for months. Other patients may tolerate rupture of chordae tendineae surprisingly well. This is probably due to a number of factors, including the type and location of chordae that have ruptured and the presence or absence of previous left ventricular disease.

Rupture of chordae attached to the posterior mitral leaflet can cause a murmur which radiates to the "aortic area" and even to the carotids and may lead to confusion with the murmur of aortic stenosis. The regurgitant jet in this instance is directed toward the posterior left atrial wall which is adjacent to the spine, accounting for the unusual transmission of this murmur. Chordal rupture may be secondary to chest trauma, rheumatic valvulitis, bacterial endocarditis, myxomatous degeneration of the mitral apparatus, and "idiopathic."

DIFFERENTIATION. — The systolic murmur of mitral regurgitation must be differentiated from other systolic murmurs of maximum intensity at the apex. Not many murmurs, fortunately, other than mitral regurgitation, are maximal at the apex — and very few of these are high pitched. Murmurs having their origin in the aortic valve, and possibly in the first part of the aorta, are usually well heard at the apex; and in older patients with deep chests or emphysema, the murmur is often louder at the apex than in the second right intercostal space (p. 111).

Analysis of an apical systolic murmur depends, therefore, on the findings in the aortic area. If no systolic murmur is heard in the second right intercostal space, a high-pitched systolic murmur of maximum intensity at the apex is almost surely due to mitral regurgitation. If a systolic murmur is heard in the second right intercostal space, an apical systolic murmur must be interpreted more cautiously. This is discussed on page 113.

Apical systolic murmurs that are medium pitched and rough, rather than high pitched and usually not holosystolic, present a problem. (1) Many of these murmurs have their origin in the aortic region. This is true even when on first examination there appears to be no murmur in the second right intercostal space. A careful reexamination of the aortic region, with the patient sitting and holding his breath in expiration, may reveal a faint systolic murmur that has the same pitch and timing as the apical murmur. (2) A careful check will occasionally show that the murmur is actually louder medial to the apex or along the left border of the sternum. Such a murmur should be studied for the characteristics of an innocent systolic murmur (p. 121). (3) Some medium-pitched apical systolic murmurs may be due to mitral regurgitation, but other evidence should be sought for confirmation. Loud murmurs of mitral regurgitation may be somewhat harsh but are almost always holosystolic. (4) Some rough apical systolic murmurs may represent an early stage in the development of muscular subaortic stenosis (p. 116). These murmurs are often of maximum intensity at the apex or just within the apex. (5) Some of these medium-pitched murmurs are best labeled as of unknown origin.

The Systolic Murmur of Tricuspid Regurgitation

The murmur of tricuspid regurgitation begins with the first sound and, when faint, is rather short and decrescendo. Louder murmurs are holosystolic. The *point of maximum intensity* is to the left of the lower end of the sternum (see Figs 7–1 and 12–5, p. 199). When the murmur is faint, it is heard only in this area. Louder murmurs, associated with right ventricle enlargement, may be heard as far laterally as the anterior axillary line. The point of maximum intensity, however, remains between the left border of the sternum and the midclavicular line. Loud murmurs are transmitted to the right of the sternum, but fade rapidly toward the base of the heart.

The *pitch* and *quality* of the murmur are similar to those of the murmur of mitral regurgitation—high pitched and blowing. Louder murmurs tend to be somewhat harsh. The murmur is best heard with the *diaphragm chest piece.*

Respiration has a characteristic effect on the murmur of tricuspid regurgitation. The murmur increases in loudness, often quite markedly, with deep inspiration and usually with normal inspiration. In some patients, the murmur will be heard only during inspiration, or a faint, short murmur on expiration may become louder, holosystolic, and rarely even "honking" on inspiration. Augmented filling of the right ventricle during inspiration probably produces this phenomenon. With marked tricuspid regurgitation and a loud murmur, the effect of respiration on the intensity of the murmur may not be evident. This is true especially in the presence of right ventricular failure and increased systemic venous pressure. Inspiration may not be able to augment the filling of the right ventricle under these conditions. Inspiratory splitting of the second sound may be absent for the same reason.

The *first heart sound* in the tricuspid area may be increased, normal, or somewhat decreased, depending on the pathology of the valve and on masking.

Differentiation of the systolic murmurs of mitral and tricuspid regurgitation can usually be made on the basis of the effect of respiration and the difference in the points of maximum intensity. Mitral murmurs are unchanged or diminished on inspiration, and the point of maximum intensity is at the apex or, in large hearts, lateral to the apex. Tricuspid murmurs increase in loudness on inspiration, and their point of maximum intensity is closer to the sternum. The sign classically associated with tricuspid regurgitation—systolic expansion of the neck veins and liver—is usually associated with right heart failure and need not be present for the diagnosis to be made. Pressure on an enlarged liver may increase the intensity of a tricuspid regurgitant murmur.

Relative tricuspid regurgitation as a result of right heart failure is common. In patients with right heart failure, it is impossible to determine whether the tricuspid regurgitation is due to organic involvement of the valve, relative tricuspid regurgitation, or both. In the absence of evidence of increased pressure in the right ventricle, tricuspid regurgitation can be recognized on the basis of the characteristic murmur alone and can be assumed to be of organic origin (see Fig 12–5, p. 199).

In patients with a transvenous pacemaker in place, the development of a systolic murmur usually indicates tricuspid regurgitation possibly due to interference of tricuspid valve closure by the pacemaker cable.

There is a rough correlation between the intensity of the murmur and the degree of regurgitation, but a marked regurgitation may be present with practically no murmur. In right heart failure, a decrease in the intensity of the murmur is a good indication of the effectiveness of therapy. With more severe grades of regurgitation, a right-sided third heart sound and middiastolic murmur may occur.

In acute pulmonary embolism, the temporary occurrence of the murmur of tricuspid regurgitation (usually not very loud) has not been given the attention it deserves.

The Systolic Murmur of Aortic Stenosis and Aortic Valvular Deformity

Aortic stenosis must involve more than 50% of the opening before changes in the pulse wave and blood pressure occur. Minor grades of deformity may produce a systolic murmur with little or no change in the circulatory dynamics. Many murmurs may represent roughening or perhaps mild deformity of the valve without any significant stenosis; one hesitates, therefore, to call this murmur the murmur of aortic stenosis. It is in these cases that the term *aortic valvular deformity* is used.

TIMING AND DURATION. — The murmur of moderately severe and severe aortic stenosis builds up to a peak in midsystole and then decreases; it is absent by the time the aortic second sound occurs. The murmur recorded on phonocardiograms, therefore, has a diamond shape (Fig 7–8). With lesser degrees of aortic deformity, the murmur may be shorter and reach a peak earlier in systole.

PITCH AND QUALITY. — Faint murmurs are rough and of medium pitch; louder murmurs are harsh and often associated with a thrill. Either chest piece may be used satisfactorily. At

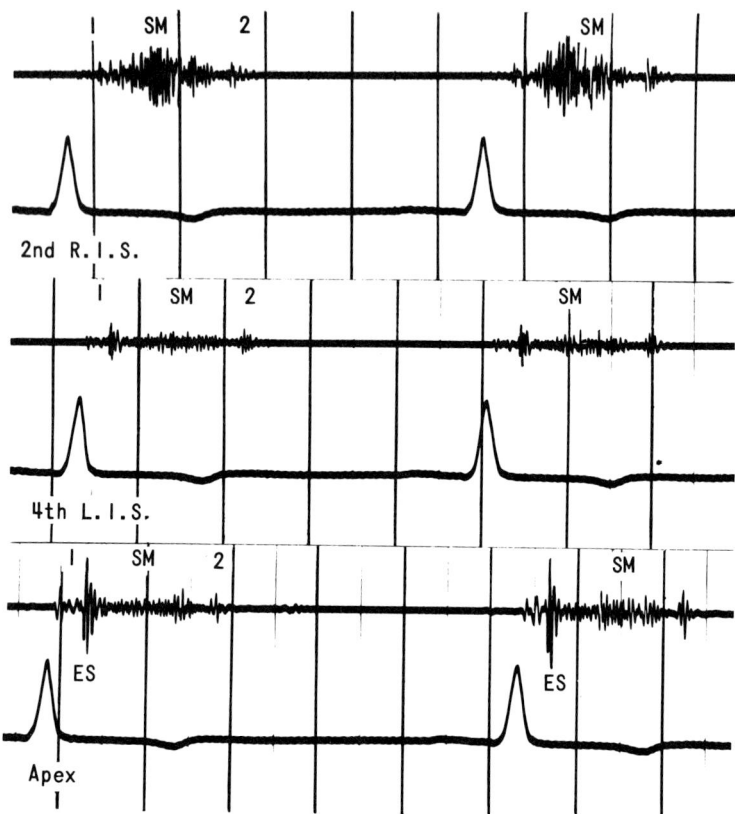

Fig 7–8.—Murmur of aortic stenosis. This murmur *(SM)* is loudest in the second right intercostal space *(upper tracing),* and in this area it often shows its characteristic diamond shape on the phonocardiogram. Note that the murmur stops well before the second heart sound and that if a second heart sound is present it can usually be heard, although if the murmur is very loud, there may still be some masking. The murmur is heard well at the apex *(lower tracing)* and in this area has a quality similar to that in the second right intercostal space. In the fourth left intercostal space *(middle tracing)* the murmur is not as loud as it is at the apex. Faint murmurs may be heard at the second right intercostal space and at the apex and not be evident along the left border of the sternum. Note the ejection sound *(ES)* is best heard at the apex.

times, the murmur is so loud that it can be heard with the stethoscope away from the chest wall.

POINT OF MAXIMUM INTENSITY AND AREA OF TRANSMISSION. —The point of maximum intensity is usually in the second or first right intercostal space (Figs 7–1 and 7–9). A murmur

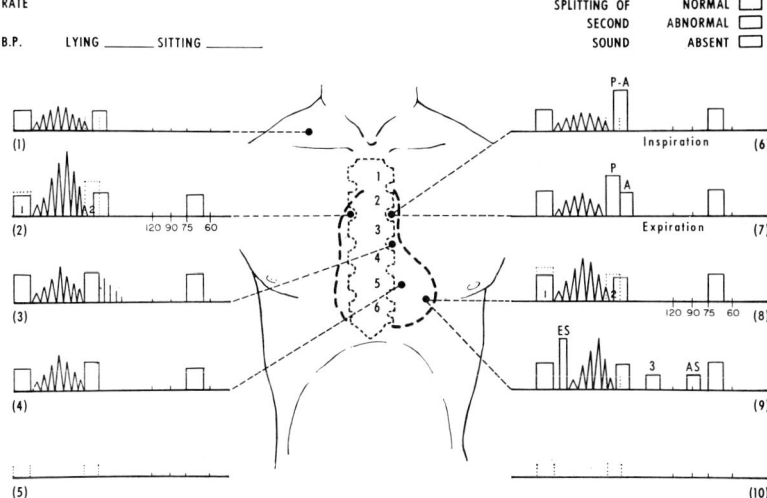

Fig 7–9.—Systolic murmur of aortic stenosis. (The figures in parentheses refer to the lines on the chart.) This is a harsh systolic murmur which reaches its peak in midsystole and then decreases in intensity so that it is gone before the second sound. It is of maximum intensity in the first and second *(2)* right intercostal spaces. It is well heard at the apex *(8)*. Along the left border of the sternum *(3)* the murmur is often less intense than it is at the apex. The murmur is well heard in the neck *(1)*. An aortic ejection sound *(ES)* is usually heard in congenital aortic stenosis *(9)*. A fourth sound will be heard if there is a marked left ventricular-aortic gradient and consequent left ventricular hypertrophy *(9)*. A third heart sound may be heard at the apex and suggests ventricular dilatation and possible early left ventricular failure *(9)*.

Paradoxical splitting of the second heart sound occurs if the aortic stenosis is severe and an aortic second sound can be heard. The splitting is more evident on expiration *(7)* than on inspiration *(6)*.

In this chart, a faint, high-pitched early diastolic murmur (slight aortic regurgitation) is shown in the third left intercostal space *(3)*. This is frequently heard in patients with aortic stenosis.

well heard in the first right intercostal space is likely to be of aortic origin. Murmurs of only moderate intensity are usually well transmitted to the apex and the neck. When the murmur is very loud, it is heard over the entire thorax and as far down as the olecranon process of the ulna. In older patients with deep chests and in the presence of emphysema, the murmur is often louder at the apex than in the second right interspace. In transmission from the base to the apex, there is often an area along the left border of the sternum where the murmur is less intense than it is at the apex or base (see Fig 7–8). The murmur may sound somewhat higher pitched and less harsh at the apex than at the base. The question of two separate murmurs may, thus, be posed; and, at times, it may be difficult to decide this point. Usually, however, the rather characteristic quality, pitch and timing of the aortic murmurs will still be recognizable at the apex.

POSITION OF THE PATIENT. — The murmur is heard best with the patient sitting up and leaning forward, and with the breath held in expiration.

CHANGES IN HEART SOUNDS. — With advanced degrees of aortic valvular stenosis, the second heart sound may be entirely absent in the second right intercostal space; with lesser degrees, it may be normal or diminished. Even when no second sound is heard at the base, a second sound of aortic origin may, at times, be heard at the apex, indicating a masking of the sound at the base. In congenital aortic stenosis, a normal or even increased aortic second sound may be present.

An accentuated pulmonic second sound may occasionally account for a second sound heard in the second right intercostal space. When both aortic and pulmonic second sounds are heard, either normal splitting, no inspiratory splitting, or paradoxical splitting (see Figs 4–7 and 4–8, pp. 48 and 49) may occur.

A fourth sound, when present, indicates significant stenosis (p. 60). A third heart sound may be present indicating even more advanced disease in an adult. An aortic ejection sound is present in most patients with congenital aortic stenosis (see Fig 5–6, p. 65).

RELATION OF INTENSITY OF MURMUR TO SEVERITY OF LESION. — Several factors disturb this relationship.

1. In persons with deep chests or with emphysema, the intensity of all sounds at the base may be diminished, and severe aortic stenosis may exist with a faint murmur which is easily overlooked. The murmur in these patients may be better heard at the apex and mistaken for that of mitral regurgitation. The quality and timing of the murmur at the apex are clues to listen more carefully at the base. The quality of the pulses and the presence of a loud bruit over the carotid arteries are additional clues.

2. In the presence of marked or moderate aortic regurgitation, the amount of blood flowing through the valve during systole is increased and flows by the deformed valve at an in-

creased velocity. This velocity of blood flow may increase the loudness of the murmur beyond what would be expected from the degree of stenosis.

3. With the onset of failure, arrhythmia or shock, the murmur may decrease markedly in loudness.

OCCURRENCE. — Rheumatic fever is the most common cause of aortic valvular deformity and aortic stenosis. Calcific aortic stenosis occurs in an older age group and may be of congenital origin. Congenital aortic stenosis is a common deformity. Other congenital lesions include supravalvular and discrete subvalvular stenosis but are much less common. Muscular subaortic stenosis is considerably more common than was previously thought (p. 116), and a few cases of systolic ejection murmurs due to muscle bands lower in the ventricle have been described.

Organic aortic systolic murmurs are also heard in bacterial, nonbacterial (marantic) endocarditis, verrucous (Libman-Sacks) endocarditis, as well as with dissecting hematoma of the aorta.

DIFFERENTIATION. — Differentiation from the more common basal systolic murmur associated with arteriosclerosis and hypertension is given on page 115. When a murmur of mitral regurgitation is present alone, its recognition is *usually* no problem. Difficulty arises when a classic murmur of aortic stenosis is present, and one must decide whether there is also a murmur of mitral regurgitation. The murmur of aortic stenosis is well transmitted to the apex, whereas the murmur of mitral regurgitation is poorly transmitted to the aortic region. The presence of a murmur of similar quality in the two areas, therefore, usually leaves little doubt that there is an aortic lesion. It may be difficult or impossible, however, to rule out by auscultation the simultaneous presence of mitral regurgitation. The following differential features may be helpful. (1) When the aortic murmur is not loud and the murmurs are of different quality, both lesions probably are present. (2) The harsh systolic murmur of aortic stenosis may be present at the apex, or within the apex, while a holosystolic murmur of higher pitch may be evident lateral to the apex. (3) If the murmur definitely stops before the second sound, only an aortic murmur *may* be present. The aortic second sound is often very faint and it may not be possible to tell whether the murmur stops before the second sound. It is important not to mistake a loud third heart sound for the second heart sound; otherwise, a holosystolic murmur may not be recognized. (4) In the presence of atrial fibrillation or premature contractions, the variation in intensity of the systolic murmur with the length of diastole is usually greater with an aortic murmur than with mitral regurgitation (see Fig 6–2, p. 89). This was discussed on page 88. (5) Amyl nitrite may be of some value (p. 252).

The Basal Systolic Murmur Associated with Arteriosclerosis and/or Hypertension

A basal systolic murmur is probably the most common murmur heard in older persons and is frequently associated with other evidence of arteriosclerosis or hypertension. The aorta is often widened and tortuous. The murmur is of maximum intensity in the second right intercostal space (Fig 7–10). It is of medium pitch and rough, rather than harsh like the murmur of aortic stenosis. The murmur is not usually very loud and does not get as loud as the murmur of aortic stenosis,

Fig 7–10.—Basal systolic murmur associated with arteriosclerosis. This murmur *(SM)* is best heard in the second and first right intercostal spaces. It is often transmitted to the apex. It is usually not as long a murmur as that of aortic stenosis and it reaches a peak earlier in systole.

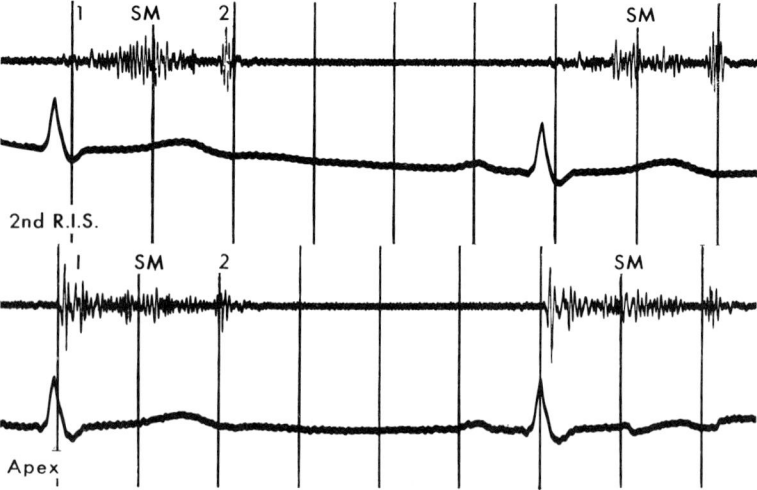

but an overlap occurs both in intensity and in quality. The murmur is best heard when the patient is sitting up and leaning forward. Either the diaphragm or the bell chest piece may be used.

The murmur is often well *transmitted to the apex,* and it may be difficult to decide in these patients whether an apical systolic murmur is transmitted from the aortic area, or whether it represents a mitral regurgitation. If the aortic systolic murmur is moderately loud and the apical systolic murmur is not holosystolic and does not have the high pitch and blowing quality of mitral regurgitation murmur, the murmur should usually be considered as having been transmitted from the aortic area. Since all the sounds may be faint at the base because of emphysema or a deep chest, the murmur may be louder at the apex than at the base. Transmission into the neck occurs but is not marked, possibly because the murmur is usually not very loud. The second sound is of normal or increased loudness.

Factors that may play a part in the production of this murmur are: (1) arteriosclerotic roughening of the aorta; (2) fibrosis and calcification at the base of the aortic valves producing protrusions into the vessel; and (3) relative aortic stenosis resulting from dilation of the aorta.

This murmur will not be confused with that of aortic stenosis when the latter is loud and harsh. When the murmurs are of moderate intensity, the following factors help to distinguish the two:

1. The age group in general is different, although calcific aortic stenosis often occurs in the same group.

2. The presence of a dilated or tortuous aorta, hypertension, or arteriosclerosis favors the diagnosis of relative aortic stenosis. The presence of other murmurs (indicating aortic regurgitation or mitral stenosis) favors the diagnosis of organic aortic stenosis.

3. The second aortic sound is of normal or increased loudness in patients with arteriosclerosis or hypertension and is often diminished or absent in patients with organic aortic stenosis.

4. A prominent fourth sound is more likely to be heard with significant aortic stenosis, especially in patients under age 40.

Subaortic Stenosis

This entity is felt to be genetic in origin and transmitted as an autosomal dominant trait. In some individuals of an affected family, the disease remains latent throughout life. In others the typical murmur appears if certain forms of stress are applied to the left ventricle, such as systemic hypertension, aortic valvular stenosis or chronic inhalation of isoproterenol.

With idiopathic hypertrophic subaortic stenosis (IHSS) a

Fig 7–11.—Murmur of muscular subaortic stenosis. The murmur in this patient was loudest at the apex *(lower tracing)* although it may, in other patients, be loudest in the apicosternal area. It was faint in the second right intercostal space *(upper tracing)* and was not heard at all in the neck. The murmur started with the first sound but faded off before the second sound. It was very harsh in quality. A fourth sound *(AS)* was noted at the apex and could also be heard in the fourth left interspace *(middle tracing)*.

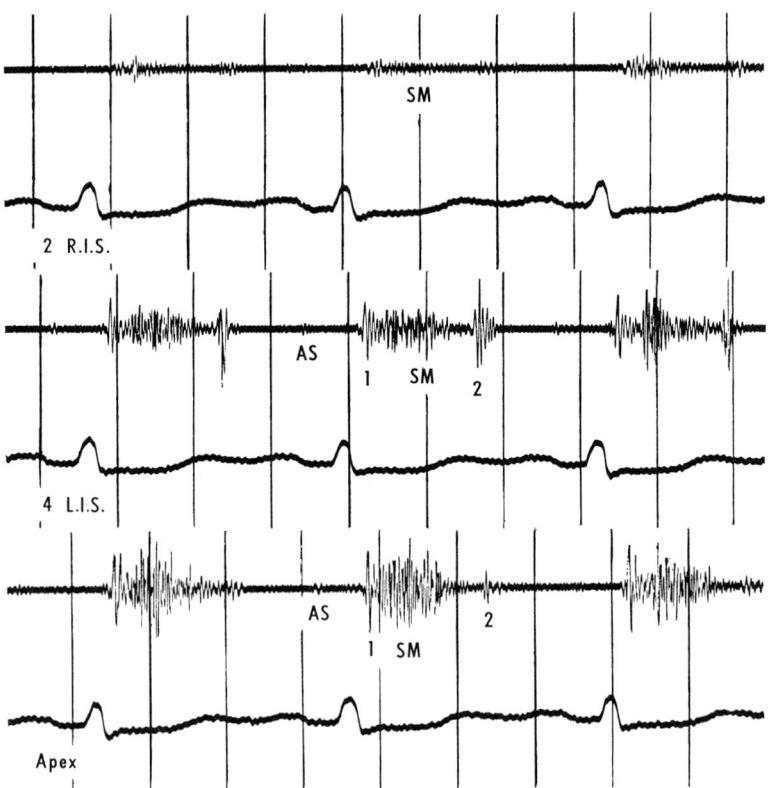

rough or harsh systolic murmur develops over a period of years. Mitral regurgitation is present in some and evidence of marked left ventricular hypertrophy (LVH) may develop. The electrocardiographic evidence of LVH is more than would be expected from mitral regurgitation alone. Occasionally prominent septal Q-waves suggest previous infarction.

Certain physical findings are characteristic of IHSS (Fig 7–11). The murmur may vary greatly in loudness in the same individual and at times may be absent altogether. It is poorly transmitted to the second right interspace and very rarely to the neck. It usually ends before the second heart sound but it is not necessarily diamond shaped. The aortic second sound is usually normal and well heard at the apex. It is common to hear a fourth sound and not infrequently a third sound. Aortic ejection clicks are very rare and aortic regurgitation does not occur. When mitral regurgitation is an associated lesion, a holosystolic murmur may be present at the apex.

It is ordinarily not difficult to separate this condition from aortic valvular stenosis. The main differences are in location and radiation of the murmur (see p. 110), and the character of the peripheral pulse is distinctly different. With valvular aortic stenosis, the pulse is small, shows a slow rise and fall, and may have an anacrotic notch. In IHSS, the rise and fall are brisk and may be bisferiens, and the pulse volume is normal (Fig 7–12).

A helpful technique for distinguishing these two conditions is to have the patient perform the Valsalva maneuver. During the straining phase the murmur of aortic valvular stenosis is unchanged or becomes less intense. The murmur of IHSS often increases in intensity and becomes harsher.

The response to a ventricular premature contraction (VPC) is another point of differentiation. In IHSS the contraction following a VPC occurs with greater than usual vigor, causing momentarily an increased stenosis in the subvalvular region and a louder murmur. In valvular aortic stenosis, the left ventricular-aortic pressure gradient following an extrasystole is also moderately increased but not to the degree seen in IHSS. In the beats following an extrasystole in IHSS, the first heart sound is also markedly increased.

The murmur of IHSS may be confused with that of ventricular septal defects. The Valsalva effect has value in this situa-

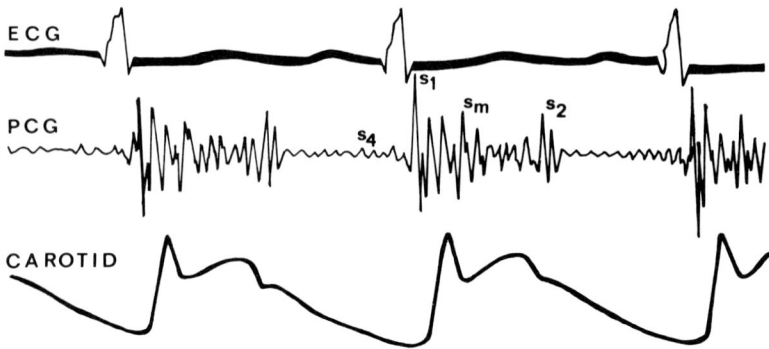

Fig 7–12.—Muscular subaortic stenosis. This patient had severe left ventricular outflow obstruction with a subvalvular peak gradient of 150 mm Hg. The murmur is harsh, ejection in type and indistinguishable from that of valvular aortic stenosis, except that it is transmitted poorly to the neck. Note, however, the abrupt rise in the carotid pulse tracing (unlike that in valvular stenosis) followed by a slower second wave corresponding to the period of maximal obstruction in mid and late systole.

tion since it tends to obliterate the murmur of a ventricular septal defect.

It is sometimes more difficult to distinguish the systolic murmur of IHSS from the loud, harsh murmur of chordal rupture producing severe mitral regurgitation. Both murmurs are extremely harsh but that of mitral regurgitation tends to be best heard at the apex. The murmur of mitral regurgitation in these cases usually extends to the aortic second sound and may partially mask it, whereas the murmur of IHSS frequently ends before the second sound. The difference in behavior of the two murmurs after a long diastole is of great diagnostic value; this was described on page 88. A third heart sound is more common in severe mitral regurgitation, whereas a fourth sound is common in IHSS; paradoxical splitting of the second sound suggests IHSS.

A striking feature of the murmur of subaortic stenosis is its response to changes in body position. Squatting, for example, promptly diminishes or obliterates it. The physiologic effect is to increase peripheral vascular resistance and venous inflow to the heart, thereby relaxing the muscular stenosis and reducing the left ventricular-aortic pressure gradient. Sudden standing, on the other hand, tends to accentuate the murmur and fourth sound. Inhalation of amyl nitrite lowers peripheral vas-

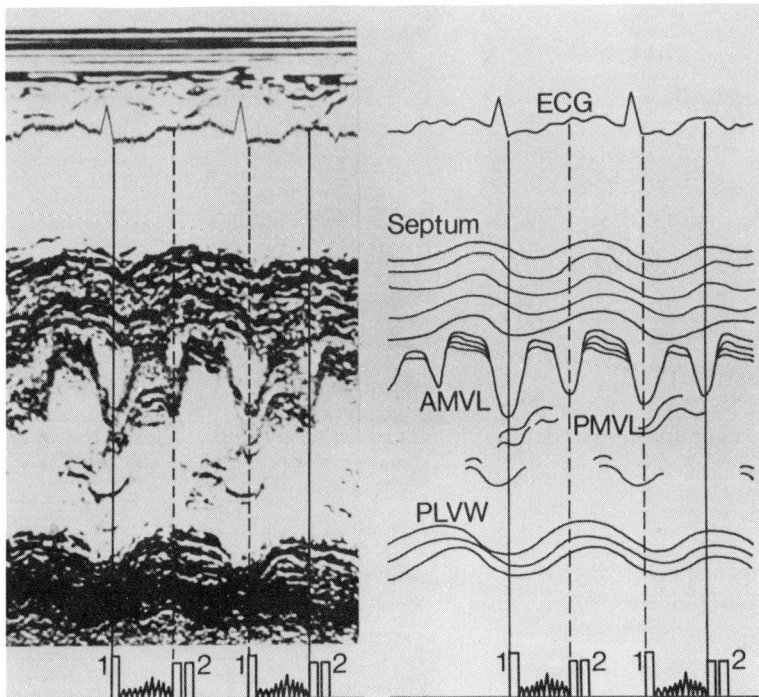

Fig 7–13.—Mitral valve echocardiogram in a patient with muscular sub-aortic stenosis. In diastole the anterior mitral valve leaflet *(AMVL)* moves in a normal direction (toward the interventricular septum) while the posterior mitral valve leaflet *(PMVL),* which is not well seen, moves toward the posterior left ventricular wall *(PLVW).* In systole, however, contrary to the normal situation, the anterior leaflet again moves toward the interventricular septum, narrowing the outflow tract of the left ventricle. This obstruction results in an ejection systolic murmur, which in this instance begins shortly after the first heart sound and ends with the second sound. The murmur's peak intensity coincides with the period of maximum subvalvular obstruction. This abnormal motion of the anterior leaflet of the mitral valve may result in mitral valve regurgitation, which commonly occurs in this entity.

Echocardiography has been of considerable diagnostic value in muscular subaortic stenosis. In addition to that described above, a discrepancy in the thickness of the interventricular septum when compared to the posterior left ventricular wall, as well as an abnormal anterior displacement of the mitral valve in the left ventricular chamber, are helpful diagnostic findings. Both are present in this illustration.

cular resistance and is a convenient bedside method for increasing the loudness of the murmur. Inotropic agents such as epinephrine, isoproterenol and digitalis will also increase the intensity of the murmur; whereas peripheral vasoconstriction with neosynephrine or methoxamine reduces it.

Echocardiography has been of considerable help and certain features may be diagnostic of IHSS (Fig 7 – 13).

Severe, long-standing valvular aortic stenosis may be complicated by gradual thickening of the interventricular septum, causing muscular subaortic obstruction. This obstruction may be unmasked by operation on valvular aortic stenosis. Persistence of a loud systolic murmur following operation suggests residual subaortic stenosis.

Innocent Systolic Murmurs

As used here, the term *innocent systolic murmurs* refers to a clear-cut group of murmurs with definite characteristics that permit their recognition. The term does not include murmurs that are clearly recognized as being produced in some valve or congenital defect, but are innocuous ("innocent") in that there is no other evidence of cardiac involvement. Nor is the term to be used as a catchall for murmurs of which the origin is unknown but which do not have the characteristics of the murmurs to be described. Innocent systolic murmurs are also called *accidental murmurs* and *physiologic murmurs*. Frequently, they are called *functional murmurs*. Because the term *functional* is ambiguous and often misleading, it is best not to use it.

The innocent systolic murmurs are the most common systolic murmurs heard in children, and their main importance is that they must be separated from those murmurs that indicate organic valvular pathology or congenital heart disease. Some studies of children demonstrate that as many as 90% may show an innocent murmur at one time or another. These murmurs may persist for years or disappear quickly.

Innocent systolic murmurs may be separated into two groups: (1) those of maximum intensity in the apicosternal region and (2) those of maximum intensity in the second left intercostal space. The apicosternal group is the more important. The exact mode of production of these murmurs is not known.

The innocent systolic murmurs of maximum intensity in the second left interspace are probably produced by flow into the pulmonary artery.

INNOCENT SYSTOLIC MURMURS OF MAXIMUM INTENSITY IN THE APICOSTERNAL REGION*

In this group, localization of the exact point of maximum intensity may at times be difficult because the murmur may be of almost equal intensity over much of the apicosternal area (Fig 7 – 14). The point of maximum intensity will vary somewhat with the position of the patient and is about one intercostal space lower when the patient sits up. *These murmurs are not of maximum intensity at the apex.*

AREA OF TRANSMISSION. — A very interesting and important differentiating characteristic of the apicosternal murmurs is that these murmurs, considering their intensity, are heard in a wide area from the point of maximum intensity. A murmur of moderate intensity and maximum in the third left intercostal space may be heard at the apex, in the aortic area, and usually into the neck. Many innocent systolic murmurs are especially well transmitted into the neck, actually much better than most organic murmurs, e.g., the murmur of patent ductus arteriosus. Because they may be heard at the apex, they will be recorded as apical systolic murmurs if the precordium is not carefully investigated to determine the point of maximum intensity. These murmurs are almost always heard in the pulmonic area, no matter where they may be most intense. This is not true of the systolic murmur of mitral regurgitation.

TIMING AND DURATION. — These murmurs occur in early and midsystole. Late systole is quiet. They are usually crescendo-decrescendo in form (Fig 7 – 15).

PITCH AND QUALITY. — Innocent systolic murmurs are of medium pitch, rough, and not usually harsh. They are *not* high pitched. The term *vibratory* has been used and is descriptive of the quality of many of the innocent systolic murmurs heard in the apicosternal region (see Fig 7 – 15). To realize the true

---

*We have arbitrarily used the term *apicosternal* to indicate the area from the left sternal border to the apex, *excluding the apex* but including the left sternal border. The mesocardiac area is the area between the left sternal border and the apex, excluding both the left sternal border and the apex.

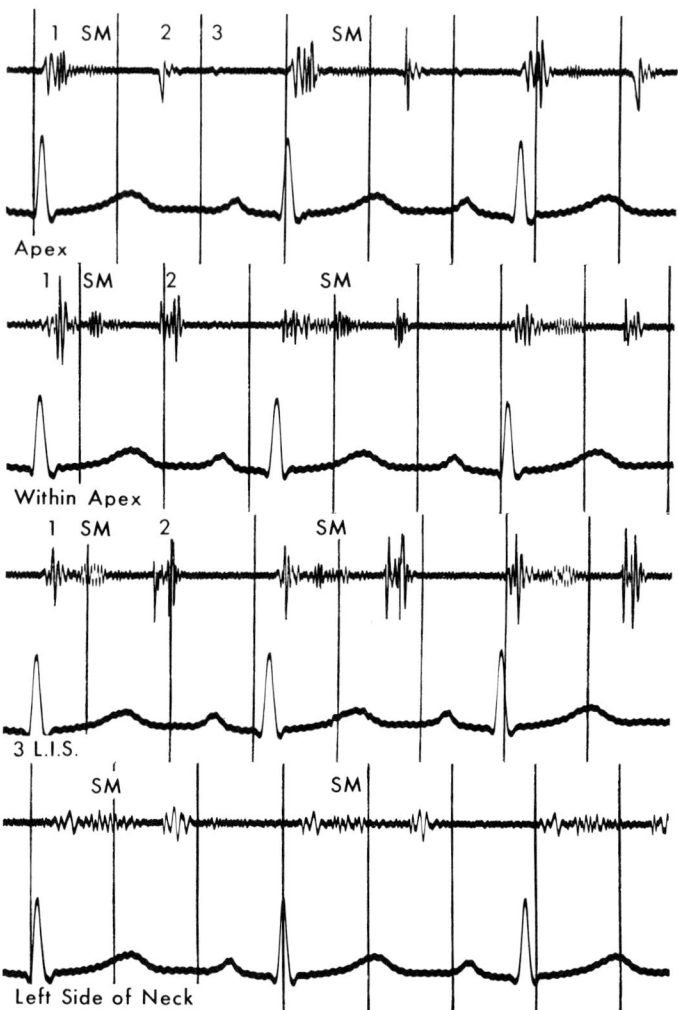

Fig 7–14.—Innocent systolic murmur. This murmur was of maximum intensity between the apex and the left border of the sternum, although it can be noted that the intensity within the apex *(second tracing)* and in the third left intercostal space *(third tracing)* is similar, and it would be difficult to say that the murmur was louder in one area than in the other. It was definitely not loudest at the apex *(first tracing)*. Note the intensity in the left side of the neck *(fourth tracing)*.

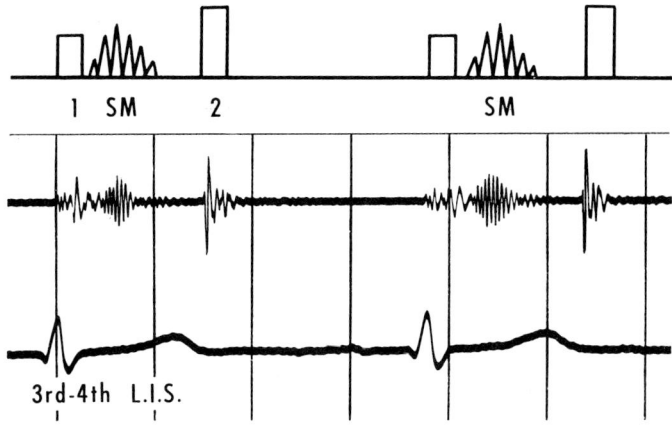

Fig 7–15.—Innocent systolic murmur. Note the uniform vibrations that are characteristic of those innocent systolic murmurs that have a "vibratory" quality. Also note that the murmur is short and that it is mainly in the first half of systole.

quality of the murmur, one must listen to it with a bell chest piece applied lightly. With heavy pressure on the bell, the murmur is usually greatly diminished, but often some high-pitched components remain, which may resemble the murmur of mitral regurgitation. The diaphragm chest piece may also be misleading with regard to the quality of the murmur.

LOUDNESS. — Some of the innocent murmurs may be quite loud in children. Exercise, as it does for most murmurs, increases the loudness of innocent murmurs and is of no value in differentiating them from other murmurs. Fever and tachycardia will increase the loudness of a murmur, and often a murmur will be heard only when these conditions are present.

POSITION OF THE PATIENT. — Innocent systolic murmurs are usually best heard when the patient is lying down but may occasionally be heard better when the patient is sitting up. The murmur will often increase at the apex in the left lateral position in a manner suggesting the murmur of mitral regurgitation; however, the murmur will usually be found to have also increased in intensity along the left border of the sternum and will be louder in that region than at the apex.

EFFECT OF RESPIRATION. — Held expiration will usually increase these murmurs.

CHANGES IN THE HEART SOUNDS. — With innocent systolic

murmurs there are no changes in the heart sounds. The clear-cut presence of heart sound changes, especially an abnormally split or accentuated second sound, should therefore, make one consider the possibility of a congenital heart murmur.

DIFFERENTIATION. — The differentiation of these murmurs from the murmurs produced by rheumatic heart disease is usually easy and depends on the *point of maximum intensity, quality*, and *transmission*, which, as has been indicated, are quite different from those of the murmurs described up to this point. In doubtful cases, the presence of a clear-cut diastolic murmur is helpful in deciding whether the murmur is innocent or organic. However, innocent murmurs may occur in the presence of organic murmurs and can often be recognized as such. In some normal children, after exercise, the third heart sound at the apex may be prolonged and give the impression of a middiastolic murmur. If this sound is mistaken for a middiastolic murmur, an innocent systolic murmur may be given more importance than it deserves.

An innocent systolic murmur of maximum intensity in the third or fourth left intercostal space should be differentiated from the murmur of a small ventricular septal defect or a very mild infundibular stenosis. This is discussed on page 179.

INNOCENT SYSTOLIC MURMURS OF MAXIMUM INTENSITY IN THE SECOND LEFT INTERCOSTAL SPACE

These murmurs are localized and do not show the wide transmission of the apicosternal murmurs. They are rough in quality and are best heard when the patient is in the recumbent position. Held expiration increases the intensity, and there are few children in whom a faint systolic murmur will not be heard in the pulmonic area if the child expires forcibly and stops breathing for 10 to 15 seconds. There are no changes in the heart sounds.

This murmur sounds very much like the murmur of an atrial septal defect or a mild pulmonary valvular stenosis. The presence of a widely split second sound in these latter two conditions is the most helpful differentiating point.

Cardiopulmonary Murmur

The cardiopulmonary murmur is frequently mentioned in the literature, but it does not seem to occur commonly, although it may be that it is so easily recognized that one soon learns to ignore it. Along the borders of the heart, where the respiratory sounds can be heard along with the heart sounds, the inspiratory sound will seem at times to be broken up and heard only during systole. It gives the impression of a faint, high-pitched murmur resembling the murmur of mitral regurgitation. This apparent murmur occurs only during inspiration or, at least, is much louder during inspiration. Having the patient hold his breath does away with the murmur and is the most important means of recognizing the murmur if there is any doubt. The heart action against the adjacent lung tissue may account for the production of this apparent murmur.

CHAPTER 8

Diastolic Murmurs

The Diastolic Murmur of Mitral Stenosis

TIMING AND DURATION.—The murmur of mitral stenosis is produced by the flow of blood into the ventricles during diastole and is more intense when the velocity of flow is greatest. Normally, when the left ventricular pressure at the end of systole drops below that in the left atrium, the mitral valve opens and the blood that has collected in the left atrium flows rapidly into the left ventricle. This is the phase of rapid filling, and it occurs with a small pressure gradient between the left atrium and the left ventricle (see Fig 5–1, p. 54). By the time of the atrial contraction, most of the ventricular filling has occurred and comparatively little is added by atrial contraction. If the mitral valve becomes mildly stenotic, there is usually a significant left atrial-left ventricular pressure gradient during the phase of rapid filling, and a murmur is heard. The gradient falls as the ventricle fills. (Fig 8–1, A). Since the murmur occurs an appreciable time after the second sound, it has been called a middiastolic murmur. A murmur may occur with atrial contraction at this stage, especially at more rapid rates, since atrial contraction now occurs before ventricular filling is complete; at slow rates, only the middiastolic murmur may be present.

As the degree of stenosis increases, the filling of the ventricle is slower and the murmur becomes longer. A significant left atrial-left ventricular pressure gradient is usually present throughout diastole. Toward the end of diastole, further narrowing of the mitral orifice, associated with the increase in velocity of blood flow produced by atrial contraction, results in a murmur (Fig 8–1, B). This murmur is called *presystolic* and is crescendo in character, ending in the first sound.

As the stenosis increases, the middiastolic and presystolic components blend into one murmur (Fig 8–2). At rapid rates, the two murmurs telescope, so that the murmur is shorter and mainly presystolic. In atrial fibrillation only the middiastolic component is usually present. However, a presystolic crescendo murmur is occasionally heard and more often recorded phonocardiographically. Recent studies have shown that the presystolic murmur can at times result from mitral leaflet approximation in late diastole associated with beginning mitral valve closure, even in the absence of atrial contraction.

Echocardiography has been a sensitive tool in the detection of mitral stenosis, especially in those instances where the physical findings are minimal or atypical. The echocardiogram usually demonstrates leaflet thickening, manifested by multiple, reduplicated echoes from the mitral leaflets, a reduction in the slope of the posterior drift of the anterior leaflet in diastole, and anterior motion of the posterior leaflet in diastole as opposed to the normal posterior motion (Fig 8–3). A left atrial myxoma can readily be recognized by the appearance of multiple echoes behind the mitral leaflets usually seen in diastole. The Austin Flint murmur (see Fig 8–6) likewise can be distinguished from that of mitral stenosis by echocardiography.

It is important to repeat that the earliest murmur of mitral stenosis is nearly always a middiastolic murmur, although occasionally only a presystolic murmur can be heard. However, it is always dangerous to make the diagnosis of mitral stenosis on what appears to be a presystolic murmur alone, since other sounds occurring at the time of the first sound can give the impression of a presystolic murmur, e.g., an atrial sound, a split first sound, or an ejection sound.

MAXIMUM INTENSITY AND AREA OF TRANSMISSION. — The murmur of mitral stenosis is of maximum intensity just within and above the apex (see Fig 7–1, p. 97). It is generally confined to a rather small area, even when the murmur is quite loud in this area. It usually corresponds closely to the point of maximum impulse. With enlargement of the right ventricle, the left ventricle and atrium may be pushed laterally and pos-

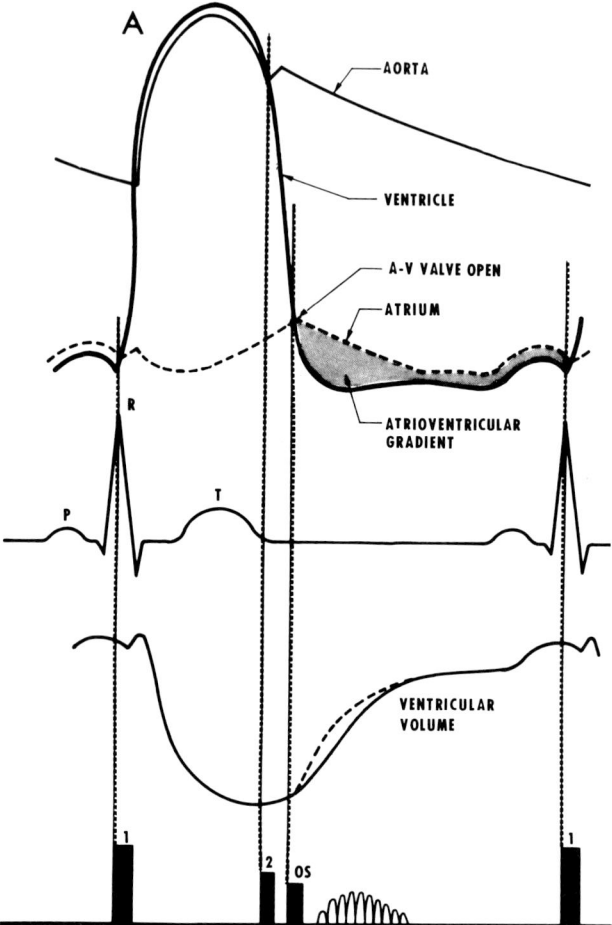

A

AORTA

VENTRICLE

A-V VALVE OPEN

ATRIUM

ATRIOVENTRICULAR
GRADIENT

R

P   T

VENTRICULAR
VOLUME

1   2 OS   1

Fig 8–1.—Mitral stenosis—relation of pressures, electrocardiogram, and ventricular volume to the heart sounds and murmurs.

A, early mitral stenosis. Because of changes in the mitral valve, the intensity of the first heart sound is increased and the opening of the mitral valve produces a sound *(OS)*. When the pressure in the atrium is still essentially normal, the first heart sound occurs at the normal time, which is usually at the peak of the R-wave of the electrocardiogram. The interval between the aortic second sound and the opening snap is the time it takes for isometric relaxation. Because of the mitral stenosis, ventricular filling is somewhat delayed (normal filling indicated by dotted line) and there is, during early diastole, a gradient between the left atrium and left ventricle. A murmur is produced during rapid ventricular filling when this gradient exists. Because the stenosis is mild, ventricular filling, although somewhat slowed, is adequate and if the heart rate is slow, the ventricles are full by the time atrial

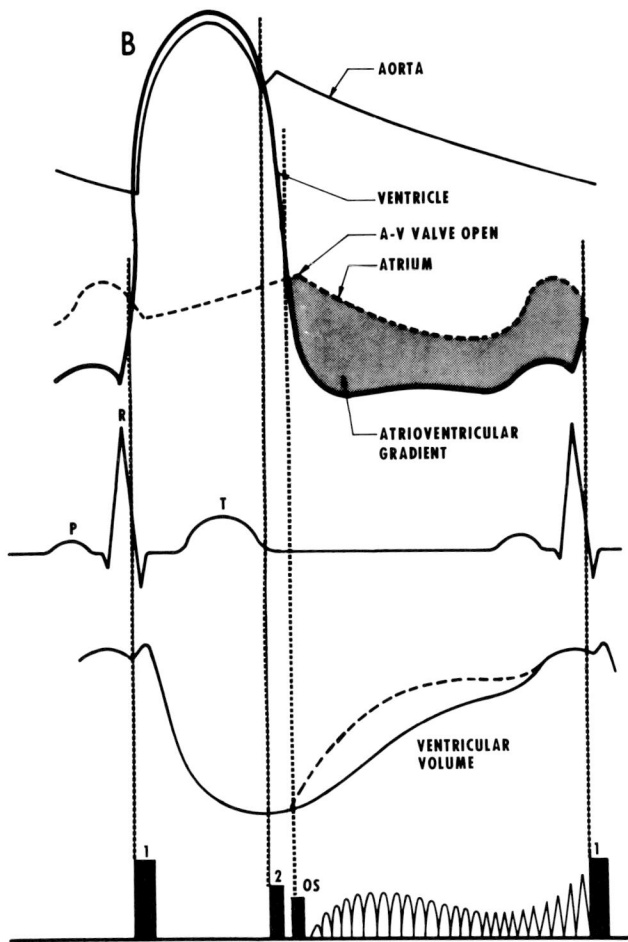

contraction occurs. If atrial contraction produces no gradient, then there will be no presystolic murmur. If it does produce a gradient, there may be a presystolic murmur.

B, severe mitral stenosis. Left atrial pressure is increased. The first heart sound is accentuated and is delayed because it takes the ventricle some time to build up a pressure equal to the increased atrial pressure. The onset of the first sound is after the peak of the R-wave. Because of the delay in the first sound, systole is shortened. The opening snap is loud and is closer to the aortic second sound because isometric relaxation is shorter due to the high pressure in the atrium. The murmur starts with the opening of the mitral valve and persists throughout diastole. At the time of atrial contraction, the ventricles are still not full and atrial contraction increases the flow and produces a rough presystolic murmur which ends with the accentuated first heart sound.

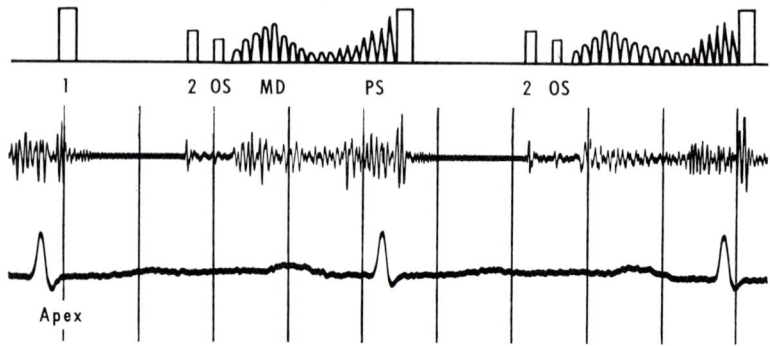

Fig 8–2.—Diastolic murmur of mitral stenosis. The second sound is followed by a faint opening snap *(OS)*. Diastole is long, and the middiastolic murmur *(MD)* begins to fade before atrial contraction produces the presystolic murmur *(PS)*.

teriorly, and the murmur in these cases will often be heard in the anterior or midaxillary line.

PITCH AND QUALITY.—When faint or moderately loud, the middiastolic murmur is low pitched and rumbling. As it becomes louder, it becomes more rough. Because the murmur is low pitched, it is best heard with the bell applied very lightly to the skin; in fact, when the murmur is faint, it will be heard only with the bell applied lightly. The use of the diaphragm chest piece or heavy pressure on the bell will completely obliterate a faint murmur that is clearly heard with the bell applied lightly (see Fig 2–4, B, p. 14). Since even faint middias-

Fig 8–3.—**A,** echocardiogram of a young woman with pure mitral stenosis. The heavy reduplicated echoes of both leaflets of the mitral valve indicate marked thickening. Two features are of diagnostic value: (1) In diastole the posterior leaflet *(PMVL)* moves toward the interventricular septum, as does the anterior leaflet *(AMVL)*, whereas normally the leaflets move in opposite directions. (2) There is loss of the normal posterior drift of the anterior leaflet after its maximal diastolic motion toward the septum. This indicates a continued gradient of pressure between left atrium and ventricle throughout diastole, due to the stenotic valve orifice. Note that the opening snap *(OS)* coincides with the movement of maximal anterior excursion of the thickened leaflets. The presystolic component of the murmur occurs as the leaflets are approximating in late diastole, resulting in increased blood flow velocity. **B,** echocardiogram of the same patient following mitral commissurotomy. The leaflets remain thickened and the posterior leaflet *(PMVL)* motion in diastole remains abnormal. Note, however, that in diastole, following its maximal ex-

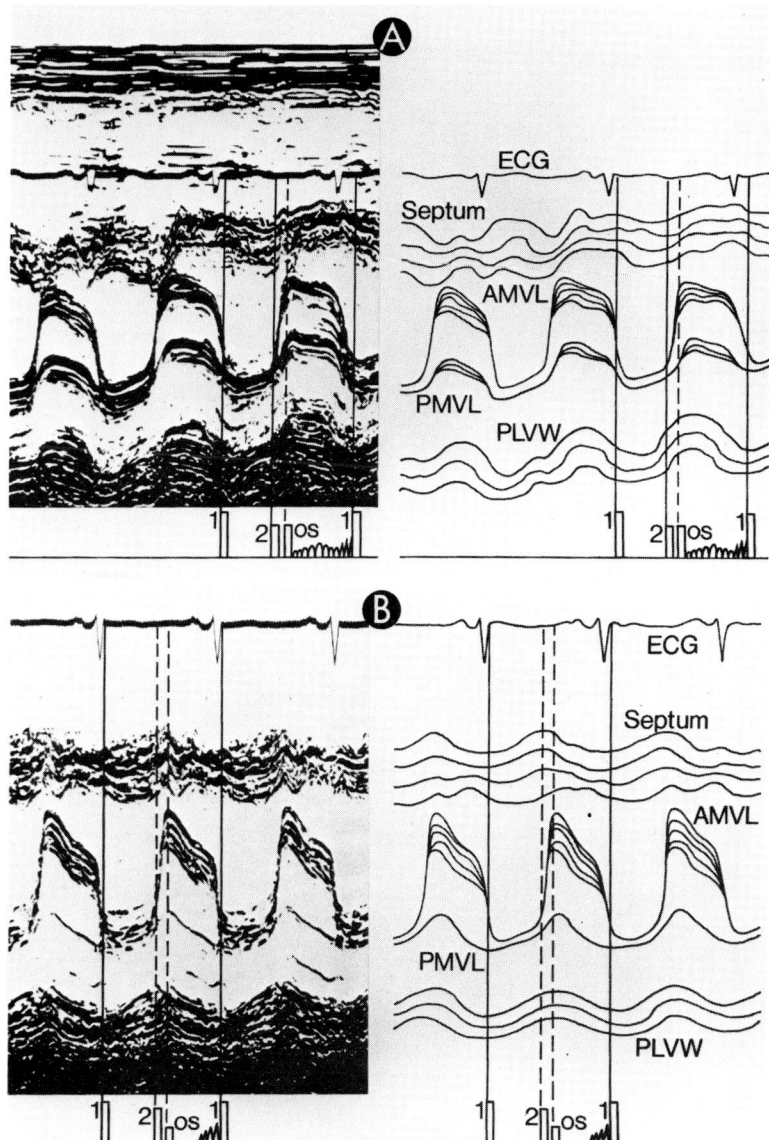

cursion toward the septum, the anterior leaflet *(AMVL)* drifts more rapidly toward the posterior left ventricular wall *(PLVW)*, indicating a reduction in the pressure gradient between left atrium and ventricle. The opening snap is less prominent and only the presystolic component of the diastolic murmur remains.

tolic murmurs are highly significant, the skilled use of the bell is an important asset in auscultation. As the murmur becomes louder, it becomes more rough and may be heard equally well with the bell or diaphragm. The presystolic murmur is usually somewhat rough and is heard almost equally well with the bell or diaphragm.

POSITION OF THE PATIENT. — The murmur is best heard when the patient is in the recumbent position; even when the murmur is loud in this position, it may not be heard at all in the upright position. To listen to the patient only in the upright position, therefore, is to ignore one of the most important murmurs in cardiac auscultation. The murmur is usually heard better in the left lateral decubitus position and is usually increased for a few beats just as the patient is turned from recumbent to the left lateral position, or from the left lateral to the recumbent position. It is, therefore, important to listen while turning the patient.

EFFECT OF RESPIRATION. — The murmur is either unchanged by respiration or somewhat diminished on inspiration.

CHANGES IN HEART SOUNDS. — Mitral stenosis is usually associated with an accentuated first heart sound (p.37). When the first sound is loud, there is usually an opening snap of the mitral valve (p. 69). If the valve and chordae tendineae are markedly fibrosed and the cusps are immobile, the first sound is diminished in loudness, and usually there is no opening snap of the mitral valve. The second heart sound may be accentuated in the pulmonic area, but this accentuation is due to an increase in pulmonary artery pressure and is a late change. The presence or absence of an accentuated pulmonic second sound gives information regarding pulmonary artery pressure and not regarding the presence or absence of mitral stenosis. The frequent occurrence of an opening snap of the mitral valve accounts for the common impression that the second heart sound is abnormally split in mitral stenosis. The splitting is usually of normal degree.

A third heart sound at the apex is rarely heard if there is a significant degree of mitral stenosis. The production of a third sound depends, in part, on rapid ventricular filling (p. 76). This cannot occur with tight mitral stenosis. The presence of a third heart sound at the apex, therefore, accentuates the importance of a systolic murmur and indicates that mitral regurgitation is the predominant lesion. A right-sided third heart sound may occur in mitral stenosis with right ventricular failure; however, this third sound will not usually be mistaken for that heard in mitral regurgitation. Since an opening snap of the mitral valve can occur in the presence of mild mitral stenosis, it may occasionally be heard in the presence of mild stenosis with fairly marked mitral regurgitation and a third heart sound.

EFFECT OF EXERCISE.—Since exercise increases the cardiac output and the speed of blood flow, it will increase the intensity of the murmur of mitral stenosis or will bring out a murmur not evident when the patient is at rest. Since even a faint murmur brought on by exercise is significant, it is important, if there is any suspicion of mitral stenosis, that the patient be exercised.

RELATION OF INTENSITY OF MURMUR TO SEVERITY OF LESION.—To make any correlation, the following factors must be considered:

1. The general intensity of all the sounds and murmurs must be compared, since a heavy chest wall or emphysema may dampen a loud murmur. In marked emphysema, a significant mitral stenosis may be present with a very faint murmur, which, because of the voluminous lungs, is heard much closer to the sternum than normally.

2. The cardiac output, mainly as judged by heart rate, must be considered. The increase in heart rate that occurs with excitement, exercise, thyrotoxicosis, and fever is associated with a marked increase in intensity of the murmur. A decrease in output, such as occurs in decompensation, may make the murmur much less evident or may make it disappear. The murmur is less evident at rest and in hypothyroidism. For comparison of the murmur on different occasions, it is best to use the intensity at rest.

3. When an enlarged right ventricle pushes the left atrium and the left ventricle laterally and posteriorly, the murmur is heard faintly in the midaxillary line and may be completely overlooked.

4. When a stenosis becomes very marked, the stream producing the murmur may be small and the murmur actually less evident.

5. Mitral stenosis without a murmur is a rare occurrence but
has been seen with severe degrees of narrowing of the mitral
orifice usually associated with marked calcification and immo-
bility of the mitral leaflets, in conjunction with very low cardiac outputs. A marked decrease in the cardiac output may
render a murmur of mitral stenosis inaudible even in the presence of mobile leaflets.

6. The murmur produced by a given degree of mitral stenosis will be increased by a significant degree of mitral regurgitation. A significant degree of mitral regurgitation implies, of
course, that the stenosis is not marked. In mitral regurgitation,
the flow through the mitral valves is increased, since there
must be enough flow during each diastole to make up for what
is to be regurgitated on the next beat. There is also an increase
in the size of the left ventricle in mitral regurgitation, which
would make the stenosis relatively greater. In the presence,
therefore, of mitral regurgitation, a murmur of mitral stenosis
is increased out of proportion to the degree of stenosis.

7. For stenotic valve openings of similar size, most males
will have louder murmurs than females. Males are generally
larger and have a greater cardiac output and, therefore, a greater blood flow through the valve.

Despite the many factors influencing the relation between
the intensity of the murmur and the degree of mitral stenosis,
there is usually a rough correlation.

DURATION OF THE MURMUR. — This should be given as
much attention as the intensity, since it is closely correlated
with the degree of stenosis and may be subject to fewer modifying factors.

DIFFERENTIATION. — The murmur of mitral stenosis can be
separated from the early diastolic murmurs of aortic and pulmonary regurgitation with no difficulty. The main problem is
differentiating it from the murmurs of tricuspid stenosis and
those of relative mitral stenosis. These will be discussed in
the following section.

The Diastolic Murmur of Tricuspid Stenosis

The diastolic murmur of tricuspid stenosis usually has the
same timing and much the same pitch and quality as that of

mitral stenosis; often, however, the murmur seems higher pitched and earlier in diastole, and may somewhat resemble the early diastolic murmur of aortic and pulmonic regurgitation. The murmur is best heard with the patient in the recumbent position, using the bell chest piece. The first sound is less commonly accentuated than in mitral stenosis.

Tricuspid stenosis practically always occurs in association with mitral valvular lesions, which may overshadow it. However, the presence of a tricuspid stenosis usually can be recognized, even in the presence of mitral stenosis, by the *characteristic location* of the murmur and its *reaction to respiration*. The murmur is best heard just to the left of the lower end of the sternum (see Fig 7–1, p. 97). It is usually fairly well localized and does not extend far to the left, even when loud and when the right side of the heart is quite enlarged. If the murmurs of mitral stenosis and tricuspid stenosis are both present, two areas of maximum intensity can often be determined—one close to the sternum and the other at the apex. With cardiac enlargement, both areas may be shifted somewhat to the left.

Like the murmur of tricuspid regurgitation, the murmur of tricuspid stenosis is markedly increased in loudness with inspiration. It may be several times as loud on inspiration as on expiration and may be heard only on inspiration. The murmur of mitral stenosis will be essentially unchanged or slightly decreased on inspiration.

Tricuspid regurgitation will increase the loudness of the murmur of mild tricuspid stenosis. This effect results from the increased flow through the tricuspid valve during diastole and the relative stenosis produced by the dilation of the right ventricle; stretching and distortion of the valve have also been implicated. With marked tricuspid regurgitation, a diastolic murmur can occur even in the absence of stenosis. Since some tricuspid regurgitation is nearly always associated with tricuspid stenosis, caution must be exercised in estimating the degree of tricuspid stenosis from the loudness of the diastolic murmur.

A large A-wave, which increases on inspiration, is present if the patient is in sinus rhythm. At times it may be palpable and synchronous with the presystolic portion of the murmur.

The Diastolic Murmur of Aortic Regurgitation

TIMING AND DURATION.—The maximum intensity of the diastolic murmur of aortic regurgitation occurs immediately after the second sound; as the pressure in the aorta falls and the ventricles fill, the murmur decreases in intensity (Fig 8–4). Since the murmur is loudest in early diastole, it is considered an early diastolic murmur even though it may last throughout diastole. Phonocardiograms occasionally show that the murmur has a short period of crescendo and then becomes decrescendo; the ear can occasionally distinguish this sequence, but, essentially, the murmur can be considered decrescendo. The murmur may be very short or may last throughout diastole.

PITCH AND QUALITY.—The murmur is high pitched and blowing and usually remains so even when loud. When aortic regurgitation is very severe, the murmur may be harsh and surprisingly short for the degree of regurgitation. A loud, high-pitched, musical murmur may occur when the regurgitation is associated with a retroverted cusp.

Fig 8–4.—Diastolic murmur of aortic regurgitation. The high-pitched diastolic murmur *(DM)* starts with the second sound. It is loudest early in diastole and in this case is heard throughout diastole in diminishing intensity. In the diagrammatic representation of this murmur, it is shown louder than on the phonocardiogram. This is because this is a high-pitched murmur and high-pitched murmurs seem louder to the ear than when recorded on the phonocardiogram. A moderately loud, medium-pitched systolic murmur is present in this patient. There is an ejection sound *(ES)*. The second sound is normal or slightly accentuated.

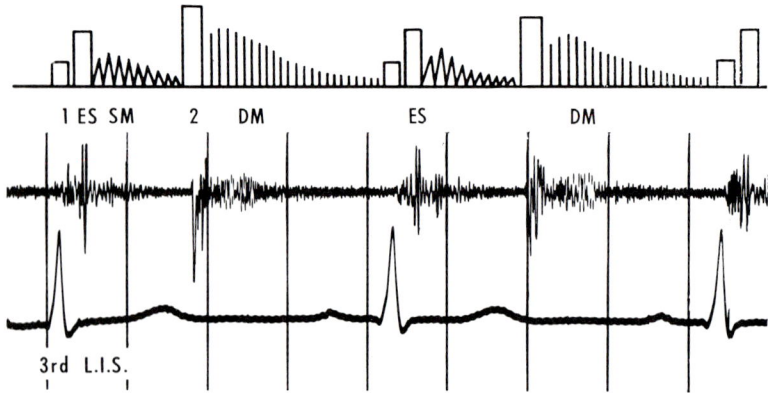

Since the murmur is high pitched, the diaphragm chest piece is essential when the murmur is faint. The room must be quiet, and attention must be directed at early diastole. A normal or accentuated second sound may mask a faint murmur unless the latter is carefully sought.

POINT OF MAXIMUM INTENSITY. — This is usually in the third left intercostal space next to the sternum, and when the murmur is faint, it may be heard only in this area (see Fig 7–1, p. 97). When the aorta is dilated, the murmur may be loudest in the second right intercostal space. Occasionally, when all sounds are faint at the base, the murmur may be most intense to the left of the lower end of the sternum or at the apex.

Unusual causes of aortic regurgitation, such as aortic dissection, lues, and some cases of ruptured aneurysms of the sinus of Valsalva, result in a murmur often best heard in the right third and fourth intercostal spaces. The atypical transmission of these murmurs is felt to be due to the severe dilatation of the proximal portion of the ascending aorta.

AREA OF TRANSMISSION. — When the murmur is loud, it may be heard over most of the precordium. In some cases, when the left ventricle is quite enlarged, the murmur may be loudest along the left border of the sternum, but is also very well heard in an area above the apex in the anterior axillary region (Fig 8–5). Between these two areas, the murmur may not be heard at all or may be only faintly heard. With transmission, the murmur loses some of its characteristic high pitch but is not difficult to recognize because of its timing.

When the aortic regurgitation is marked and associated with a moderately loud systolic murmur of aortic stenosis, an unusual auscultatory phenomenon may occasionally be heard in the left anterior axillary region. In this area the transmitted systolic and early diastolic murmurs combine with an apical middiastolic murmur, due to relative mitral stenosis (p. 141), to give the impression of a continuous murmur similar to that heard in arteriovenous fistulae. The lowered pitch of the early diastolic murmur resulting from transmission favors this impression.

POSITION OF THE PATIENT. — Older patients should sit up and lean forward, with respiration held on expiration. In younger patients, the murmur is often as well, or better, heard when they are in the recumbent position.

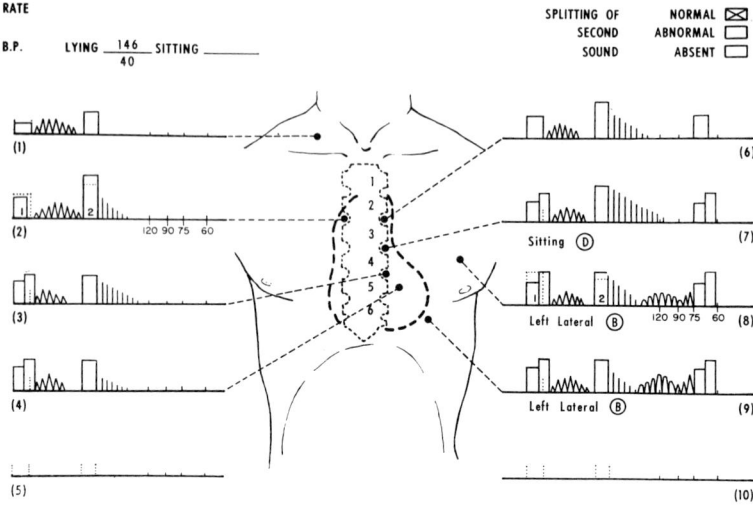

Fig 8–5.—Severe aortic regurgitation. A mild mitral stenosis or an Austin Flint murmur is also present. The numbers in parentheses refer to the lines on the chart. The following features are shown:

a. A high-pitched, diastolic murmur starting with the second sound and diminishing in intensity is the characteristic finding. The murmur is loudest in the third left intercostal space *(7)* and is usually well heard in the fourth left intercostal space *(3)*. When loud, it is heard to a lesser degree in other areas of the precordium. It is occasionally loudest in the second right intercostal space.

b. When the heart is very large, the early diastolic murmur is often well heard in the anterior axillary line above the apex *(8)*. It is often of greater intensity in this area than it is in any other area, except the third left intercostal space.

c. At the apex and laterally from the apex, a rumbling middiastolic murmur and a presystolic murmur are present *(8) (9)*. These middiastolic and presystolic murmurs may represent a mild degree of organic mitral stenosis or may be an Austin Flint murmur. If the cardiac lesion is due to rheumatic fever, one must assume that the middiastolic murmur is probably due to mitral valve involvement.

d. A rough systolic murmur is usually present in the second right intercostal space *(2)*. This may occur even in the absence of aortic stenosis and may be due in part to roughening of the aortic valves, and in part to a *relative* aortic stenosis produced by some aortic dilation and by the marked increase in flow through the aortic valve.

e. Although the heart sounds are often unchanged, an ejection sound may be present which gives the impression of a split first sound (see text, p. 63, and Figs 5–7 and 8–4).

CHANGES IN HEART SOUNDS. — The aortic second sound is frequently increased in aortic regurgitation (pp. 44–45). With syphilitic involvement of the aorta, the second sound may also have a resonant or tympanitic quality. If rheumatic aortic stenosis is present with calcification, the aortic second sound is usually diminished.

An ejection sound is often present and is usually most evident at the apex, where it gives the impression of a split first sound because the ejection sound, instead of having a high-pitched quality, resembles the first sound.

RELATION OF INTENSITY OF MURMUR TO SEVERITY OF LESION. — When the regurgitation is mild, a faint murmur may be the only evidence of the lesion. When the lesion is severe enough to produce peripheral signs of aortic regurgitation, the murmur is usually more intense and prolonged. This is not, however, always the case, and at times the murmur may be deceivingly faint in the presence of significant aortic regurgitation. On occasion, marked peripheral evidence of regurgitation may be associated with a very short harsh murmur.

OCCURRENCE. — The diastolic murmur of aortic regurgitation is most commonly heard in association with rheumatic heart disease. Syphilitic aortic regurgitation is becoming less frequent. Faint murmurs are occasionally heard in hypertension and become louder in proportion to the diastolic blood pressure. The sudden appearance of this murmur in a patient with hypertension and acute chest pain should lead one to consider a dissecting aortic aneurysm, especially if the point of maximum intensity is to the right of the sternum. Aortic regurgitation occurs rather frequently with all types of congenital aortic stenosis (p. 185) and with bicuspid aortic valves. It is occasionally associated with high ventricular septal defects.

A loud, high-pitched, musical murmur, associated with a retroverted cusp, or possibly a ruptured cusp, occurs primarily in syphilitic aortitis but is also heard occasionally in rheumatic aortic regurgitation or bacterial endocarditis and, rarely, in arteriosclerosis. This loud, musical murmur ("sea gull" or "cooing") may persist for years, or gradually be replaced by the usual murmur of aortic regurgitation.

Rupture of the sinus of Valsalva may occur in association with subacute bacterial endocarditis and rarely in unexplained situations. Rupture may occur into the atria or ventricles, producing a decrescendo diastolic murmur. Rupture into the right atrium or right ventricle is associated with a continuous murmur. Other causes of aortic regurgitation include Marfan's disease, Marie Strümpell's disease (rheumatoid spondylitis), and dissecting hematoma of the aorta.

Apical Diastolic Murmurs Not Associated with Organic Mitral Stenosis

Murmurs resembling the murmur of mitral stenosis in quality and timing occur in a number of conditions in which organic mitral stenosis is not present. In general, one or both of two conditions are present when these murmurs are found: an increase in the size of the left ventricle or an increased flow of blood through the mitral valve. A normal mitral valve may be relatively stenotic if there is a markedly enlarged left ventricle. An increased flow through the mitral valve occurs in such conditions as patent ductus arteriosus, ventricular septal defect, and mitral regurgitation. Poor tone of the muscle of the left ventricle may, at times, play a part, e.g., in rheumatic carditis.

A similar murmur may be heard in relative tricuspid stenosis when the same factors are present, e.g., atrial septal defect.

The murmur is most often heard in children, and this is probably due in part to the fact that blood flow through the mitral valve in children seems more likely to produce sound. Phonocardiograms in normal children may show a few vibrations during diastole in association with a third heart sound.

The *timing* of the murmur is similar to that of the murmur of mitral stenosis. Since the mitral valve is widely opened, most of the ventricular filling is completed before atrial contraction, so that atrial contraction may produce no murmur. A presystolic murmur will, therefore, usually not be present if the heart rate is slow. When the rate is rapid, atrial contraction is superimposed, in part, on rapid ventricular filling, and a presystolic murmur is heard (see Fig 11–5, p. 181). Since similar murmurs may be produced at both the mitral and the tricuspid valve, these murmurs are heard over a fairly wide area. The point of maximum intensity is commonly just medial to the apex and between the apex and sternum.

The middiastolic murmurs are low pitched, with a rumbling quality, and are best heard using the bell chest piece with the patient in the recumbent or left lateral position. When produced at the tricuspid valve, they may be louder with inspiration.

OCCURRENCE AND DIFFERENTIATION

1. AORTIC REGURGITATION. — Since Austin Flint, in 1862, described a diastolic murmur at the apex in patients with aortic regurgitation, there has been much difference of opinion as to the cause of this phenomenon, its frequency, and the exact nature of what is heard. Considered unusual by some physicians, it has been heard frequently by others; the murmur has been described as presystolic, middiastolic, or both middiastolic and presystolic; it has even been considered an auditory illusion. Whatever the background may be, not infrequently patients with aortic regurgitation and no mitral involvement have a diastolic murmur at the apex which, to the ear, is indistinguishable from that of mitral stenosis (see Fig 8–5). There may be a rumbling middiastolic component, a presystolic component, or both.

Much of the controversy regarding the occurrence of an Austin Flint murmur has resulted from the fact that the presence of a middiastolic or presystolic murmur may be simulated by changes in the heart sounds, the presence of extra sounds, and changes in the early diastolic murmur that occur on transmission to the apex. Accentuated third heart sounds, atrial sounds, and split first heart sounds might be mistaken for a rumbling middiastolic murmur and presystolic murmur but, in most instances, do not give the characteristic sound of the murmur of mitral stenosis. The early diastolic murmur of aortic regurgitation, in transmission to the apex, may become lower pitched. If careful attention is not paid to timing, the murmur may be considered middiastolic, especially if the heart rate is somewhat rapid.

The apical murmur has been considered to be the murmur of relative mitral stenosis, resulting from the enlargement of the left ventricle. It has, however, been reported in hearts showing very little enlargement. The rather commonly seen presystolic component is also somewhat unusual in relative mitral stenosis. The hypothesis has been advanced that the anterior cusp of the mitral valve may be partially closed by the regurgitant aortic stream, with production of a functional stenosis. Other causes that have been advanced to explain the Austin Flint murmur include turbulence produced by the striking together of the mitral inflow stream and the aortic regurgitant stream, late diastolic mitral regurgitation due to left ventricular dilatation, and mitral orifice narrowing in late diastole due to a rapidly rising left ventricular enddiastolic pressure associated with increased velocity of flow across the mitral valve.

Differentiation depends on the history and findings of syphilitic aortitis on the one hand, and of rheumatic fever on the other. If the patient has had a clear-cut episode of rheumatic fever, the murmur should be considered as resulting from mitral stenosis. An accentuated first heart sound is more likely to occur with true mitral stenosis. An opening snap of the mitral valve is helpful if present. Pharmacologic maneuvers that may be useful in distinguishing these murmurs are described in Chapter 17. As mentioned, echocardiography may be of diagnostic value (Fig 8–6).

2. ACUTE RHEUMATIC CARDITIS. — A middiastolic rumbling murmur will not infrequently be heard in children in their first attack of rheumatic carditis. Cardiac enlargement is usually, but not always, present; mitral regurgitation is usually present. Since mitral stenosis takes years to develop, the occurrence of a middiastolic murmur during the early phases of rheumatic fever would indicate that it was not due to organic mitral stenosis. In a child with active carditis, the diagnosis of organic mitral stenosis should not be made on a middiastolic murmur alone. Stiffening of the cusps and irregularity of their surfaces resulting from inflammation may play a part in the production of the murmur (Carey Coombs murmur). A presystolic component is unusual, even when the middiastolic component is loud. These murmurs disappear as the inflammation subsides and the heart decreases in size.

The differentiation of organic mitral stenosis from relative mitral stenosis during an episode of acute rheumatic carditis is often complicated by the fact that it is difficult to be sure whether that attack being witnessed is the first attack or

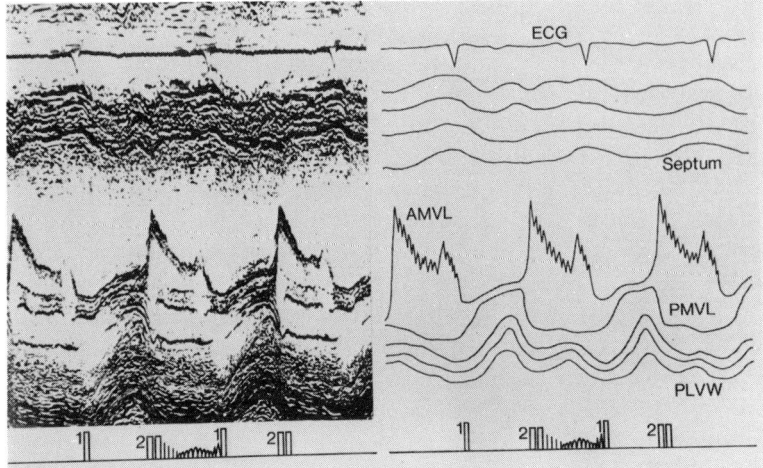

Fig 8-6.—Echocardiogram of a patient with severe aortic regurgitation and an Austin Flint murmur. Despite the presence of a murmur suggesting mitral stenosis (superimposed on an aortic regurgitant murmur), the echocardiogram of the mitral valve shows: (1) no evidence of leaflet thickening, (2) a normal slope for the posterior drift of the anterior leaflet *(AMVL)* in early diastole, (3) normal posterior motion of the posterior leaflet *(PMVL)* in diastole, and (4) fluttering of the anterior leaflet of the mitral valve due to the regurgitant jet from the aorta impinging on the opened valve. The echocardiogram is frequently the most useful diagnostic procedure in excluding mitral stenosis in the presence of severe aortic regurgitation.

whether there has been scarring of the valves from previous attacks.

3. CONGENITAL HEART DISEASE.—Apical diastolic murmurs can occur in several forms of congenital heart disease. Their occurrence in patent ductus arteriosus and ventricular septal defects causes no difficulty in diagnosis if it is realized that these murmurs may be part of the picture. The other characteristic findings usually make the diagnosis apparent. The murmur probably results from the increased flow through the mitral valve and the enlargement of the left ventricle.

Since atrial septal defects do not have a very characteristic murmur, it is important to recognize that apical diastolic murmurs can occur in this condition; otherwise, the diagnosis of organic mitral stenosis may be made. In most patients considered to have Lutembacher's syndrome (atrial septal defect and organic mitral stenosis), the condition has probably been misdiagnosed on this basis. The murmur probably results from the increased flow through the tricuspid valve and from the increase in the size of the right ventricle. In atrial septal defects, the murmur is heard along the left border of the sternum and out toward the apex, and consists mainly of a middiastolic component, but may at more rapid rates have both middiastolic and presystolic components (see Fig 11–5, p. 181). Differentiation from mitral stenosis on the basis of auscultation is discussed on page 184.

4. INACTIVE RHEUMATIC HEART DISEASE WITH MARKED MITRAL REGURGITATION.—A patient with marked mitral regurgitation and a large left ventricle may have a middiastolic murmur in the absence of any mitral stenosis (Fig 8–7). Patients with marked regurgitation and very mild stenosis may have a middiastolic murmur out of all proportion to the degree of the lesion. This is especially true in children. The murmur

Fig 8–7.—Middiastolic murmur in a patient with mitral regurgitation. *Upper tracing:* The first sound is followed by a systolic murmur *(SM)*. The second sound is of normal intensity. A moderately loud middiastolic murmur *(DM)* is present. *Lower tracing:* In a slightly different area at the apex and with a different method of recording, it is evident that there is a loud third sound (3) followed by a diastolic rumble *(DM)*.

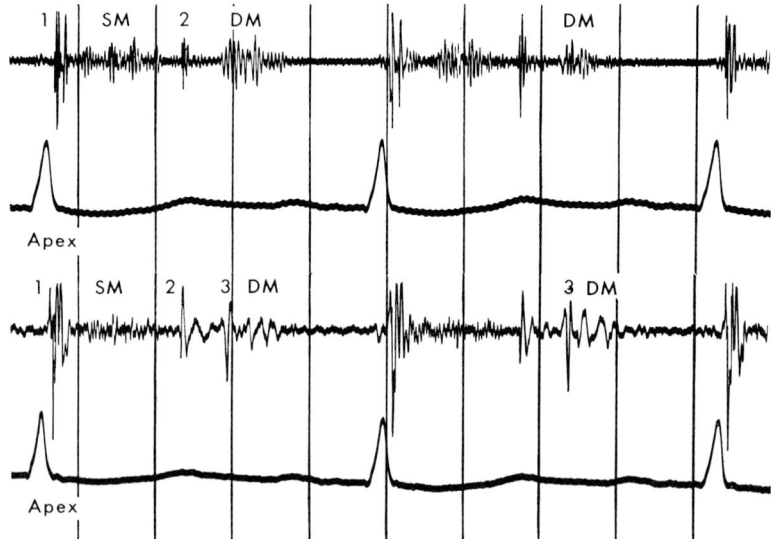

results from the increased flow through the mitral valve and the enlargement of the left ventricle. It may be distinguished from the murmur of organic mitral stenosis on the following bases:

a. The presence of marked mitral regurgitation, especially with a systolic expansion of the left atrium, indicates that there cannot be any important degree of mitral stenosis.

b. The murmur, at slower rates, is nearly always limited to middiastole, even when the murmur is loud and the rhythm regular. A presystolic component may occur at rapid rates.

c. The first sound is not accentuated.

d. An opening snap of the mitral valve is rarely present. It is occasionally heard in the presence of moderate mitral regurgitation associated with moderate stenosis.

e. A third heart sound is often present (see Fig 8–7). It may be mistaken for the second heart sound or may be masked by the middiastolic murmur. When a third heart sound is present, the murmur may have an unusual contour in that it starts and is loudest immediately after the third heart sound and fades rapidly.

f. In the presence of a large left ventricle, the diagnosis of significant mitral stenosis must be made with hesitancy, even in the presence of a middiastolic murmur.

5. LEFT VENTRICULAR ENLARGEMENT. — Middiastolic murmurs are occasionally heard in conditions showing only marked left ventricular enlargement. The cause of the enlargement may be hypertension, coronary artery disease, or diffuse myocardial disease other than rheumatic. Differentiation is usually not difficult, since the murmur is not especially marked and the condition producing the cardiac enlargement is evident. In cardiac enlargement associated with severe anemia, a middiastolic murmur may be heard. The increased blood flow associated with the anemia is probably an additional factor in this condition.

The Diastolic Murmur of Pulmonary Regurgitation

GRAHAM STEELL MURMUR

This murmur has the same timing, pitch and quality as the murmur of aortic regurgitation. The *point of maximum inten-*

sity is in the second or third left intercostal space. *Transmission* is down the left border of the sternum, but the murmur is not transmitted far unless quite loud. Because this murmur is high pitched, the *diaphragm chest piece* is preferred. Since pulmonary hypertension is almost always present, the second heart sound is usually accentuated and masking may occur; it is, therefore, important to direct attention to the period immediately after the second sound. A pulmonary ejection sound may be present (p. 65).

Pulmonary regurgitation is occasionally due to rheumatic fever, congenital deformity, aneurysm, carcinoid syndrome or bacterial endocarditis, the latter finding being more common with the increasing incidence of right-sided endocarditis. It is most commonly associated with pulmonary hypertension and/or dilation of the pulmonary ring. Any condition producing pulmonary hypertension may be associated with this murmur-mitral stenosis, left heart failure, idiopathic or primary pulmonary hypertension, pulmonary hypertension secondary to lung changes, such as emphysema, and pulmonary hypertension associated with congenital heart diseases.

This murmur may be a valuable clue to the patient's clinical condition. In patients with pulmonary hypertension associated with lung changes, marked variations in the degree of hypertension occur and depend on the status of the lungs. In such patients, an early diastolic murmur may come and go, depending on the degree of pulmonary hypertension.

Following surgery for pulmonary valvular stenosis, marked pulmonary regurgitation may be present. The murmur in these patients is often short, rough and diamond shaped. A short interval may be present between the second sound and the onset of the murmur.

Differentiation of the murmur of pulmonic regurgitation from that of aortic regurgitation presents difficulties when the peripheral vascular signs of aortic regurgitation are not clearcut. The following factors may help:

1. If other evidence of rheumatic heart disease is present, it is best to assume that the murmur is that of mild aortic regurgitation, unless the evidence in favor of pulmonary hypertension is strong.

2. The presence of a systolic murmur of aortic stenosis

should usually be considered as evidence that the murmur is due to aortic regurgitation.

3. If a loud pulmonic second sound is present and there is no evidence of rheumatic heart disease, the murmur may be considered due to pulmonary regurgitation.

4. A loud murmur with no peripheral evidence of aortic regurgitation may favor the diagnosis of pulmonary regurgitation.

5. Wide transmission favors aortic regurgitation. The murmur of pulmonary regurgitation is not heard in the second right intercostal space.

6. In some patients with pulmonary regurgitation, the murmur is louder on inspiration than on expiration. This respiratory effect is usually not evident and, when present, it is not as evident as it is in the case of tricuspid murmurs. The murmur of aortic regurgitation is usually louder on expiration.

7. If the regurgitation is of significant degree, fluoroscopy may help by indicating whether it is the aorta or pulmonary artery that shows evidence of increased pulsation. A large pulsating pulmonary artery favors pulmonary regurgitation.

8. The effect of drugs may occasionally be of value (p.256).

Other Causes of Diastolic Murmurs

While some investigators have described innocent diastolic murmurs, such a finding is rare and should lead one to careful investigation for cardiac pathology. Diastolic murmurs have occasionally been heard in association with coronary artery stenosis, usually affecting the left anterior descending coronary artery and usually indicating a relatively mild degree of narrowing of this vessel. Diastolic murmurs have been described in association with the straight back syndrome where they are believed to represent a very mild degree of pulmonary regurgitation.

CHAPTER 9

Pericardial Friction Rub; Venous Hum; Extracardiac Auscultation

Pericardial Friction Rub

THE PERICARDIAL FRICTION RUB is produced by the parietal and visceral surfaces of the roughened pericardium rubbing on each other. Three sounds may occur: (1) a presystolic component due to atrial contraction; (2) a systolic component due to ventricular contraction; and (3) a diastolic component associated with rapid filling of the ventricle (Fig 9–1). The sound often resembles that produced by squeaky saddle leather and may be described as scratching, grating or rasping; at times, it may be musical. The rub seems closer to the ear than the heart sounds. It may be so loud that it masks all other cardiac sounds. Occasionally, a rub may so closely resemble a murmur that it is difficult to be sure whether a pericardial rub or a murmur is present. Continued observation over several days is usually decisive.

The rub is most commonly heard between the apex and the sternum but may be very widespread. It is usually fairly well localized and persists only for a day or two in cases of myocardial infarction. It is much more widespread and may last longer in idiopathic pericarditis and often in rheumatic pericarditis. It is commonly heard postoperatively in patients who have had heart surgery. In these patients, it is usually loudest in the third or fourth left intercostal space.

A characteristic feature of the pericardial rub is its variability. The intensity or even the presence of the rub may vary

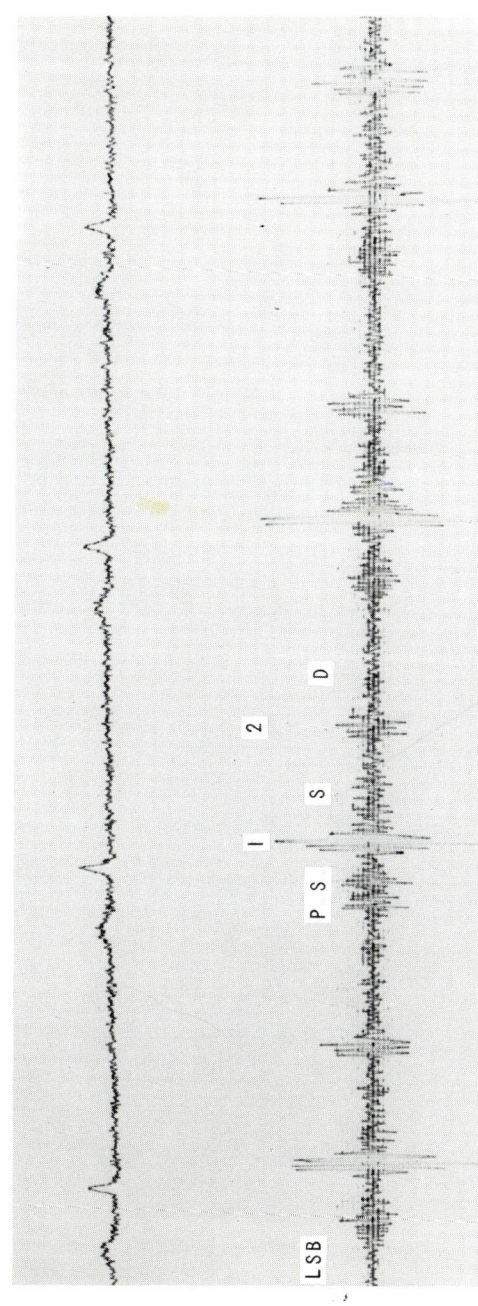

Fig 9–1. – A pericardial friction rub heard in a 58-year-old man three days after an extensive anterior wall myocardial infarction (see text). *PS*, presystolic component; *S*, systolic; *D*, diastolic; *LSB*, left sternal border.

from moment to moment. It is markedly influenced by position and may be more evident with the patient in the upright position. When looking for a pericardial rub, one should check the patient in many different positions, including the standing-flexion position. In most patients, the rub varies in intensity with respiration and is usually *louder on inspiration.* If the patient takes a moderately deep breath and holds it, the rub increases in loudness; this is especially true of those rubs best heard along the left border of the sternum. It seems probable that the increased loudness is due to increased filling of the right atrium and ventricle with inspiration, since, if the patient continues to hold his breath, the rub gradually decreases in loudness. In some patients, pressure over the liver or right upper quadrant of the abdomen will accentuate a rub. Often, pressure with the stethoscope on the chest wall will increase the rub or make the rub more evident by decreasing the intensity of the heart sounds.

Free air in the mediastinum can produce a systolic "crunch" (Hamman's sign) along the left sternal margin that may be confused with a pericardial rub. It differs from a rub in having a high-pitched, crackling quality that is usually confined to systole. Conditions producing this entity include thoracotomy, esophageal rupture and pneumomediastinum associated with parturition.

Venous Hum

The venous hum is a continuous, low-pitched hum heard in the neck and upper part of the chest in many children and in some adults (Fig 9–2). The point of maximum intensity is usually just above the clavicle, in the angle between the insertion of the sternocleidomastoid muscle and the clavicle. However, it is often heard at the base of the heart and, rarely, may be heard far down the sternum. The hum is heard on both the right and the left side but is more common on the right. It is heard better with the patient sitting up than with the patient lying down and is accentuated on the right by having the patient turn the head to the left and lift the chin. It is louder in diastole. Normal respiration may not affect the intensity or may increase it during inspiration. A Valsalva maneuver usually stops the hum.

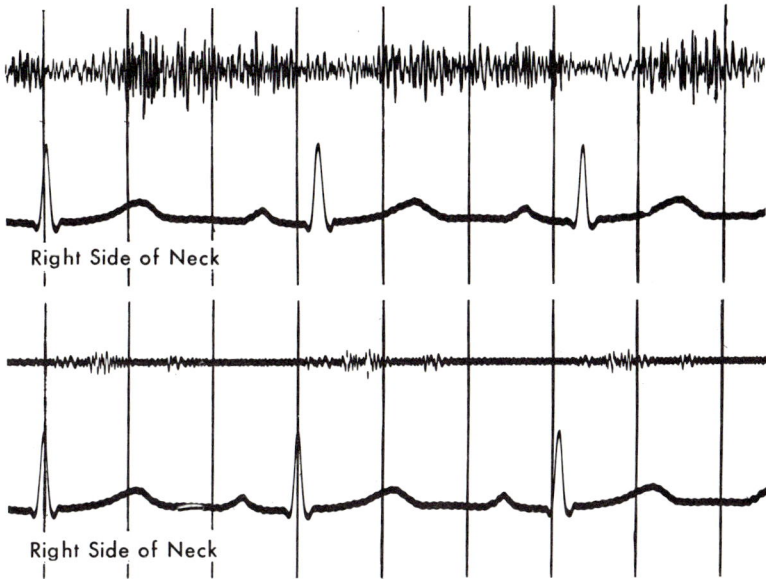

Right Side of Neck

Right Side of Neck

Fig 9–2.—Venous hum. This record was taken on the same patient whose innocent systolic murmur was shown in Figure 7–14. In an attempt to get a tracing from the right side of the neck, the patient was instructed to turn her head to the left. She did this and raised her chin; immediately the loud hum was heard *(upper tracing)*. Note that the hum is loudest during diastole. Also note the similarity to the tracing of a murmur of patent ductus arteriosus (see Fig 11–1). The lower tracing was obtained by placing the finger over the jugular vein above the microphone. Nothing else was changed. The hum disappeared, leaving only a systolic murmur. The innocent systolic murmur was somewhat less intense than it was in the left side of the neck (see Fig 7–14).

The hum is produced by turbulence in the blood flow in the internal jugular vein, possibly where it enters the innominate vein. It can, therefore, be stopped by placing a finger on the internal jugular vein in the neck between the trachea and the sternocleidomastoid muscle at about the level of the thyroid cartilage.

The incidence of the hum is increased in conditions associated with increased blood flow, e.g., thyrotoxicosis and anemia.

When the hum is well heard at the base of the heart, it must be differentiated from the murmur of patent ductus arteriosus. The main point in differentiation is to remember the possibility of a venous hum, since it is easily recognized, if considered and can be stopped by neck pressure.

Extracardiac Auscultation

PRODUCTION OF ARTERIAL MURMURS

Murmurs may be heard over arteries and veins outside the thorax and may yield very helpful information. Murmurs are heard over the arteries in the following conditions:

1. *Murmurs produced in the heart* may be transmitted outside the thorax. Such murmurs are most commonly heard in the neck but may occur in the upper abdomen and back. Murmurs produced by aortic valve lesions and basal systolic murmurs associated with arteriosclerosis and hypertension (p. 114) are commonly carried into the arteries of the neck. Some murmurs of aortic stenosis are exceptionally well transmitted and are audible in such distant sites as the skull and the elbow.

2. *Pressure with the stethoscope or a finger* on an artery may produce a murmur due to narrowing of the artery. It is important not to mistake a murmur produced by pressure of the stethoscope for a murmur due to pathology. Light pressure with a finger on a normal artery will produce a short systolic murmur; somewhat heavier pressure will produce a sound rather than a murmur in many cases. This sound disappears if the pressure is increased. If the flow through an artery is excessive, light pressure may produce a much more prolonged murmur, which may actually extend into diastole.

3. *Atheromatous changes* in a peripheral artery may produce a murmur. This may result from the projection of a plaque into the artery, without significant stenosis, or from the presence of stenosis of the artery.

4. *Increased blood flow* due to hyperkinetic states, such as exercise, anemia, thyrotoxicosis, and pregnancy, can produce murmurs in normal arteries or accentuate faint murmurs due to arterial pathology. The increased blood flow in aortic regurgitation during early systole can also produce a murmur. When there is an increased blood flow and tortuosity of a vessel, murmurs are especially likely to occur. Whether tortuosity alone can result in a murmur is not clear. Kinking of an artery can produce a murmur.

5. *Arteriovenous fistulae* are associated with murmurs that are usually continuous but may, at times, be only systolic.

The continuous murmur has a systolic accentuation, and a palpable thrill occurs at the site of the lesion.

6. The *pressure gradient* across an obstruction determines the velocity of blood flow past the obstruction. The higher the pressure gradient, the greater is the velocity of blood flow, and the more likely a murmur is to be produced. The gradient depends on the following factors:

a. The degree of stenosis. The greater the stenosis, the greater will be the gradient. As the gradient increases, the murmur becomes longer, louder, higher pitched and reaches a peak intensity later. If, however, the stenosis becomes very severe, the flow may be so low that the murmur becomes faint or may actually disappear. The murmur disappears with complete occlusion of the artery. When a carotid artery is so severely stenosed that only a fine trickle of blood gets through, the absence of a murmur may mislead one into overlooking an operable lesion.

b. The blood pressure proximal to the obstruction. During systole, the pressure is high and the gradient is large; during diastole, the gradient is usually small unless the stenosis is marked. Thus, most arterial murmurs occur only during systole. If the systemic blood pressure falls, a continuous murmur may become systolic only, or a systolic murmur becomes fainter and disappears.

c. The diastolic pressure distal to the stenosis. If this is close to normal, there is little gradient during diastole and no murmur; if it is low, there is a diastolic gradient and a murmur. The diastolic pressure distal to the stenosis depends on the *collateral circulation* and the *runoff* into the tissues. In the presence of a marked stenosis, there is a balance between the collateral circulation and the runoff. If the runoff is normal and the collateral circulation is adequate, the diastolic pressure is maintained, the gradient during diastole is small, and no diastolic murmur is heard. A comparatively poor collateral circulation may maintain the diastolic pressure if the runoff is poor due to involvement of vessels peripheral to the stenosis. If the runoff is normal or increased (e.g., by exercise) and the collateral circulation is inadequate, the diastolic pressure is low, and a diastolic murmur will be present. A *continuous murmur heard over a peripheral artery indicates, therefore, that there is marked stenosis, an inadequate collateral cir-*

culation, and a good runoff. If the runoff is prevented by increasing venous pressure with tourniquets, a continuous murmur becomes shorter and less intense; it may become systolic only.

TRANSMISSION OF ARTERIAL MURMURS

In a stenotic peripheral artery, the murmur is most evident at the point of stenosis and is very well transmitted peripherally. On the other hand, it is only transmitted centrally for 1 or 2 cm. A murmur produced by a stenosis of a carotid artery may be transmitted into the cranium, where occasionally it can be heard over the eye on the involved side. Some bruits are occasionally perceived by the patient himself as a "rushing"sound in the head. If the internal carotid artery is stenosed within the cranium, no murmur is usually heard in the neck, but a murmur may be heard over the eye on the involved side. A loud aortic systolic murmur may be transmitted along the carotid arteries into the cranium and may be heard over both eyeballs. If such a murmur is heard over one eye and not the other, it may indicate an occlusion of the carotid artery on the side on which the murmur is absent.

MURMURS OCCURRING IN THE HEAD AND NECK

In children and young adults, murmurs are frequently heard over the carotid arteries. Short, faint, rather low-pitched, systolic murmurs may be present in the supraclavicular region and sometimes extend higher in the neck. The mechanism of their production is not clear. As has been noted on page 121, one of the characteristics of the innocent systolic murmur in children is that it is commonly heard in the neck. Aortic valve lesions and arteriosclerotic involvement of the ring area and ascending aorta will produce systolic murmurs which may be transmitted into the carotid and subclavian arteries. In the absence of cardiac murmurs, however, it is not common to hear a murmur over the carotid arteries in normal adults. In listening for a murmur in the neck, the patient should be told to stop breathing because the respiratory sounds may be mistaken for a murmur or they may mask a murmur.

Arteriosclerotic involvement of the carotid arteries will often result in murmurs which, by their location, transmission, and response to carotid compression, give valuable information. The common carotid artery and the internal carotid artery, at the point of bifurcation of the common carotid artery, are frequently involved. The murmur is most likely to be significant if its point of origin along the artery can be localized by carefully tracing changes in intensity as the stethoscope is moved along the artery. Poor transmission centrally and good transmission peripherally are important. Significant murmurs are also more likely to be harsh or of high pitch. Since the internal carotid arteries are connected through the circle of Willis, collateral circulation is good and, with unilateral involvement, the murmur is usually only systolic. If a systolic murmur produced by a stenosis is heard over the common carotid artery or its bifurcation, compression of this artery below the stenosis will stop the murmur. However, if one compresses the carotid artery on the other side, the murmur may become louder and even continuous. This occurs because the collateral circulation is removed and the diastolic pressure distal to the stenosis is decreased (p. 153).

If an internal carotid artery is completely occluded by disease, the murmur should disappear and usually does, but in a number of cases, a murmur may persist due to stenosis of the external carotid artery at its origin. Occasionally, with complete occlusion of one carotid artery, the opposite carotid artery may develop a murmur. This can occur in the absence of any stenosis of the patent carotid artery, and is apparently due to an increased blood flow resulting from the greater peripheral bed which the artery now has to supply. This murmur due to increased blood flow has been called an *augmentation murmur* or *bruit* (Fisher) and may be heard at times over the eye on the same side. A similar murmur over the carotid artery can be heard in some patients having an increased blood flow for other reasons, such as a large intracranial angioma or a carotid-cavernous sinus fistula. The presence of even a mild stenosis will accentuate such a flow murmur, and light pressure on the artery with a finger or stethoscope may produce a continuous murmur.

Cranial murmurs are common in infants and may occur in children. They are rare in normal adults. Murmurs produced in the cranial cavity are usually transmitted to the orbit and can be heard over the eye. They may be transmitted to the cranium. Transmission to the eye is determined by putting the bell of the stethoscope on one closed eye, while the other eye remains open and gazes at a fixed object. The breath should be held.

Carotid-cavernous sinus fistulae produce a continuous murmur with systolic accentuation which is heard over the orbit and the cranial bones. Intracranial angiomas also may produce continuous murmurs which can be heard over one or both orbits and the cranium. Orbital murmurs may occasionally be heard in Paget's disease, ruptured saccular aneurysm, meningioma, and anemia, and, at times, with no obvious cause.

In patients with thyrotoxicosis, a continuous murmur may occasionally be heard over the thyroid gland because of the marked increase in the vascularity of the gland.

In the aortic arch syndrome, the ostium of one or more of the vessels coming off the arch may be narrowed or occluded by atherosclerotic involvement or by an arteritis (Takayasu's disease). Systolic or continuous murmurs over the subclavian, innominate or carotid arteries may be heard. The radial pulse may be absent in one or both arms, hence the designation of *pulseless disease*. Occasionally, a subclavian murmur may occur with a thoracic outlet syndrome.

MURMURS OCCURRING IN THE DESCENDING AORTA AND ITS BRANCHES

Murmurs can occur over any part of the descending aorta as a result of a constriction or a sudden dilation (aneurysm). The renal, mesenteric, iliac, or femoral arteries may have murmur-producing obstructions. Spinal cord angiomas can produce murmurs heard over the spinal column. Rarely, solid tumors such as hepatoma are associated with a systolic bruit.

Murmurs may be produced in the renal arteries in some patients with hypertension. These are most commonly heard by listening 1 or 2 inches above the umbilicus to the right or left of the midline. The murmur is usually best heard on expiration. If the murmur is also heard in the flank and is loud and continuous, it is almost definitely due to renal stenosis. If the murmur is only systolic but is loud and high pitched, it is often due to renal stenosis even if it is heard only anteriorly.

The *mammary souffle of pregnancy and lactation* is heard in some women in the latter months of pregnancy or during the postpartum period, if lactation occurs. It is usually maximum in the second or third intercostal space and shows very little radiation. It may be heard on the right or left side, or both sides. It may be systolic or systolic with some diastolic element, and is usually of fairly high pitch. The intensity varies from time to time and the murmur is most obvious when the patient is lying flat; it often disappears if the patient sits up. Pressure with the stethoscope or with a finger will obliterate the murmur, and this maneuver avoids confusing the mammary souffle with the murmur of patent ductus arteriosus. Its characteristics suggest that it is of arterial origin, and it may be related to an increased blood flow in the internal mammary and intercostal arteries. The *uterine souffle* is a continuous murmur heard over the lower abdomen of pregnant patients during the last trimester. It is produced in the uterine arteries and is of no clinical significance.

In aortic regurgitation and conditions characterized by large pulse pressure and increased blood flow, the murmur produced by compression of a large artery is louder than that produced under normal conditions, and often both a systolic and a diastolic murmur can be heard. This double murmur has been called the *sign of Duroziez*. It is heard in aortic regurgitation and thyrotoxicosis, and occasionally in hypertension and in fevers. A "pistol shot" sound over the femoral and larger arteries may be present in aortic regurgitation. The sound is loud and short and is produced by the sudden and marked expansion of the almost collapsed artery.

VENOUS HUMS

The venous hum that is heard in the neck and may be heard in the precordium has already been described (p. 150). In some patients with cirrhosis of the liver and portal hypertension, a continuous high-pitched hum may be heard near the xiphoid and in the epigastric region. This venous hum results from the formation of anastomoses between the portal and systemic circulations, especially those involving the paraumbilical veins. A venous hum may rarely be heard over an enlarged spleen.

CHAPTER 10

Cardiac Arrhythmias

THE DEFINITIVE DIAGNOSIS of a rhythm disturbance of the heart requires an electrocardiogram. However, careful examination of the patient will frequently yield clues to the nature of the cardiac arrhythmia (dysrhythmia) and occasionally obviate the need for electrocardiography where the irregularity is clearly benign. In the following discussion, therefore, only the most commonly encountered disturbances of the cardiac rhythm will be considered. It is assumed that the reader is familiar with the mechanisms and electrocardiographic characteristics of the arrhythmias, so none of the latter information is included.

The cardiac arrhythmias can be characterized according to heart rate and regularity. While there is no such thing as a "normal heart rate," a rate of less than 50 beats per minute is generally defined as bradycardia and one above 100 beats per minute as tachycardia. The rhythm may be regular or irregular. Irregular rhythms may be totally irregular, transiently irregular, or rhythmically irregular (in which case the irregularity is recurrent and predictable).

The examination (Table 10–1) should include the arterial and venous pulse, auscultation of the heart with regard to rate and heart sounds, response to exercise, "vagal maneuvers" (e.g., carotid massage, Valsalva maneuver), response to drugs, and the general clinical setting in which the arrhythmia has occurred. Vagal maneuvers and the use of pharmacologic agents should be done with electrocardiographic monitoring whenever possible.

TABLE 10-1.—PHYSICAL SIGNS OF CARDIAC ARRHYTHMIAS

RHYTHM	VENTRICULAR RATE	REGULARITY	JVP°	HEART SOUNDS S_1 INTENSITY	SPLITTING†	RESPONSE TO CSM‡
Sinus tachycardia	100–180	Regular	Normal	Constant	Normal	Gradual slowing with return to previous rate
Paroxysmal atrial tachycardia (PAT)	140–200	Regular	Normal or regular A-cannon waves	Constant	Normal	No effect or abrupt termination
Paroxysmal junctional tachy-cardia (PJT)	140–200	Regular	Regular cannon A-waves	Constant (variable with AV dissociation)	Normal	No effect or abrupt termination
Atrial flutter (usually with 2:1 block)	120–180	Regular or ir-regular	Flutter waves	Constant	Normal	Abrupt slowing with prompt return to previous rate
Atrial fibril-lation (untreated)	100–200	Totally irregular	No A-waves	Variable	Normal	Gradual slowing with return to previous rate
Multifocal atrial tachycardia (MAT)	100–200	Totally irregular	A-waves detect-able	Variable	Normal	No effect or gradual slowing with return
Ventricular tachycardia	120–200	Regular or slightly irregular	Irregular cannon A-waves	Variable	Abnormal	None
Complete heart block	<50	Regular	Irregular cannon A-waves	Variable (atrial sounds frequently audible)	Normal (with nar-row QRS) or abnor-mal	

°JVP = jugular venous pulse.
†Aberrant conduction will result in abnormal splitting with any arrhythmia.
‡CSM = carotid sinus massage.

159

1. SPLITTING OF THE HEART SOUNDS. — Normally, no splitting or fine splitting of the first heart sound is present (p. 29). The second heart sound is usually not split on expiration and only mildly to moderately split on inspiration. An abnormal degree of asynchrony in contraction of the ventricles will result in abnormal splitting of the first sound, second sound, or both sounds. Such asynchrony will occur with several conditions: *(a) Right bundle branch block.* The first heart sound can usually, but not always, be recognized as abnormally split along the left border of the sternum and in the apicosternal area. Instead of the normal, fine splitting, the two components are clearly separated. The second heart sound is abnormally split on expiration and the split increases with inspiration (p. 47). *(b) Left bundle branch block.* Splitting of the first heart sound is not ordinarily evident (p. 38); the second heart sound shows paradoxical splitting (p. 47). *(c) Ventricular premature contractions and ventricular tachycardias.* If the abnormal beat originates in the left ventricle, the first and second heart sounds are almost always abnormally split (Fig 10 – 1). Since the majority of ventricular tachycardias and ventricular premature contractions originate in the left ventricle, the first and second sounds are usually split. The degree of splitting will correlate to some extent with the width of the QRS complex.

2. VARYING INTENSITY OF THE FIRST HEART SOUND. — The first heart sound varies in intensity in the presence of atrioventricular dissociation. The varying intensity of the first heart sound in complete heart block was described and discussed in detail on page 34 (see Fig 4 – 4). In ventricular tachycardia, there is also usually a dissociation of the atrial and ventricular contractions, and a variation in the intensity of the first sound occurs.

3. JUGULAR VENOUS PULSATIONS. — With training, it is possible to recognize the A-wave in the jugular pulse when the heart rate is not too rapid. This is done best by observing the jugular vein while listening at the apex and feeling the opposite carotid artery. For a study of jugular pulsations, the lighting must be good and a back rest which can be tilted to the desired angle should be available. With rapid heart rates and less than ideal conditions, recognition of the A-wave is quite difficult and of limited value. However, when there is a disso-

ciation between atrial and ventricular contractions, some of the atrial contractions occur when the tricuspid valve is closed during ventricular systole. This produces a markedly accentuated A-wave, which has been called a giant or cannon A-wave. An irregularly occurring cannon A-wave, like the varying intensity of the first heart sound, indicates atrioventricular dissociation.

4. CAROTID SINUS MASSAGE OR VALSALVA MANEUVER. — These procedures are used to increase vagal influence and to slow the heart. They are of value in separating some of the rapid rhythms. The breath is held after a deep inspiration and the patient is told to "bear down."

5. EXERCISE. — This is used to decrease vagal influence and to increase the heart rate. Its main value is in atrial flutter and in heart block.

6. THE CLINICAL SETTING. — The age of the patient, evidence of other cardiac involvement, and other pertinent clinical information should be used in making the diagnosis. These factors are not discussed in this section.

Regular Rhythms with Rapid Heart Rate

DIFFERENTIATION OF VENTRICULAR AND SUPRAVENTRICULAR RHYTHMS. — This may be accomplished by the determination of the presence or absence of (a) abnormal splitting of the heart sounds and (b) atrioventricular dissociation, as indicated by the presence of varying intensity of the first sound and irregularly occurring cannon A-waves. *If the sounds are normally split, the tachycardia is probably of supraventricular origin.* With some exceptions, ventricular tachycardias have abnormally split sounds, and the splitting may be more marked than in any other condition. In the apicosternal area, the impression obtained, because of the rapid rate, is one of multiple sounds, and it may be difficult to decide which sound represents which event. Summation sounds may occur and play a part in the auditory impression of multiple low-pitched sounds. Splitting of the second sound is heard best in the second left intercostal space. In both supraventricular and ventricular tachycardias, blood pressure may be low and the intensity of the second heart sound diminished, so that splitting of the second heart sound may not be clearly evident.

Unfortunately, in the presence of atrioventricular dissociation (variation in the intensity of the first heart sound and irregularly occurring cannon A-waves) the ventricles may be controlled by a focus in the atrioventricular junction (producing a wide or narrow QRS) or the ventricle itself (producing a wide QRS), with the former being more common than the latter. These two situations, which have somewhat different clinical implications, can be distinguished only by electrocardiogram.

A supraventricular tachycardia with bundle branch block or aberrant conduction may also manifest abnormal splitting of the heart sounds and can be distinguished from ventricular tachycardia only by absence of signs of atrioventricular dissociation (Fig 10–1). This criteria fails in the presence of ventricular tachycardia with atrial fibrillation, or ventricular tachycardia with retrograde conduction to the atria—two not very common conditions. Ventricular tachycardia may show slight irregularity but the irregularity is not easily detected by auscultation. Generally speaking, clinical deterioration occurs more rapidly with ventricular than with supraventricular tachycardia at equivalent rates.

Because differentiation of ventricular from supraventricular tachycardias is so important, it is worthwhile summarizing the above (see Fig 10–1).

1. If the heart sounds are single or normally split, the tachycardia is, in all probability, supraventricular.

Fig 10–1.—Heart sounds (in apicosternal area), electrocardiogram, and jugular venous pulsation in patients with supraventricular tachycardia, ventricular tachycardia, and supraventricular tachycardia with right bundle branch block. With supraventricular tachycardia, the heart sounds are not split and there is no variation in the intensity of the first heart sound; the QRS interval of the electrocardiogram is of normal width; the jugular venous pulse shows no cannon A-waves. With ventricular tachycardia, the heart sounds are split and there is a variation in the intensity of the first sound which depends on the relation of the atrial contraction (P-wave) to the ventricular contraction; the electrocardiogram shows wide QRS complexes and independent atrial activity as indicated by the P-waves; the jugular venous pulse shows a cannon A-wave when atrial contraction occurs simultaneously with ventricular contraction. With supraventricular tachycardia with right bundle branch block, the heart sounds are split but the first heart sound does not show any variation in intensity; the electrocardiogram shows broad QRS complexes and, as is often true, no P-waves are discernible; the jugular venous pulse does not show any cannon A-waves.

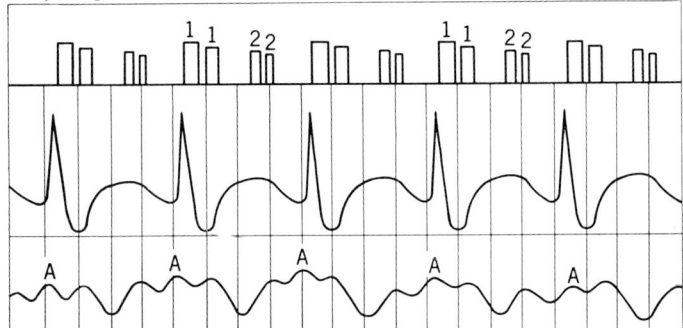

SUPRAVENTRICULAR TACHYCARDIA

Synchronous Ventricular
Contraction
No Splitting of Heart Sounds

No A-V Dissociation
No Variation in First Heart Sound
No Cannon A-Waves

VENTRICULAR TACHYCARDIA

Asynchronous Ventricular
Contraction
Splitting of Heart Sounds

A-V Dissociation
Variation in First Heart Sound
Cannon A-Waves

SUPRAVENTRICULAR TACHYCARDIA WITH RIGHT BBB

Asynchronous Ventricular
Contraction
Splitting of Heart Sounds

No A-V Dissociation
No Variation in First Heart Sound
No Cannon A-Waves

Fig 10–1.—Legend on facing page.

163

2. If abnormal splitting of the heart sounds is present and there is atrioventricular dissociation (variation in the intensity of the first heart sound and irregularly occurring cannon A-waves), the tachycardia is most often of ventricular origin.

3. If abnormal splitting of the heart sounds is present and there is no atrioventricular dissociation, supraventricular tachycardia with bundle branch block or with aberrant conduction is probably present, but there are exceptions.

DIFFERENTIATION OF THE SUPRAVENTRICULAR TACHYCARDIAS. — *Carotid sinus massage or Valsalva maneuver* may help in the separation of these rhythms. If carotid sinus massage is effective in *sinus tachycardia,* it slows the heart gradually, and the heart then returns gradually and smoothly to its original rate. Unfortunately, when this procedure would be of most value, the sinus tachycardia may be quite unaffected by carotid sinus massage. Sinus tachycardia is not likely to be present with persistent rates of over 160 in the resting adult. In *atrial flutter,* carotid sinus massage and Valsalva maneuver are possibly of most value because they are quite likely to produce a sudden break in the rate as the rhythm drops from a 2:1 block to a 3:1 or 4:1 block. This sudden change and "jerky" return to the original rate can be most helpful in making the diagnosis. A fixed rate of about 130–140 which does not vary with moderate exercise is most likely to be an atrial flutter with a 2:1 block. Tachycardias with rates of 180–200 in adults are, in the absence of medication, unlikely to be due to atrial flutter. *Atrial tachycardias* are not slowed by carotid sinus massage but may be stopped; unfortunately, this does not occur often enough to be a clear-cut diagnostic maneuver. *Atrial tachycardias with block* behave like an atrial flutter in response to carotid sinus massage. When there is a 1:1 response, this arrhythmia belongs in the group of tachycardias. When there is a 2:1 block, it falls in the group with normal rates. In many patients, the block varies and the rhythm is irregular. *Nodal tachycardias,* like atrial tachycardias, are not slowed by carotid sinus massage, but may occasionally be stopped. Nodal tachycardias may have regular cannon A-waves due to the occurrence of atrial contraction at the same time as ventricular contraction. Ventricular tachycardias are not supposed to be affected by carotid sinus massage, but even a ventricular tachycardia may, on rare occasion, be stopped.

Regular Rhythms with Normal Heart Rate

Atrial flutter with 3:1 or 4:1 block, and sinus or atrial tachycardia with 2:1 block, are the most common conditions, other than sinus rhythm, that fall into this group. *Exercise* is the most valuable method for differentiating them. With *atrial flutter,* the heart rate will suddenly increase with a marked jump and may then continue regular or become irregular at a higher rate. In *sinus tachycardia with block,* exercise will usually only mildly and gradually increase the rate, although sometimes the block may disappear and there will be a sudden doubling of the rate. The converse occasionally occurs, where with an increase in sinus rate, 2:1 atrioventricular block appears with an abrupt fall in ventricular rate. Such a paradoxical response may occur following administration of intravenous atropine to patients with a slow sinus rhythm and atrioventricular junctional disease. An atrial sound may be heard at times with the blocked atrial contraction; and if the P-R interval of the conducted beat is prolonged, the first sound is dull and an atrial sound may be heard before the first sound. *Atrial tachycardia with 2:1 block* behaves like atrial flutter on exercise, and the rate may double to a rapid rate, usually in the 150–190 range. Cannon A-waves may occur with 2:1 block if the blocked atrial contraction occurs during ventricular systole. In atrial flutter or atrial tachycardia with block, examination of the jugular venous pulse will commonly reveal flutter waves or A-waves at a rate considerably faster than the arterial pulse.

In association with acute ischemic heart disease and rarely in the presence of digitalis intoxication, an accelerated idioventricular rhythm ("slow ventricular tachycardia") may develop. This common rhythm disturbance is manifested by the appearance of a ventricular focus, which appears with slight slowing of the atrial focus. The rate is in a normal range, 50–100 beats per minute, but occasionally may accelerate to a more rapid rate. With the appearance of this rhythm disturbance there are accompanying signs of atrioventricular dissociation. Cannon A-waves appear and the first heart sound becomes progressively louder as the P-R interval shortens and then abruptly becomes softer as the P-wave moves into the QRS complex. The first heart sound becomes split during the dominance of the ventricular focus.

Regular Rhythms with Slow Heart Rate

A slow, regular rate under 40 may be due to *sinus bradycardia, complete heart block, or partial heart block with a 2:1 or 3:1 conduction.* The variation in the first heart sound, the presence of cannon A-waves, and the effect of exercise are helpful in differentiation. In complete heart block, the first heart sound will show the characteristic variation previously described (p. 34) and cannon A-waves are present. Atrial sounds can also often be heard during diastole. Sinus bradycardia and second-degree heart block do not show this variation in the first heart sound or the presence of cannon A-waves. Exercise will increase the heart rate in sinus bradycardia but will ordinarily not change the rate in complete heart block, although at times there may be a slight increase, especially in congenital complete heart block. The rate in partial heart block with 2:1 conduction will increase, but to a lesser extent than in sinus bradycardia, unless there is a sudden jump in heart rate due to loss of the block. In partial heart block, the first heart sound may be faint, and atrial sounds may be heard.

A common error is to record a regular slow pulse on palpation at the wrist, without confirmation by auscultation. Bigeminal rhythms are frequently associated with a 50% pulse deficit, which can be verified only by listening for the alternating premature contractions.

Rhythmically or Transiently Irregular Rhythms with Normal Heart Rate

SINUS ARRHYTHMIA. — The rhythmic variation in the heart rate associated with respiration is usually easily recognized. The rate increases during inspiration, and the arrhythmia is usually exaggerated by slow, deep respirations. It disappears or decreases as the heart rate increases with exercise, fever or drugs. It is rare in adults with heart rates over 100 and is more commonly seen in children and young adults. The rhythmic variation in vagal tone resulting from respiration affects the rate of impulse formation by the sino-atrial node.

VENTRICULAR PREMATURE CONTRACTIONS AND ATRIAL PREMATURE CONTRACTIONS. — These represent the most important arrhythmias in this category. They are usually super-imposed on a sinus rhythm, but ventricular premature contractions can occur in atrial fibrillation or in any of the supraventricular arrhythmias. Ventricular premature contractions are more common than atrial premature contractions, and both occur more commonly in older age groups. Both, and especially the ventricular premature contractions, tend to diminish in frequency if the heart speeds up with exercise, fever, etc. In patients with coronary artery disease, however, exertion may produce myocardial ischemia and ventricular premature contractions. To differentiate ventricular premature contractions from atrial premature contractions, electrocardiography is essential but the following observations are of value.

1. The pause following an atrial premature contraction is usually shorter than that following a ventricular premature contraction because of the full compensatory pause associated with the latter. In ventricular premature contractions, the normal beat that would follow the premature contraction usually drops out, giving an abnormally long or compensatory pause. Compensatory pauses associated with atrial premature contractions are thought to be due to sino-atrial node suppression associated with premature atrial discharge, and they are occasionally quite long, especially in the presence of sinus node disease.

2. The heart sounds are usually abnormally split in ventricular premature contractions and not split in atrial premature contractions. Because prematurities are commonly random and infrequent, this distinction may be very difficult to make. Furthermore, atrial prematurities are frequently aberrant, resulting in abnormal splitting of the first sound.

3. The intensity of the first sound is generally more accentuated with atrial premature contractions than with ventricular premature contractions. The second sound is diminished in both situations and may be entirely absent if the prematurity fails to open the semilunar valve.

4. Since an atrial contraction is commonly superimposed on the premature ventricular contraction, ventricular premature contractions are usually associated with cannon A-waves. Atrial premature contractions may be associated with cannon A-waves when the P-wave occurs during the preceding mechanical systole, in which case the cannon A-wave occurs

immediately prior to the first sound of the premature beat.

WENCKEBACH TYPE OF SECOND-DEGREE BLOCK.—With Wenckebach-type second-degree heart block the sounds may seem regular except for the dropped beat, although occasionally a slight acceleration of the rate prior to the pause may be detected, and a rhythmically varying intensity of the first sound may occur. This finding of repetitive "group beating" is highly suggestive of the Wenckebach phenomenon.

Transiently Irregular Rhythms with Rapid Heart Rate

These are composed mainly of atrial and junctional tachycardias and atrial flutter with ventricular premature contractions.

Transiently Irregular Rhythms with Slow Heart Rate

Sinus bradycardia with atrial or ventricular premature contractions and partial or complete heart block with occasionally conducted (captured) beats or ventricular premature contractions fall into this catagory. Complete heart block may be recognizable by the varying intensity of the first heart sound and cannon A-waves.

Absolutely Irregular Rhythms

Any number of rhythms can give the impression of being absolutely irregular, and only the electrocardiogram can help distinguish the more unusual forms. Of main interest to us are atrial fibrillation, treated and untreated, multifocal atrial tachycardia, usually associated with chronic obstructive lung disease, and sinus arrhythmia of the aged. Atrial flutter can also fall into this group.

Atrial fibrillation is usually a rapid rhythm in untreated patients; it will be slow in the presence of digitalis or intrinsic atrioventricular block. If it is extremely rapid, the irregularity is not too obvious and it can occasionally be mistaken for a rapid regular rhythm. Carotid sinus massage or Valsalva maneuver will slow the rate and often bring out a rather striking irregularity. When the rate is slow, it may be difficult to recognize total irregularity and distinguish it from a regular rhythm with frequent ventricular premature contractions. This differentiation may often be made on the following criteria: (1) When the rate is increased by exercise, the irregularity due to ventricular premature contractions tends to disappear, whereas the irregularity due to atrial fibrillation tends to increase. (2) The occurrence of a number of beats (three to five or more) in rapid succession points to the presence of atrial fibrillation. Since ventricular premature contractions are nearly always followed by compensatory pauses, it is unusual to have more than two beats, rarely three, in rapid succession. (3) By the same reasoning, two long pauses should not follow each other if the irregularity is produced by ventricular premature contractions, because two compensatory pauses should not follow each other.

The intensity of the first sound in atrial fibrillation varies with the position in diastole of the ventricular contraction. If diastole is very short and ventricular contraction occurs during the phase of rapid ventricular filling, the intensity of the first heart sound is increased (p. 36). In mitral stenosis with atrial fibrillation, the intensity of the first heart sound often varies with the length of the previous diastole (p. 36).

The second sound is often diminished due to a lowering of the closing pressure because of the weak beats. If diastole is very short, the semilunar valves may not be opened and there will be no second sound. The jugular venous pulse, of course, fails to show A-waves.

Multifocal atrial tachycardia (chaotic atrial rhythm) differs from atrial fibrillation in that there is an atrial contraction preceding each ventricular beat. A-waves can usually be detected in the jugular venous pulse, especially after longer pauses. The rhythm, however, is totally irregular. It is seen almost exclusively in the presence of advanced chronic obstructive lung disease with hypoxia and can rarely be distinguished with certainty from atrial fibrillation without an electrocardiogram. Like atrial fibrillation, it may slow with carotid sinus massage.

Sinus arrhythmia of the aged usually occurs with a normal rate, and the rhythm may be absolutely irregular, although, not infrequently, there is a bigeminy. When the rhythm is totally irregular, differentiation from slow atrial fibrillation is extremely difficult. This rhythm should be considered in an older person presenting a totally irregular rhythm with a slow or normal rate if no digitalis has been taken.

A peculiar irregularity affecting the sinus node is seen in older people. It includes a spectrum of rhythm disturbances generally referred to as the *sick sinus syndrome.* A normal rhythm may alternate with periods of total irregularity or runs of marked bradycardia or tachycardia. This is due to sinus pauses, sinus arrest, sinus bradycardia and periodic runs of supraventricular tachycardia. Many patients show evidence of atrioventricular disease. Electrocardiographic analysis is essential.

Atrial flutter may be totally irregular due to variable Wenckebach-type conduction via the atrioventricular node. But it often still may be recognized by a rather abrupt slowing in rate which results from carotid massage, or, if slow, by the abrupt increase in rate and regularity which results from exercise. When atrial flutter shows a varying P-R interval and is irregular, there may be a varying intensity of the first heart sound.

Partial or complete heart block with frequent ventricular premature contractions and occasional conducted contractions may give a totally irregular rhythm which is difficult to recognize.

CHAPTER 11

Congenital Heart Disease

THE DISCOVERY OF A cardiac murmur is usually the event that directs attention to the presence of acyanotic congenital heart disease. In many acyanotic patients, a single defect is present which produces auscultatory findings so characteristic as to be diagnostic. In cyanotic patients, however, several defects are usually present, and the auscultatory findings show variations, depending on the combination of septal, arterial and valvular lesions.

A systolic murmur that disappears within a week or two may normally be present at birth. Persistence of a significant murmur usually indicates some congenital malformation.

Patent Ductus Arteriosus

The characteristic murmur of patent ductus arteriosus is a continuous murmur with systolic accentuation (Fig 11–1). The murmur starts with the first sound, increases in intensity to the second sound, and then decreases in intensity during diastole, reaching a minimum at the time of the next first sound. Many of the murmurs are not actually continuous, in that they start a little after the first sound and fade away somewhat before the beginning of the next first sound. A thrill can usually be felt when the murmur is loud. The intensity of the murmur is increased by exercise. Occasionally, in an adult at rest, the murmur may be so short that it appears to be entirely systolic; on exercise, a typical continuous murmur develops. The intensity of the murmur shows only a rough correlation with the size of the lesion.

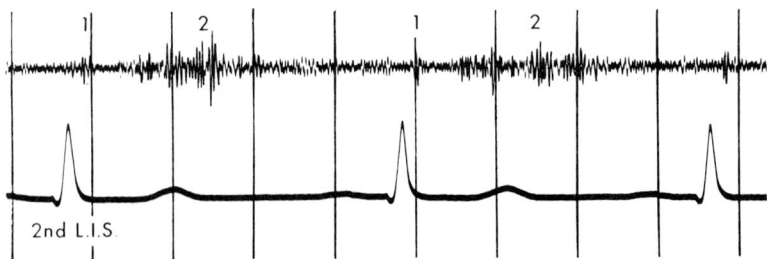

Fig 11–1. – Murmur of patent ductus arteriosus. This is a continuous murmur which reaches its peak at about the time of the second heart sound and often masks the second heart sound, even though the latter may be accentuated. It diminishes during diastole.

A characteristic continuous murmur is present in many children in the first few months of life and in the majority by the end of the first year. Often during the first year, however, the murmur may be only systolic or extend only into early diastole. Many of these later develop into typical murmurs. The shortened murmur is likely to occur when the shunt is large and when some increase in pulmonary resistance persists; as the systemic pressure increases and the pulmonic resistance decreases, the typical murmur develops. A short murmur is often heard with a large patent ductus and cardiac failure.

The *point of maximum intensity* of the murmur is almost always in the second left intercostal space next to the sternum; occasionally, it may be in the first left intercostal space. When the murmur is faint, it may be limited to this area; with increased intensity, the systolic component is much better transmitted than the diastolic component and can be heard along the left border of the sternum and occasionally at the apex (Fig 11–2). When the murmur is loud anteriorly, the systolic component may be heard in the interscapular region, especially in children. Transmission to the neck is not especially good.

The murmur has the same *quality* during systole and diastole and tends to show a marked variation in intensity from moment to moment during both systole and diastole. There may be bursts of medium-pitched vibrations which resemble heart sounds. The roughness and the varying intensity during the cycle give the murmur its characteristic "machinery-type" quality – a very descriptive term. The murmur is well heard with either the bell or the diaphragm.

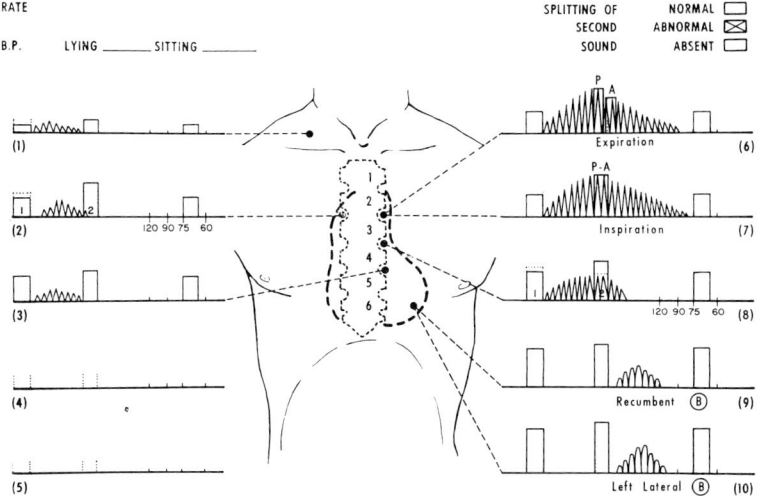

Fig 11–2.—Murmur of patent ductus arteriosus. The figures in parentheses refer to the lines on the chart. The following features are shown:

a. Murmur is usually of maximum intensity in the first or second left intercostal space *(7)*.

b. The murmur is rather harsh. It starts with the first sound, reaches a maximum at the time of the second sound, and then diminishes during diastole.

c. If the murmur is loud, the systolic component may be transmitted down along the left border of the sternum *(8)* and somewhat into the neck *(1)* and right side of the sternum *(2)*. The murmur is not especially well transmitted to the neck.

d. An apical middiastolic murmur that is low pitched and rumbling is often present at the apex *(9) (10)* if there is a large shunt. This is best heard with the bell and when the patient is in the recumbent or left lateral position.

e. With large shunts, there may be paradoxical splitting of the second sound so that only a single sound is heard on inspiration *(7)* whereas a split sound is heard on expiration *(8)*. Usually, when the shunt is large enough to produce paradoxical splitting, the murmur may be so loud as to mask the second sound.

Since the murmur is most intense at the time of the *second sound,* this sound is often somewhat masked and may not be obvious even when accentuated. If the shunt is marked, the increased output of the left ventricle over the right ventricle will increase the ejection time of the left ventricle, and paradoxical splitting of the second sound occurs. The first heart sound is usually unchanged. A third heart sound may be heard at the apex in children and may be just a normal third heart sound or an accentuated sound due to the increased flow into the left ventricle.

A low-frequency apical diastolic rumble is very common in those cases where the flow through the lungs is at least twice the systemic flow. The factors in the production of these murmurs have been discussed (p. 140). The murmur disappears with repair of the ductus.

Some patients with patent ductus arteriosus develop pulmonary hypertension. This may occur at any age. The pulmonary hypertension first decreases the flow through the ductus during diastole; the diastolic component of the murmur disappears, and only the systolic component remains (Fig 11–3). With further increase in pulmonary artery pressure, the mur-

Fig 11–3.—Patent ductus arteriosus with pulmonary hypertension. The following features are shown:

a. The continuous murmur previously present disappears and a rough systolic murmur may be heard along the left border of the sternum *(6) (8)*. Sometimes no systolic murmur at all is present.

b. Pulmonic second sound is markedly accentuated *(6) (7)* and, because the pulmonic sound is much louder than the aortic second sound, splitting is often not evident. The degree of splitting is usually decreased.

c. Usually pulmonary regurgitation develops with the production of a high-pitched, early diastolic murmur heard along the left border of the sternum *(3) (6) (7) (8)*.

d. A tricuspid regurgitation often develops. This is recognized by a high-pitched, systolic murmur of maximum intensity to the left of the lower end of the sternum. This murmur is louder on inspiration *(5)* than on expiration *(4)*.

e. Frequently, an ejection sound *(ES)* is heard in the second or third left intercostal spaces. The ejection sound is louder on expiration *(6)* than on inspiration *(7)*.

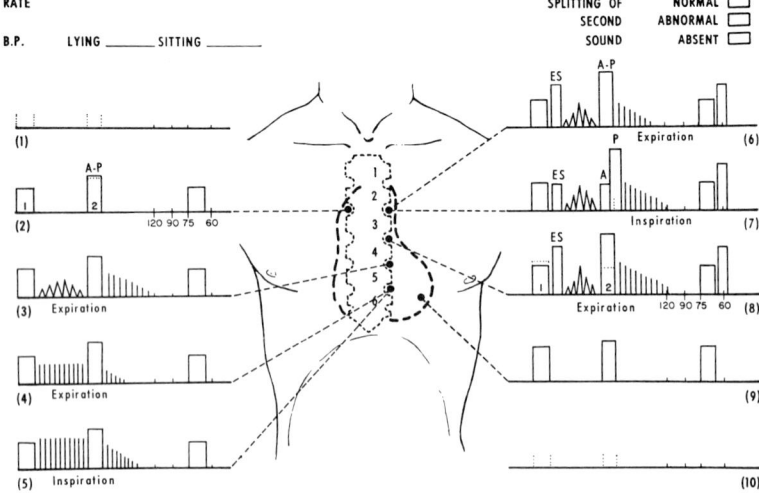

mur may disappear or become insignificant. Some of these patients will develop the early diastolic murmur of pulmonary regurgitation. The pulmonic second sound is accentuated, and a pulmonary ejection sound is often present. The murmur of tricuspid regurgitation is commonly present. A middiastolic murmur, if previously present, becomes less evident or disappears. The thrill usually leaves.

The peripheral pulse is characteristic in patent ductus arteriosus. It resembles the pulse in aortic regurgitation in having an increased volume and rapid rise and fall. Palpation of the precordium reveals a brisk left ventricular impulse. This information is especially important in the newborn since congestive heart failure due to a ductus may develop in the neonatal period without the typical continuous murmur.

Following the successful closure of a patent ductus arteriosus, the continuous murmur always disappears, and often no murmur at all remains. Occasionally, a systolic murmur in the pulmonary region may persist; even this murmur may disappear over a period of months or years.

DIFFERENTIATION. — 1. When the murmur of a patent ductus·arteriosus in an infant is entirely systolic, it is often difficult or impossible to separate it from the murmur of a *ventricular septal defect*. The heart is small, and the difference in point of maximum intensity is not great enough to be of importance. Brisk arterial pulses favor the diagnosis of patent ductus arteriosus.

2. A *venous hum* can be confusing only if one does not consider the possibility of its presence. The hum will be loudest above the clavicle, usually on the right, and can be stopped by correct pressure on the neck.

3. A small *aortopulmonary septal defect,* a defect between the aorta and pulmonary artery just above their origin, produces a murmur almost identical with that of patent ductus arteriosus in timing and quality. The majority of these defects are, however, large and in these patients pulmonary artery pressure is equal, or nearly equal, to systemic arterial pressure. The murmur is not continuous but systolic in time. The point of maximum intensity of the murmur may be in the third intercostal space and may be somewhat more medial than that of patent ductus arteriosus. The pulmonic second sound is markedly accentuated. A large aortopulmonary septal defect

can be differentiated from a large ventricular septal defect only with difficulty. Perforation of an aortic sinus into the pulmonary artery will give a similar murmur.

4. In a *tetralogy* with severe stenosis or atresia of the pulmonary artery and no patent ductus arteriosus, the blood reaches the lungs through markedly dilated and tortuous bronchial arteries. In such a condition, one may hear a continuous murmur very similar in quality to that of patent ductus arteriosus. Cyanosis is present with this condition, whereas patients with patent ductus arteriosus and cyanosis lack the continuous murmur. The murmur is much more diffusely heard than that of patent ductus arteriosus and is usually better heard in the back. The murmur is apparently produced by vibrations of the tortuous bronchial arteries. A single second sound is heard in this condition.

5. The murmur that occurs after a successful *shunt* operation for congenital heart disease is also similar to that of patent ductus arteriosus. The location will vary with the location of the shunt.

6. Other conditions producing a continuous murmur include: *(a)* Perforation of an aortic sinus into the right ventricle or right atrium. The maximum intensity of the murmur is lower than in patent ductus arteriosus and may be in the fourth left or right intercostal space. Congestive heart failure occurs rapidly in one not previously known to have heart disease. *(b)* Arteriovenous fistulae of any of the vessels in the thorax — bronchial, pleural, pulmonary, coronary or intercostal. A coronary arteriovenous fistula may drain into the cardiac cavity. This murmur is usually loudest in the apicosternal area. *(c)* Total anomalous drainage of the pulmonary veins. *(d)* A pulmonary artery branch stenosis. The murmur may be systolic only or continuous and is often widely heard through the chest, but may be loudest in the axilla and back. An atrial septal defect is often associated with this condition. *(e)* A small atrial septal defect with tight mitral stenosis produces a continuous murmur due to the build-up of pressure in the left atrium and the flow through a small atrial septal defect. *(f)* Rarely, a continuous murmur may be heard at the base of the heart following a massive pulmonary embolus. *(g)* Pulmonary arteriovenous fistula produces a murmur often heard over the

lung bases. Some cyanosis and clubbing develop if the size of the shunt is of any consequence. *(h)* Truncus arteriosus. Cyanosis is present and the murmur is usually to and fro rather than continuous.

Ventricular Septal Defects

The murmur of ventricular septal defects is usually holosystolic (Fig 11–4), although when the murmur is not very loud, the ear may have difficulty recognizing this. The murmur may be of equal intensity throughout systole but commonly shows some peaking during systole and may be diamond shaped. With small ventricular septal defects and possibly when they are in the muscular septum, the murmur is often diamond shaped and ends before the second sound. It is possible that the septal defect may be closed during the latter part of systole by ventricular contraction. When the murmur is faint or moderately loud, it tends to be high pitched with only mild harshness, but louder murmurs are harsh. The murmur may be very loud. A thrill is present with the louder murmurs.

The point of maximum intensity is most often in the third or fourth intercostal space to the left of the sternum. Rarely, very high septal defects give a murmur that is most intense in the second left intercostal space when the patient is lying down. Transmission depends mainly on the intensity; the more intense murmurs may be heard over the entire precordium and posteriorly but are poorly heard in the neck.

The first sound is usually not remarkable. In some of the moderate defects there is an abnormal degree of splitting of the aortic and pulmonic components of the second sound. This is not usually impressive but is interesting, since both ventricles are handling the same amount of blood. It may be that the left ventricle handles the additional load better than does the right ventricle. Loud murmurs may partially mask the aortic second sound. When the defect is small, the second sound is normally or finely split. With large defects and greater flow into the pulmonary circuit, splitting of the second sound is usually close or absent. A third heart sound is often heard at the apex.

When the shunt is fairly marked, a rumbling apical middia-

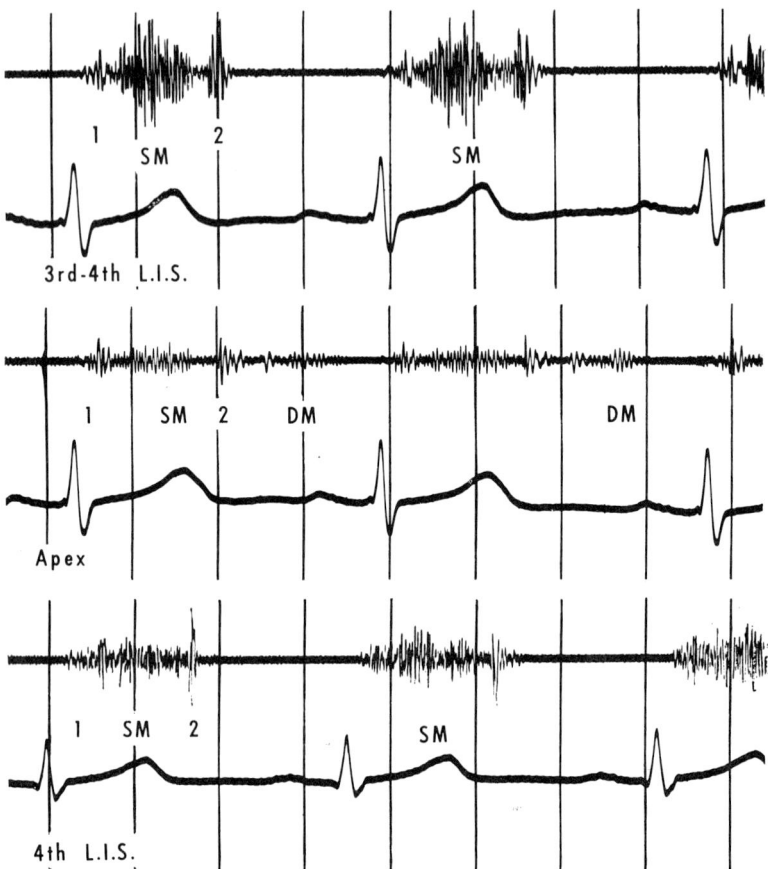

Fig 11–4.—Ventricular septal defect. The *upper tracings* show a loud holosystolic murmur *(SM)* in the third and fourth left interspaces. In this patient the murmur had a diamond shape. This is not an infrequent finding, but the shape of the murmur often varies from beat to beat. The *bottom tracing,* taken from a different patient, shows a holosystolic murmur of more uniform intensity. The *middle tracing* was taken on the same patient as the upper tracing and shows a middiastolic murmur which was evident at the apex. This is often present with large shunts and indicates a relative mitral stenosis. The systolic murmur is much less intense at the apex than along the left border of the sternum.

stolic murmur may be present (see Fig 11–4). It is produced in part by the increased flow through the mitral valve and in part by left ventricular enlargement.

Communications between the left ventricle and the right atrium (ventriculo-atrial defect) produce a systolic murmur that is similar in quality to ordinary ventricular septal defects. The murmur may be heard best over the sternum or along the right sternal edge.

An occasional patient with a very high ventricular septal defect will have an incompetent medial cusp of the aortic valve, which gives an early diastolic murmur; the combination of the systolic and early diastolic murmurs may be mistaken for the continuous murmur of patent ductus arteriosus. These murmurs can usually be recognized as "to-and-fro" murmurs (p. 204), with a different quality in systole and diastole. The point of maximum intensity is usually lower than that of the murmur of patent ductus arteriosus. An apical diastolic flow murmur is also often heard in this condition.

Pulmonary hypertension often develops with the more marked shunts but is infrequent with the small shunts. It may or may not occur with moderate shunts. In more marked shunts, pulmonary vascular resistance increases with a resultant decrease in the left-to-right shunt; the murmur becomes less intense and less harsh. When pulmonary vascular resistance increases to the point at which there is a mixed shunt, the murmur may become faint and cease to be holosystolic. The pulmonic second sound becomes loud, and splitting of the second sound, with inspiration, becomes very close or may not be evident. Pulmonary regurgitation with its characteristic murmur occurs in a moderate percentage and, with failure, a tricuspid regurgitation murmur develops. Frequently, a pulmonary ejection sound is heard. An apical flow murmur which has been previously present will diminish in intensity and eventually disappear, and a previously present thrill also disappears. The auscultatory findings may now be indistinguishable from those of patent ductus arteriosus with pulmonary hypertension (see Fig 11-3).

If the murmur of the ventricular septal defect is recognizably holosystolic, there usually will be no problem in separating it from an innocent systolic murmur, the murmur of a mild pulmonary valvular stenosis, and the murmur of a mild, isolated infundibular stenosis. When, however, the differences in the timing of the murmurs are not clearly evident, other features must be considered:

Innocent systolic murmurs. — (1) If the innocent murmur has a vibratory quality, this is helpful. (2) The point of maximum intensity of an innocent systolic murmur is not as sharply localized as that of the murmur of a ventricular septal defect (p. 121). (3) Of greatest importance is the wide transmission of an innocent murmur, as compared to a murmur of ventricular septal defect of similar intensity. (4) Innocent systolic murmurs are more common.

Mild pulmonary valvular stenosis.—(1) The murmur usually has a point of maximum intensity higher than that of a ventricular septal defect. (2) The murmur is more harsh. (3) The pulmonic second sound in mild stenosis usually can be heard and is more widely split than in ventricular septal defect. (4) A pulmonary ejection sound is nearly always present in mild pulmonary stenosis and is not heard in mild ventricular septal defect. (5) A middiastolic murmur, if present. points to a ventricular septal defect, since it usually is not present in pulmonary stenosis.

Mild isolated pulmonary infundibular stenosis.—This condition may produce a murmur similar in quality and location to a ventricular septal defect, and if the increased splitting is not too great, auscultatory differentiation may be impossible. The effect of drugs on the murmur may be helpful (p. 254).

The auscultatory findings in *Eisenmenger's complex* are those of a ventricular septal defect with pulmonary hypertension.

The murmur of ventricular septal defect is decreased by amyl nitrite and the Valsalva maneuver and is increased by pressor amines (p. 251).

Some patients with otherwise unexplained systolic ejection murmurs have been found to have aneurysms of the upper interventricular system, which are thought to represent an incomplete or closed ventricular septal defect. Some may be acquired secondary to ischemic heart disease and septal infarction.

Atrial Septal Defects

Even in its milder form, an atrial septal defect is almost always associated with a systolic murmur and a widely split second sound (Fig 11–5). The murmur is due to the marked increase in blood flow through the pulmonary valve and to a relative pulmonary stenosis, resulting from enlargement of the

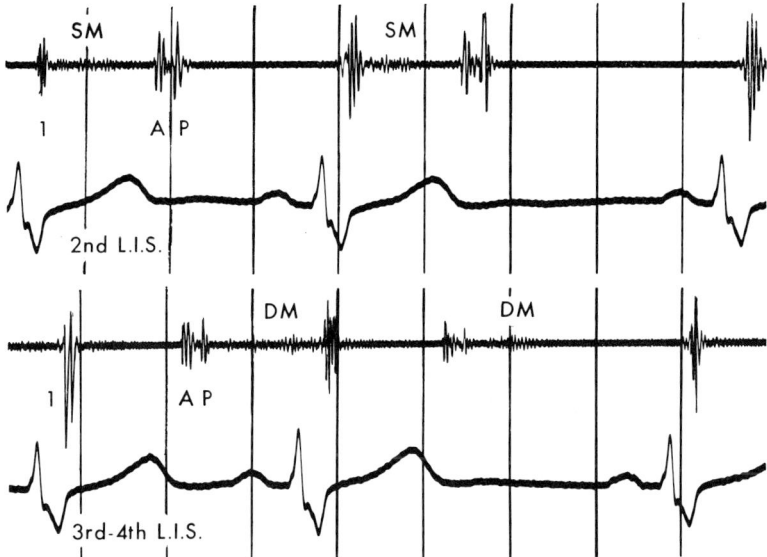

Fig 11–5.—Atrial septal defect. *Upper tracing:* The systolic murmur *(SM)* in the second left interspace is of medium pitch and not very loud. It sounds much like an innocent murmur that is of maximum intensity in the second left intercostal space. The second heart sound is clearly split on both inspiration and expiration. *Lower tracing:* In the third to the fourth left intercostal spaces, a middiastolic murmur *(DM)* is present. Although one does not expect to hear a presystolic murmur in a relative mitral or tricuspid stenosis, this tracing shows why a presystolic murmur may occur. Following the second beat, there is a long diastole; one hears only a middiastolic murmur with no presystolic murmur. However, after the first beat, diastole is shortened by the more rapid rate; atrial contraction now falls during or near the period of rapid ventricular filling and the result is a combination of a middiastolic and a presystolic murmur.

right ventricle and pulmonary artery. The shunt through the atrial septal defect does not produce an audible sound. The point of maximum intensity is usually in the second, but may be in the third, left intercostal space, and the murmur is often transmitted to the left along the second intercostal space. The murmur is of medium pitch and is rarely as harsh or as loud as that of ventricular septal defect. It may be short or extend almost to the second sound. Although a thrill is not usually present, it can occasionally be felt over the pulmonary artery in large septal defects.

The second sound is almost always split on both inspiration and expiration. The pulmonic component is not usually accentuated. The pulmonic second sound, although of normal intensity, is more widely heard than usual, and the split second sound is, therefore, evident along the left border of the sternum and often at the apex (see Fig 5–8, p. 67). With most atrial septal defects, an increase in the splitting of the second sound with inspiration is not evident to the ear (fixed splitting). At times, the splitting may not be fixed and may show some variation with respiration. Patients with small shunts, and occasionally some patients with moderate shunts, may show normal splitting. The cause of fixed splitting has been discussed (p. 48).

The degree of splitting does not appear to be related to the size of the shunt. The splitting decreases with increase in heart rate, and it is less marked in children than in adults. Following successful surgery, the splitting usually becomes normal; a mild degree of splitting may persist on expiration, but a normal inspiratory increase occurs.

Usually, only minor changes are noted in the fixed splitting following a Valsalva maneuver. This is in marked contrast to what happens normally (p. 46) where an immediate wide split rapidly decreases to a single sound. With both atria connected by the defect, there is a common reservoir; thus, a sudden load on one atrium affects the flow between the atria and results in a greater flow of blood into both ventricles, and the splitting is not appreciably affected.

In some patients, the first heart sound is increased at the apex. This has been considered to result from an increase in the intensity of the tricuspid component at the apex. The first sound may appear split at the apex. A *pulmonary ejection sound* occurs occasionally, even in the absence of pulmonary hypertension, and is probably related to the increased flow and the dilation of the pulmonary artery.

With more marked shunts, a rumbling, or rough middiastolic murmur is heard along the left border of the sternum or between the apex and the left border of the sternum (see Fig 11–5). This murmur is a tricuspid *flow murmur* produced by the marked increase in flow through the tricuspid valve, and a relative tricuspid stenosis resulting from enlargement of the right ventricle. At times a right-sided fourth sound may be heard in the same area when pulmonary hypertension is present (see Fig 5–14, J, p. 80). The middiastolic murmur and the atrial sound may increase in loudness with inspiration.

If pulmonary hypertension develops, the following changes occur: (1) the pulmonic second sound increases in loudness; (2) the pulmonary flow murmur leaves or decreases in intensity; (3) a middiastolic murmur, if present, leaves; (4) a pulmonary ejection sound nearly always develops; (5) an early diastolic murmur of pulmonary regurgitation frequently becomes evident; (6) with right ventricular failure, the systolic murmur of tricuspid regurgitation frequently is present, and may be loud; (7) if pulmonary hypertension is severe, the degree of splitting of the second sound is decreased, although some splitting usually remains. It is rare for splitting to become normal or absent. Several factors account for this loss of splitting: *(a)* the high pulmonary artery diastolic pressure results in an earlier closure of the pulmonic valve; *(b)* the hypertrophied right ventricle may be better able to handle the load; and *(c)* the shunt is decreased.

It is obvious that the auscultatory findings in atrial septal defect with severe hypertension are similar to those already described for patent ductus arteriosus and ventricular septal defect with pulmonary hypertension (see Fig 11–3). Similar auscultatory findings may occur in *primary pulmonary hypertension.*

The auscultatory findings in partial *anomalous pulmonary venous drainage* are, in general, the same as in atrial septal defect, but the tendency to fixed splitting may be less if there is no accompanying atrial septal defect.

In patients with a *persistent ostium primum (endocardial cushion defect, persistent atrioventricular canal),* the auscultatory findings may also be similar to those of an atrial septal defect. A partially or completely cleft and deformed mitral valve, however, may be present and produce the murmur of mitral regurgitation. In some instances, this mitral regurgitation murmur is quite harsh and is very well heard in the apicosternal area; it may be mistaken for the murmur of a ventricular septal defect. A ventricular septal defect is often present but appears less likely to be the cause of a murmur.

An atrial septal defect may be difficult to distinguish from a *mild pulmonary valvular stenosis* or an *infundibular stenosis,* since they have similar murmurs and split second sounds. The following distinguishing features are helpful: (1) the second sound is more likely to move with respiration in pulmonary stenosis than in atrial septal defect; (2) a pulmonary ejection sound is almost always present in pulmonary stenosis; it is much less frequent in atrial septal defect without hypertension; (3) the atrial septal defect is more likely to have a middiastolic tricuspid flow murmur.

An atrial septal defect is distinguished from an *innocent systolic murmur* by the presence of fixed splitting of the second sound.

Idiopathic pulmonary artery dilatation in many instances is due to very mild valvular pulmonic stenosis. The murmur may be similar to an atrial septal defect. The findings include an ejection sound and a soft, short midsystolic murmur in the second left interspace.

An atrial septal defect with a middiastolic murmur has to be differentiated from *mitral stenosis*. This depends on the following: (1) The diastolic murmur of mitral stenosis is loudest over the left ventricle and either does not change or decreases with inspiration, whereas the middiastolic murmur in atrial septal defect is loudest over the right ventricle and increases with inspiration. (2) An opening snap is heard only in mitral stenosis, but care must be taken not to mistake the fixed pulmonic second sound in atrial septal defect for an opening snap (p. 72). (3) The pulmonic flow murmur of atrial septal defect is not usually present in mitral stenosis.

If mitral stenosis and atrial septal defect are both present, the pressure in the left atrium cannot build up as it usually would in mitral stenosis; as a result, the diastolic murmur of mitral stenosis is less evident than the pathology would warrant, and the tricuspid flow murmur is increased.

Valvular, Discrete Subvalvular, and Supravalvular Aortic Stenosis

Subvalvular stenosis, due to a fixed stenotic band beneath the aortic valve, and supravalvular stenosis may lead to confusion with valvular stenosis. The systolic murmur in all is harsh, diamond shaped, and ends before the aortic second sound. The following considerations may be of some value in differentiation.

1. The point of maximum intensity of the murmur in valvular stenosis is usually in the second right intercostal interspace in children. Theoretically, the point of maximum intensity

should be somewhat lower in subvalvular stenosis. It is generally difficult to recognize any difference, but if the maximum intensity is in the third left intercostal space, this should suggest a subvalvular stenosis. Actually, the stenotic band is only a centimeter or less below the aortic valve, and it is easily understandable why the points of maximum intensity should be very similar. With supravalvular stenosis, the maximum intensity may be in the right side of the neck.

2. The most valuable auscultatory finding may be an aortic ejection sound. This occurs almost always, if carefully sought for, in congenital valvular stenosis, but infrequently in subvalvular stenosis, and rarely, if at all, in supravalvular stenosis.

3. Aortic regurgitation may occur in all three types, and, although it may actually be slightly more common in subvalvular stenosis, this is of no differential value.

4. The intensity of the aortic closure sound may be normal, increased, or decreased in all three, but is commonly normal or increased in valvular stenosis unless the valve is calcified, in which case it is decreased. It is usually decreased in subvalvular stenosis. The expected increase in supravalvular stenosis is not usually present. Splitting of the second sound may be normal in all three, or the sound may be single. If the stenosis is severe, a paradoxical splitting will occur.

5. A fourth sound will occur in any of the stenoses and is essentially an indication of the severity of the stenosis, since it occurs with the more significant grades of stenosis.

6. A decreased blood pressure in the left arm when compared with the right arm strongly favors the diagnosis of supravalvular aortic stenosis.

It will be noted from the above that the presence or absence of the systolic ejection sound may be the most valuable single auscultatory sign in separating valvular from other types of aortic stenosis. However, a loud murmur may mask the ejection sound which may be evident only on a phonocardiogram.

Coarctation of the Aorta

Although coarctation of the aorta occasionally produces no auscultatory findings, it usually causes a basal systolic murmur which is heard as well, or better, posteriorly in the interscapular region. Anteriorly, the systolic murmur is of maximum intensity usually in the second left intercostal space, but occasionally on the right, and rarely at the apex. It may be difficult to decide whether the murmur is louder on the left or the right, but this in itself is significant, indicating the deep origin of the murmur. The murmur may be continuous over the dorsal spine and not infrequently is both systolic and diastolic, although it is difficult to recognize this, since the heart sounds are not well heard. The murmur is rarely loud anteriorly, and the presence of a loud murmur should lead one to consider the possibility of additional defects.

The important feature of the murmur of coarctation is not that it is well heard in the interscapular region, since many loud murmurs may be heard there, but that it is often louder in the interscapular region than it is anteriorly.

A bicuspid aortic valve occurs very frequently in patients with coarctation. Varying degrees of aortic stenosis, regurgitation or both may be present. An ejection sound is usually heard and is best appreciated at the cardiac apex. Because of the increased systemic pressure, the aortic second sound may be increased. Occasionally, systolic murmurs are heard along the left border of the sternum. These may represent associated anomalies, but many of them disappear after operation. A systolic or continuous murmur or hum may be heard and a thrill felt over the ribs due to the increased flow in the dilated and tortuous intercostal arteries. It is often possible to feel a vigorous systolic pulsation in the notch above the sternum in patients with coarctation.

The diagnosis of coarctation can be made easily with the help of a few additional physical signs. Blood pressure is elevated and is always higher in the arms than in the legs. It may be absent altogether in the lower extremities. A lag between brachial and femoral pulses is the single most helpful physical sign in the diagnosis of coarctation. If a large blood pressure cuff is not available for thigh blood pressure measurement, a standard cuff can be fastened around the calf of the leg. Systolic blood pressure can be estimated with reasonable accuracy by palpation of the pedal arteries (see p. 238 and Chapter 16).

Pulmonary Valvular Stenosis with an Intact
Ventricular Septum

Pulmonary valvular stenosis with an intact ventricular septum is associated with a harsh systolic murmur of maximum intensity in the second left intercostal space, an abnormally split second sound, a pulmonary ejection sound, and often a right-sided fourth sound (see Fig 5–14, C, p. 80, and Fig 11–6).

The murmur has much the same pitch and quality as that of aortic stenosis and is also diamond shaped on a phonocardiogram. The murmur is often widely transmitted and is better heard on the left side of the neck than on the right. If the murmur is loud, a thrill is usually present. The murmur ends

Fig 11–6.—Pulmonary stenosis with an intact ventricular septum. The first heart sound is faint and followed by a long systolic murmur which reaches a peak very late and ends with a faint pulmonic second sound. The second sound is not evident on auscultation. In the second right intercostal space, the murmur is much less intense and the aortic second sound is heard before the end of the murmur. It is evident that in the second left intercostal space the aortic second sound is masked by the murmur.

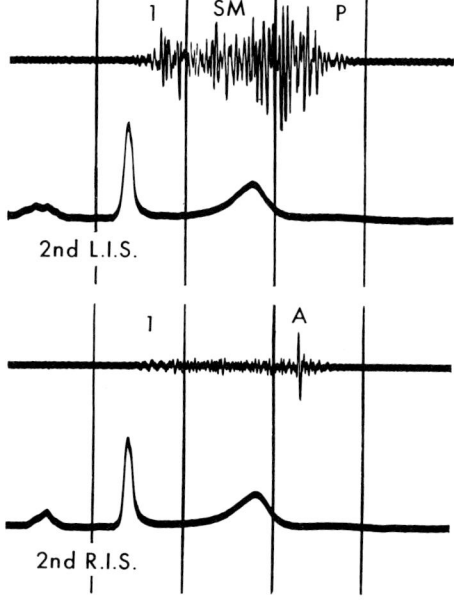

before the pulmonic second sound but may extend through the aortic second sound. When the stenosis is severe, right ventricular systole is prolonged because of the increased load. This results in a long murmur, and the duration of the murmur is related to the severity of the stenosis. With milder grades of stenosis, the maximum intensity of the murmur is earlier in systole than with more severe stenosis. With training, one can recognize whether the peak is early or late, but it is usually easier to judge by the length of the murmur. The duration of the murmur and the delay in peaking show a better correlation with the degree of stenosis than does the intensity. The murmur may be louder on inspiration than on expiration.

Since right ventricular systole is prolonged over left ventricular systole, there is an abnormal splitting of the second sound (see Fig 4–8, E, p. 49). The pulmonic second sound is fairly normal in intensity in mild pulmonary valve stenosis, but becomes faint in moderate stenosis, and is frequently not heard in severe stenosis. If one listens in the second left interspace in severe stenosis, the long murmur may extend through the aortic second sound and, since the pulmonic second sound is faint or absent, no second sound may be evident; an aortic second sound, however, may be heard at the apex and in the second right intercostal space (see Fig 11–6). If the murmur is not too loud and the pulmonic second sound is heard, the splitting is very noticeable and is often more evident in the third left intercostal space, where the murmur is not so loud and the sounds are better heard. The degree of splitting and the intensity of the pulmonic second sound are well related to the degree of pulmonary stenosis.

A pulmonary ejection sound is nearly always present, but it is less evident in more severe stenosis. It is usually heard in the second or third left intercostal space and varies with respiration (p. 64). The more severe the stenosis, the lower is the pulmonary artery pressure and the earlier is the ejection sound. Although this may sometimes be evident to the ear, it is not an especially good auscultatory method of judging severity. The ejection sound may be masked by the loud murmur and will often be heard better in the third left intercostal space. If only a single, fairly loud sound is heard, it is possible that the ejection sound and first sound are too close together to be recognized.

On inspection, in severe cases, a large A-wave is present in the jugular venous pulse. Palpation reveals a right ventricular lift along the left parasternal area. The magnitude of the lift correlates with the severity of stenosis. A systolic thrust is commonly noted at the left second interspace and is usually accompanied by a systolic thrill.

The occurrence of a right-sided fourth sound is common in moderately severe and severe pulmonary stenosis and is an indication of the severity of the stenosis.

In isolated infundibular stenosis, the point of maximum intensity of the murmur is lower (third or fourth left intercostal space) and there is no ejection sound.

Peripheral pulmonary stenosis is actually a series of narrowings of the main pulmonary artery and branches. It sometimes occurs alone as a complication of maternal rubella. More commonly it is seen with other lesions such as tetralogy of Fallot or valvular pulmonary stenosis. On examination, right ventricular enlargement may be found and the pulmonary closure sound is accentuated. The systolic murmur is characteristically widely transmitted, but may be loudest in one or both axillae. More severe degrees of stenosis result in some gradient across the stenosis, even in diastole, producing a continuous murmur.

Tetralogy of Fallot

This condition combines a severe enough pulmonary valvular stenosis (or more commonly, infundibular stenosis) and a large enough ventricular septal defect so that the shunt, except in very mild cases, is from right to left. With extremely severe grades of pulmonary stenosis or with pulmonary atresia, there may be no murmur, and it would seem that the murmur, when present, is due primarily to pulmonary stenosis. Since infundibular stenosis is most common in tetralogy of Fallot, the murmur is usually loudest in the third or fourth left intercostal space (Fig 11 – 7). There is a tendency to an inverse relationship between the loudness of the murmur and the severity of the condition; the murmur is faint or absent with severe pulmonary stenosis and becomes louder with moderate stenosis. The murmur is harsh and is not as long as the murmur of pulmonary valvular stenosis with intact ventricular

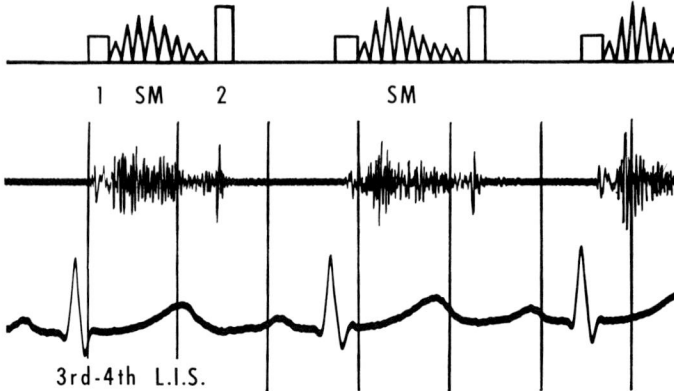

Fig 11–7.—Tetralogy of Fallot. The systolic murmur *(SM)* is faint by the time the second sound occurs. The second sound is clearly heard and shows no evidence of splitting. The second sound is produced by the aortic valve.

septum. Whereas in pure pulmonary stenosis, the right ventricle can empty itself only through a stenosed pulmonary valve, in tetralogy, the right ventricle can easily empty itself into the aorta through the ventricular septal defect. Right ventricular systole is, therefore, not prolonged and the murmur is shorter than in pure pulmonary stenosis. The systolic murmur in tetralogy fades or stops somewhat before the second sound, permitting the second sound to be well heard.

The second sound in tetralogy tends to be single, since the pulmonic second sound is faint and not usually heard (see Fig 11–7). Because of displacement of the aorta, the second sound that is heard to the left of the sternum is the aortic second sound. At the site where the murmur is loudest, the second sound is thus often clearly heard, in contrast to what is found in pulmonary stenosis with an intact ventricular septum.

When the pulmonary stenosis is severe, most of the blood is ejected through the septal defect into the aorta, and an aortic ejection sound may be present.

The differentiation of a tetralogy from a pulmonary valvular stenosis with intact ventricular septum is sometimes aided by the use of amyl nitrite (p. 254).

Other Congenital Heart Lesions

In *transposition of the great vessels,* a murmur is usually associated with the presence of a ventricular septal defect.

When this defect is not present, there may be no murmur. The second sound is often booming, and two components are present but are not often easy to recognize because of a rapid heart rate. A third heart sound is common.

In *tricuspid atresia*, the murmur may be due to the presence of a ventricular septal defect. Occasionally, the murmur of mitral regurgitation is heard.

In *Ebstein's disease*, a wide variety of findings may occur. Widely split first and second heart sounds are common because of the frequent presence of right bundle branch block. A systolic murmur may be present and is probably due to tricuspid regurgitation, but it is often more harsh than the usual tricuspid regurgitation murmur. A middiastolic and, occasionally, a presystolic murmur, probably associated with the tricuspid deformity, may occur. The murmurs may seem to be quite loud at the apex, but it should be recalled that in this condition the tricuspid valve is usually far to the left. A fourth sound may, at times, be heard along the left border of the sternum.

CHAPTER 12

Auscultatory Phenomena in Rheumatic Heart Disease

Acute Rheumatic Carditis

1. The first sound may be diminished because of prolongation of atrioventricular conduction. Myocardial involvement may, at times, play a part (p. 34).

2. Second- and third-degree heart blocks occur with more severe involvement of the conduction system (p. 34).

3. A pericardial rub may be present early (p. 148).

4. A systolic murmur with the characteristics of an innocent murmur is often heard (p. 120). This is not due to valvular involvement and may be associated with the fever and increased heart action.

5. The faint murmur of mitral regurgitation (p. 96) may be present early and remain faint or increase rapidly in loudness. If the heart size is normal, the murmur is produced by valvular deformity resulting from the acute endocarditis. Cardiac enlargement is associated with a loud systolic murmur that is usually due, in part, to relative mitral regurgitation.

6. An accentuated third heart sound may develop, especially if the heart enlarges or a loud systolic murmur is present. At rapid rates a summation sound occurs. These sounds may be of right- or left-sided origin, or both.

7. A middiastolic murmur that does not indicate organic mitral stenosis is common if the heart enlarges, but may be heard, at times, without cardiac enlargement (p. 142).

8. A faint murmur of aortic regurgitation (p. 136) is occasionally present early, often with no other murmur.

9. A pulmonary systolic murmur, rather musical in quality and often varying from day to day, occasionally occurs. Its cause and significance are not clear.

10. All the murmurs and sounds may show variation from day to day.

REGRESSION OF THE ACUTE PHASE.—1. The first heart sound improves as the atrioventricular conduction time shortens.

2. The pericardial rub disappears.

3. The middiastolic murmur disappears as the acute phase leaves or as the heart decreases in size.

4. The systolic murmur may become much less intense, and if not too loud when the heart was enlarged, it may disappear entirely or become very faint.

5. An abnormally accentuated third sound becomes less intense or leaves entirely. A summation sound leaves.

6. The murmur of aortic regurgitation usually persists but may, if it was faint, disappear. If associated with peripheral signs of regurgitation, it does not disappear.

SUBSEQUENT COURSE.—Fewer than 50% of patients who have an episode of acute rheumatic fever subsequently develop rheumatic valvulitis. The subsequent course depends on the amount of inflammation that occurred in the acute phase and on the amount of scarring that will supervene. Even more important may be recurrences of activity of rheumatic fever. *Rheumatic fever would seem to be a chronic, smoldering disease with recurrent flare-ups of subacute and subclinical severity in addition to the recognized acute incidents. Repeated insults to the valve over a period of years, rather than one injury with scarring, account for the damage.*

Mitral Valve Involvement

Figure 12–1 presents in diagrammatic form the changes that can occur in the mitral valve. As a result of an episode of acute rheumatic fever, the patient may be left with a mild mitral regurgitation. The mitral valve cusps are somewhat thickened and possibly shortened but remain flexible. The edges of the cusps may be firm and rolled. The chordae tendineae are

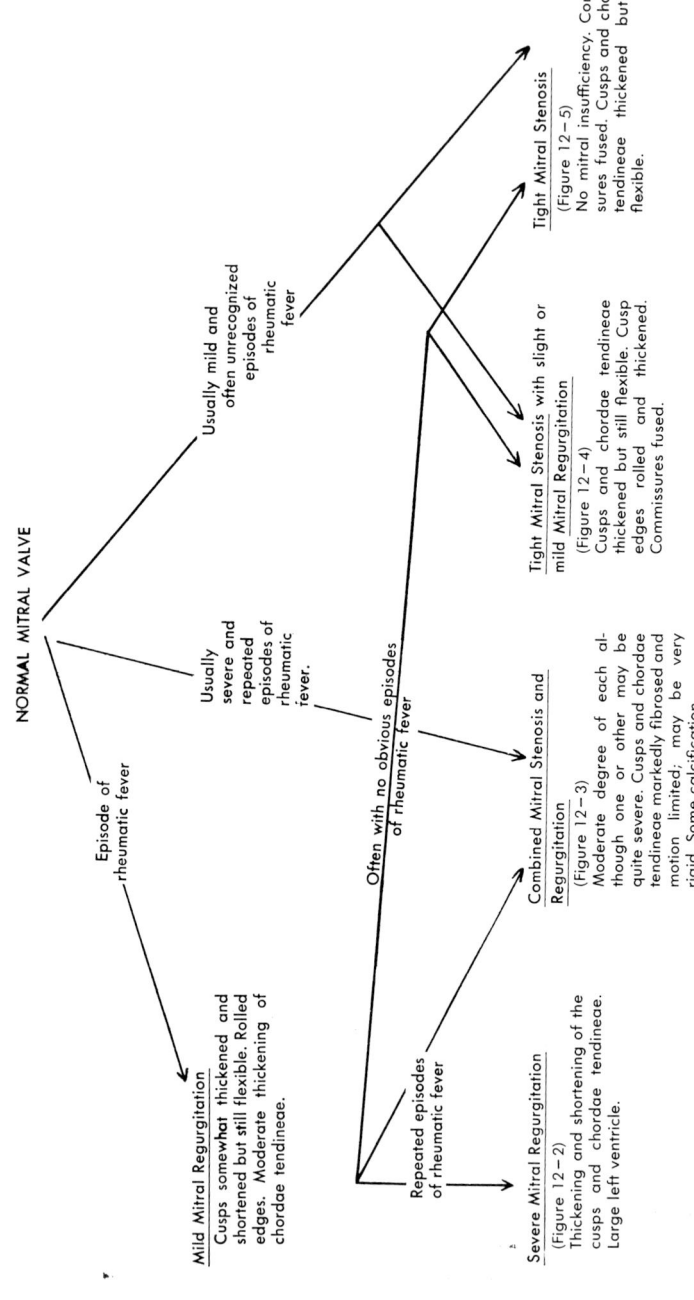

NORMAL MITRAL VALVE

Episode of rheumatic fever

Mild Mitral Regurgitation
(Figure 12–2)
Cusps somewhat thickened and shortened but still flexible. Rolled edges. Moderate thickening of chordae tendineae.

Usually severe and repeated episodes of rheumatic fever.

Usually mild and often unrecognized episodes of rheumatic fever

Often with no obvious episodes of rheumatic fever

Repeated episodes of rheumatic fever

Severe Mitral Regurgitation
(Figure 12–2)
Thickening and shortening of the cusps and chordae tendineae. Large left ventricle.

Combined Mitral Stenosis and Regurgitation
(Figure 12–3)
Moderate degree of each although one or other may be quite severe. Cusps and chordae tendineae markedly fibrosed and motion limited; may be very rigid. Some calcification.

Tight Mitral Stenosis with slight or mild Mitral Regurgitation
(Figure 12–4)
Cusps and chordae tendineae thickened but still flexible. Cusp edges rolled and thickened. Commissures fused.

Tight Mitral Stenosis
(Figure 12–5)
No mitral insufficiency. Commissures fused. Cusps and chordae tendineae thickened but still flexible.

Fig 12–1.—Changes in the mitral valve resulting from rheumatic fever.

rarely thickened or fused. The mitral regurgitation produces a typical murmur. This murmur can be recognized and the diagnosis of mitral regurgitation can be made in the absence of any other finding. The heart sounds are essentially unchanged. Occasionally, a patient may recover from acute rheumatic fever with no evidence of valvular damage and then, over a period of years, with no evidence of further rheumatic activity, develop a murmur of mild mitral regurgitation.

The involvement of the mitral valve may stop with production of a mild or moderate regurgitation, which can be recognized only by the presence of the typical murmur. Frequently, the involvement progresses even without evidence of acute rheumatic fever. Depending on the type and severity of the valvular changes, severe mitral regurgitation, mitral stenosis, or any combination of the two may result. Patients with no recognizable recurrences of acute rheumatic fever are more likely to develop mitral stenosis. Patients with repeated severe attacks of rheumatic fever are more likely to show a combination of mitral stenosis and mitral regurgitation or severe mitral regurgitation.

SEVERE MITRAL REGURGITATION. — When *severe mitral regurgitation* with little or no stenosis occurs (Fig 12–2), the valve cusps become thickened and shortened but retain some flexibility; the chordae tendineae are also thickened and may show marked shortening. Enlargement of the left ventricle as a result of the mitral regurgitation aggravates the mitral regurgitation because of relative shortening of the chordae tendineae. The result is a severe mitral regurgitation with little or no stenosis. The findings are as follows:

1. Palpation reveals an outwardly displaced, hyperkinetic left ventricular impulse. Thrills are rare.

2. The first sound is of normal or decreased intensity. A loud murmur may mask the sound, which may be seen on a phonocardiogram.

3. A loud, high-pitched, apical systolic murmur of mitral regurgitation is present. Although primarily high pitched, the murmur tends to be somewhat harsh when loud (p. 100).

4. The pulmonic second sound may be increased if there is an increase in left atrial and pulmonary arterial pressure. The degree of splitting is usually unchanged but may be increased.

5. A third heart sound is often present at the apex and may be louder than the second sound in that area.

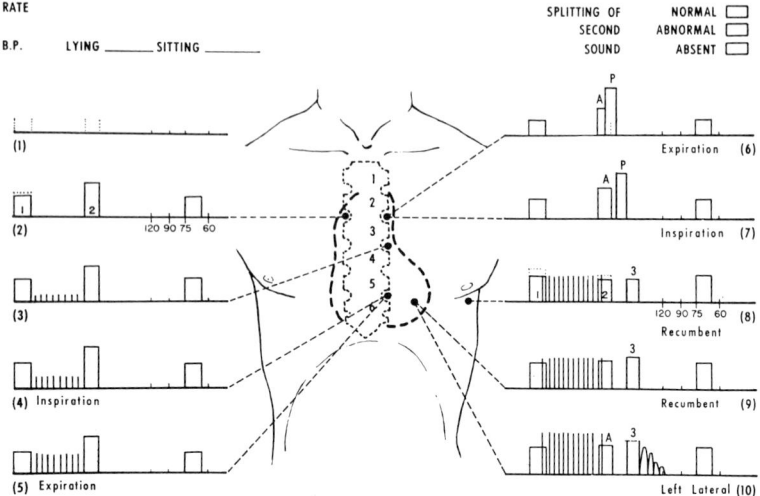

Fig 12–2.—Severe mitral regurgitation. The numbers in parentheses refer to the lines on the chart. The following features are shown:

a. A loud, high-pitched systolic murmur of maximum intensity at the apex *(9) (10)*. This murmur is well transmitted into the axilla *(8)* and is also heard medially, often up to the sternal border *(3) (4) (5)*. In this area, the murmur is louder in expiration *(5)* than in inspiration *(4)*. This murmur is heard in the aortic area only when very loud.

b. The first heart sound is diminished in intensity and masked by the loud systolic murmur *(8) (9) (10)*.

c. There is often some splitting of the second sound, even in expiration, in the second left intercostal space *(6)*. This is increased in inspiration *(7)*.

d. A third heart sound, which is often louder than the second heart sound, may be present at the apex *(9) (10)*.

e. A middiastolic murmur often follows the third heart sound *(10)*, and in some areas only the middiastolic murmur without the third heart sound may be heard.

6. <u>A middiastolic murmur is often heard.</u> This is usually of faint or moderate intensity, but in children it may be loud. A presystolic murmur is not usually present but may occur. Differentiation from the murmur of organic mitral stenosis is important (p. 145).

COMBINED MITRAL STENOSIS AND REGURGITATION.—With extensive involvement of the cusps and the chordae tendineae, a *combination of mitral stenosis and mitral regurgitation* results (Fig 12–3). The cusps and the chordae tendineae become fibrosed and rigid and there is little, if any, movement of the cusps. With severe involvement, the valve ceases to function as a valve and there is merely a funnel-shaped open-

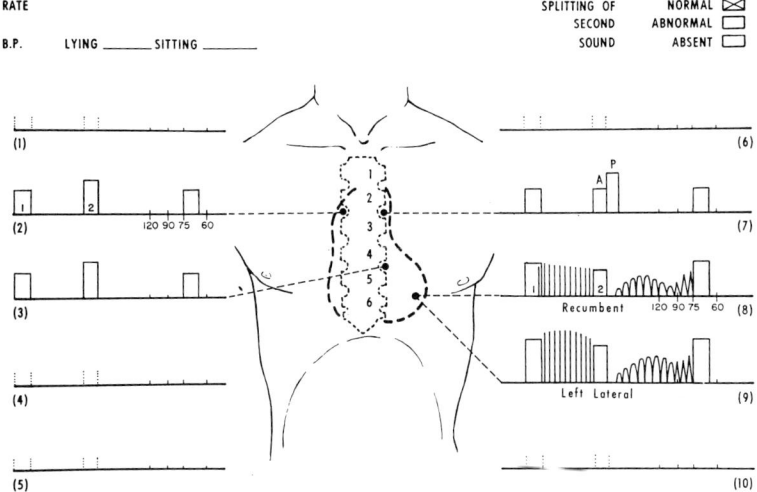

RATE

B.P.   LYING _____ SITTING _____

SPLITTING OF   NORMAL
SECOND   ABNORMAL
SOUND   ABSENT

Fig 12–3. — Combined mitral stenosis and mitral regurgitation. The following features are illustrated:

a. A systolic murmur of moderately loud or loud intensity at the apex *(8) (9).*

b. A middiastolic and presystolic rumbling murmur. This is loudest with the patient in the left lateral position in an area somewhat above the apex and with the bell endpiece *(8).*

c. A high-pitched systolic murmur. The systolic murmur is loudest with the patient in the left lateral position but usually in an area below that at which the diastolic murmur is loudest — i.e., at the apex or slightly below the apex. It is best heard with the diaphragm.

d. A normal or diminished first heart sound. It is occasionally accentuated.

e. A normal splitting of the second heart sound *(7).*

ing, which is usually somewhat larger than that of a tight mitral stenosis. During ventricular systole, free regurgitation occurs but is limited by the size of the opening. There will be a variation in the size of the opening and a corresponding reciprocal relationship between the amounts of stenosis and of regurgitation. Calcium deposits occur frequently. The involvement of the valve is often not uniform, and one commissure or cusp may be more involved than the other. The auscultatory findings are as follows:

1. Increased activity may be felt over both left and right ventricles.

2. The first sound is diminished.

3. A moderately loud or loud systolic murmur of mitral regurgitation is present.

4. An accentuated pulmonic second sound may occur if the pulmonary arterial pressure is increased. The splitting of the second sound is normal.

5. The middiastolic and presystolic murmurs of mitral stenosis are moderately loud or loud. With mitral valve openings of 1½ to 2 sq cm, both the systolic and the diastolic murmurs may be loud.

6. Neither an opening snap of the mitral valve nor a third heart sound is usually present.

TIGHT MITRAL STENOSIS. — In *tight mitral stenosis* (Figs 12–4 and 12–5) without any regurgitation or with minimal mitral regurgitation, the pathologic change is primarily a fusion of the commissures of the valve (see Fig 12–4). The leaflets are diffusely thickened and may be partially calcified. The chordae tendineae are often shortened and adherent to each other. The degree of shortening and fusion may become severe enough that the interchordal spaces are obliterated and

Fig 12–4. — Tight mitral stenosis and mild organic tricuspid regurgitation. Autopsy specimen from a 30-year-old woman who died of an arryhthmia five hours after a mitral commissurotomy. The atria have been cut away to expose both valves. The mitral valve was thickened but was quite flexible. The surgeon had fractured the valve along the anterolateral commissure *(X)* and along the posteromedial commissure *(Y).* The valve opening was originally about 9 mm long *(the dark area in the center).* The tricuspid valve shows a thickening and rolling of the valve edges that accounted for the murmur of tricuspid regurgitation.

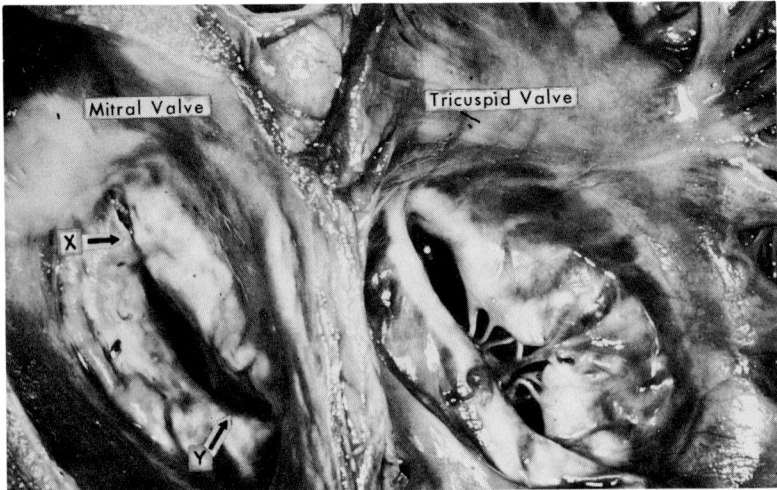

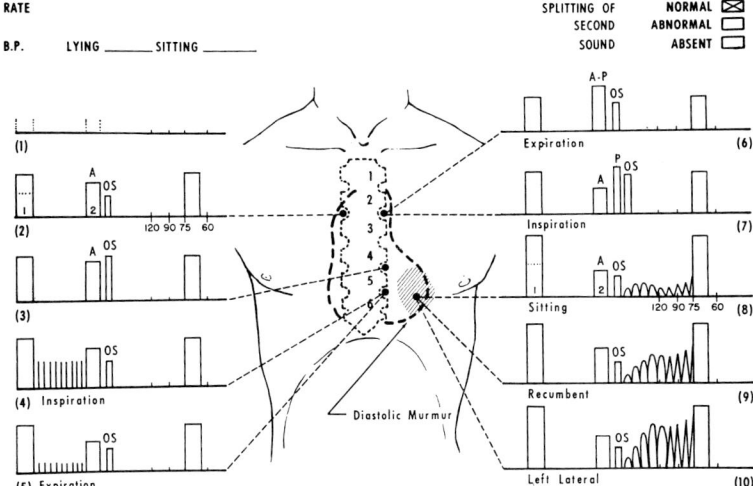

Fig 12–5. — Tight mitral stenosis with flexible valve and no mitral regurgitation. A very mild tricuspid regurgitation is present. These are the auscultatory findings for the patient whose heart valves are shown in Figure 12–4. The following typical features are shown:

a. An accentuated first sound. This is most evident at the apex *(8) (9) (10)*, but the intensity of sound is increased in other areas also.

b. A middiastolic and presystolic murmur at the apex *(8) (9) (10)*. This murmur is quite faint when the patient is in the sitting position *(8)* and is much better heard when she is recumbent *(9)*. In the left lateral position the murmur is still further accentuated *(10)*.

c. An opening snap of the mitral valve. This is loudest and most evident in the fourth left intercostal space *(3)* but is heard over the entire precordium. In the second left intercostal space, it is most evident in expiration *(6)*. In inspiration *(7)*, it follows so closely upon the pulmonic second sound that it is heard with difficulty.

d. A normally split second heart sound. The second sound is split in the second and third left interspaces in inspiration *(7)*. There is no splitting in expiration *(6)*.

e. The murmur of tricuspid regurgitation. The murmur heard to the left of the lower end of the sternum is high pitched and best heard with the diaphragm *(4) (5)*. It shows a definite increase in loudness in inspiration.

in extreme cases subvalvular stenosis may result. The edge of the cusp is rolled and thickened. Many patients with tight mitral stenosis have no history of acute rheumatic fever. The auscultatory findings are as follows (see Fig 12–5):

1. The first sound is accentuated and may be palpable.

2. The middiastolic and presystolic murmurs are moderately loud or loud.

3. An opening snap of the mitral valve is present.

4. A faint or moderately loud systolic murmur of mitral regurgitation may be present, but frequently no systolic murmur is heard.

5. The second sound is normal and shows normal splitting. What is often described as a splitting of the second sound is usually due to the presence of an opening snap of the mitral valve. The pulmonic second sound may become accentuated with increase in pulmonary arterial pressure.

With the development of atrial fibrillation, the presystolic murmur of mitral stenosis, if present, disappears. The first heart sound may or may not show the variation in intensity discussed on page 36. The findings are otherwise essentially unchanged.

TIGHT MITRAL STENOSIS WITH EARLY PULMONARY HYPER-

Fig 12–6.—Tight mitral stenosis with early pulmonary hypertension. The following features are shown:

a. An accentuated first heart sound.

b. A pulmonic second heart sound accentuated as a result of the pulmonary hypertension *(6) (7).* The degree of splitting of the second sound is normal or slightly decreased.

c. An opening snap of the mitral valve *(3).*

d. The middiastolic and presystolic murmurs of mitral stenosis *(9).*

e. A high-pitched, early diastolic murmur in the second and third left intercostal spaces *(6) (7) (8).* This is the murmur of pulmonary regurgitation.

f. Some tricuspid regurgitation. It is indicated by a high-pitched systolic murmur heard best at the lower end of the sternum, louder in inspiration *(4)* than in expiration *(5).*

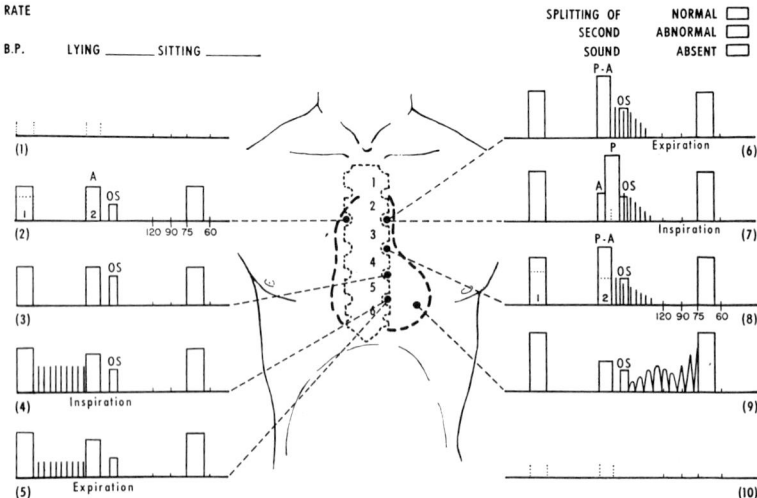

TENSION.—When severe mitral involvement is present for a number of years, pulmonary hypertension, right ventricular hypertrophy and dilation, and tricuspid regurgitation occur. These produce the following auscultatory changes (Fig 12–6):

1. Palpable right ventricular activity is present.

2. A prominent A-wave in the jugular venous pulse is seen with normal sinus rhythm.

3. The pulmonic second sound is accentuated.

4. An early diastolic murmur of pulmonary regurgitation may develop (p. 145).

5. The systolic murmur of tricuspid regurgitation is heard. This can be recognized by its location and its increased intensity with inspiration (p. 107).

6. A pulmonary ejection sound may occasionally be heard.

TIGHT MITRAL STENOSIS WITH PULMONARY HYPERTENSION AND SEVERE TRICUSPID REGURGITATION.—The auscultatory findings in tight mitral stenosis may be so changed by marked tricuspid regurgitation and right ventricular enlargement that the diagnosis of mitral stenosis is made with difficulty. The right ventricle occupies most of the anterior precordium, so that the auscultatory evidence of mitral stenosis is shifted to the axillary region. In addition, a decreased cardiac output results in a faint middiastolic murmur. The evidences of tricuspid regurgitation are dominant (Fig 12–7):

1. A palpable thrust and a shock of pulmonary valve closure are present at the second left intercostal space.

2. The jugular venous pressure is elevated and a V-wave, increasing with inspiration, can be seen.

3. The first sound is normal or somewhat diminished but is often masked by a loud murmur of tricuspid regurgitation.

4. A loud systolic murmur is heard over most of the precordium but is usually recognizable as having its origin in the tricuspid valve by the following findings:

a. The maximum intensity is at the lower end of the sternum or somewhat more lateral but usually within the midclavicular line. This murmur fades laterally, more rapidly than would a loud murmur due to mitral regurgitation in a large heart.

b. The murmur usually increases with inspiration (p. 108).

5. As one moves the stethoscope laterally over the chest, the systolic murmur fades and one hears a clear, but usually

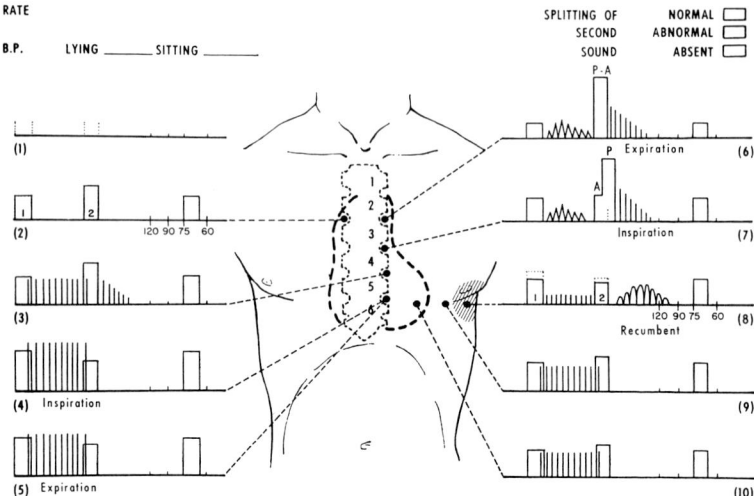

Fig 12–7.—Tight mitral stenosis with pulmonary hypertension and severe tricuspid regurgitation. The following features are shown:

a. A loud, high-pitched systolic murmur dominates the auscultatory findings. This is of maximum intensity at the lower end of the sternum or between the sternum and the apex. It is heard in diminishing loudness from its point of maximum intensity and may be heard fairly well at the apex *(10)* and even more laterally *(9)*. Because of the loudness of this murmur, changes in intensity with respiration may not be evident.

b. The murmur usually masks the first heart sound.

c. The evidences of mitral stenosis are shifted laterally to the anterior axillary and even midaxillary region *(shaded area)*. Here *(8)* the systolic murmur is faint and a rumbling diastolic murmur may be evident. It is not usually very loud.

d. The pulmonic second sound is accentuated, and the degree of splitting may be somewhat diminished *(6) (7)*.

e. A high-pitched, early diastolic murmur is heard along the left border of the sternum *(3) (6) (7)*. This murmur may be due to pulmonic regurgitation, but it is often difficult to rule out aortic regurgitation (p. 146).

rather faint, first heart sound in an area where the systolic murmur is faint or absent. This may be at the anterior or at the midaxillary line.

6. In this area where the first heart sound is heard, a faint middiastolic murmur is usually evident. Occasionally no diastolic murmur can be heard.

7. The murmur of pulmonary regurgitation is sometimes heard.

8. A pulmonary ejection sound is occasionally present and may be followed by a rough systolic murmur.

9. A right-sided third heart sound may be present and, at times, a tricuspid diastolic flow murmur.

If the condition is compensated by intensive therapy, the auscultatory pattern gradually shifts back to that of mild tricuspid regurgitation with recognizable mitral involvement (see Fig 12–6). The pulmonary regurgitation murmur and the accentuated pulmonic second sound often persist, even if the tricuspid regurgitation murmur disappears.

It is extremely important to recognize patients with tight mitral stenosis in whom the tricuspid regurgitation dominates the auscultatory findings, because these patients are often excellent candidates for surgery.

Primary tricuspid valvulitis is a rare occurrence in rheumatic heart disease and probably never occurs alone. Tricuspid regurgitation is virtually always due to right ventricular failure secondary to severe pulmonary hypertension as the result of tight mitral stenosis. The regurgitation is almost always improved following a successful mitral valve operation. Tricuspid stenosis is also present almost exclusively in patients who have mitral stenosis. The physical findings are described on page 134.

Aortic Valve Involvement

Aortic valve involvement, when due to rheumatic fever, occurs almost without exception in association with mitral valve disease. The converse is not true. In some instances of apparently isolated aortic valve disease, mitral disease is recognizable only at operation or autopsy. A faint, early diastolic murmur of aortic regurgitation sometimes occurs early in the course of acute rheumatic carditis. This murmur usually persists, but it frequently goes unrecognized because it is difficult to hear. There may be no associated systolic murmur in the aortic area. Mild to moderate degrees of aortic regurgitation may develop fairly soon after the acute episode (Fig 12–8). When the murmur of aortic regurgitation is moderately loud or loud, there is usually an associated systolic murmur in the second right intercostal space. The systolic murmur may be produced by deformity of the valve. An increased velocity of blood flow through the valve during systole can probably, in itself, produce the murmur or accentuate the murmur produced by any valvular deformity. The second heart sound may be accentuated.

A more common result than severe aortic regurgitation with little or no stenosis is the combination of regurgitation and stenosis (see Fig 12–8). This condition will give a loud systolic murmur and a moderately loud to loud diastolic murmur. The systolic murmur is often out of proportion to the degree of stenosis, again because of the increased flow due to the regurgitation. The aortic second sound is decreased. The systolic murmur is well heard at the apex and often masks the murmur of mitral regurgitation.

Severe degrees of aortic stenosis with little or no regurgitation may possibly result from a continuation of the process that produces a moderate stenosis and regurgitation. However, if calcific aortic stenosis is of rheumatic origin, it is obvious that aortic stenosis can result without a stage during which there is significant aortic regurgitation. With severe calcific aortic stenosis, the systolic murmur may be extremely loud. A diastolic murmur of regurgitation is often heard but may be quite faint. The aortic second sound is faint or absent at the base, but often when not heard at the base, it may be heard at the apex. When the aortic stenosis is severe, the peripheral pulse volume is small, the upstroke time is slow, and the impulse at the apex is forceful and sustained. The heart size remains normal in the absence of failure.

During acute rheumatic fever, a systolic murmur of medium pitch may develop in the aortic region, which may or may not be associated with a faint, early diastolic murmur. This systolic murmur may persist unchanged for years or become louder, and then usually becomes associated with some early diastolic murmur. When of moderate intensity, it may not have the harshness of a murmur of aortic stenosis, and, if no history of rheumatic fever is obtained, its significance may be difficult to determine. It is always important in this instance to make a careful search for a murmur of aortic regurgitation, even though it be of the faintest degree, because such a murmur will immediately enable the physician to make the diagnosis.

When loud systolic and diastolic murmurs are present in aortic valvular disease, they are often described as being "to and fro." This term should not be used for the continuous murmur of patent ductus arteriosus.

A middiastolic or presystolic murmur associated with aortic

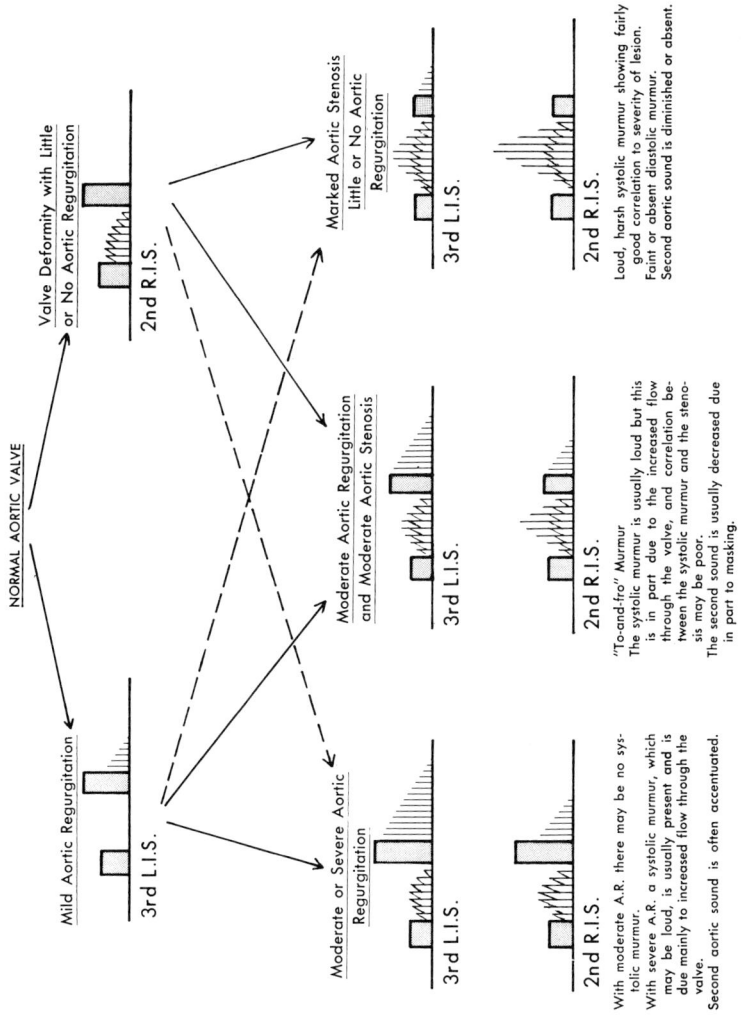

Fig 12–8.—Changes in aortic valve resulting from rheumatic fever.

regurgitation does not distinguish organic mitral involvement from relative mitral stenosis (Austin Flint murmur). Helpful features that indicate organic mitral stenosis are: (1) an accentuated first heart sound, (2) an opening snap, (3) mitral valvular calcification on fluoroscopy, (4) the amyl nitrite test (see Chapter 17) and (5) echocardiographic examination.

Selection of Patients with Valvular Involvement for Cardiac Surgery

MITRAL VALVE DISEASE. — With the wide use of open heart surgery and the availability of satisfactory prosthetic valves, the criteria for selection of patients for mitral valve surgery have changed drastically. There is some question as to whether there is still a place for the closed-heart mitral commissurotomy. In general, direct visualization and repair of the valve and subvalvular structures are the preferred approach. The added risk from cardiopulmonary bypass by an experienced team is currently negligible. Some patients may have valves that lend themselves so easily and satisfactorily to closed commissurotomy that the added risk of an open heart operation is not justified. These would be patients under 40 years of age (and the younger the better) who have a tight mitral stenosis with little or no mitral regurgitation, and who have evidence of a flexible valve. Such patients show the auscultatory findings illustrated in Figure 12–5. The long middiastolic murmur, the presystolic murmur, and the absent or faint systolic murmur indicate the presence of a tight mitral stenosis. The loud first sound and the opening snap of the mitral valve are evidence that the valve is mobile. The result of mitral commissurotomy in such a patient may be dramatic and most satisfying.

In patients over 40 years of age, even when the criteria seem ideal, open heart surgery should be considered, or at least the pump-oxygenator should be on a standby basis. Older patients may have all the criteria of a tight mitral stenosis with a flexible valve, but on operation the valve is found to be thick and leathery and it is difficult to perform a satisfactory commissurotomy. In patients with a combination of stenosis and regurgitation, open heart surgery must, of course, be done.

Patients whose condition *must* be recognized are those in

whom signs of a tight mitral stenosis are masked by the presence of tricuspid regurgitation (p. 201). In such patients, operation often gives dramatic results.

EFFECT OF MITRAL COMMISSUROTOMY ON MITRAL MURMURS. — During the first week following commissurotomy, all murmurs may be faint or absent. Thereafter, a gradual return of the diastolic murmur often occurs. The diastolic murmur does not usually disappear completely even when the results are excellent; the murmur may be faint, but it can usually be heard by listening with the patient in the left lateral position after exercise. A moderately loud diastolic murmur may persist when the clinical and physiologic results are excellent. The best results are usually associated with the greatest decrease in the intensity of the murmur. There is evidence that when the commissurotomy is done by open heart surgery, the diastolic murmur, postoperatively, is more likely to be faint or absent. It would appear that the persistence of the diastolic murmur indicates that there is a residual stenosis in most instances; some of the murmur may be due to deformity and loss of flexibility of the valves. An increased flow through the opened valve may also tend to produce more murmur. If the valve becomes stenosed again, the murmur increases in loudness.

A tight mitral valve without mitral regurgitation may be operated on without the production of any mitral regurgitation. Not infrequently, however, a faint or moderately loud murmur of mitral regurgitation will be heard after commissurotomy when none was present before. The murmur usually persists but may become less intense over an extended period. A murmur of mitral regurgitation that is present before operation usually is present after operation and may be of the same or increased intensity.

TRICUSPID COMMISSUROTOMY. — The common error is overestimation of the degree of tricuspid stenosis. Even when the signs of tricuspid stenosis are marked, the valve is rarely less than 2 sq cm in area. If a loud systolic murmur of tricuspid regurgitation is present, the diagnosis of tricuspid stenosis should be made with caution. The middiastolic murmur should be loud and the systolic murmur of tricuspid regurgitation should not be too loud.

AORTIC STENOSIS. — Aortic stenosis resulting from rheumatic fever is associated almost always with some mitral valve involvement and usually with some degree of aortic regurgitation. In a patient who is being operated on for mitral stenosis, the problem arises whether the degree of aortic stenosis is such as would make the operation on the aortic valve worthwhile. In making the decision, one finds the loudness of the murmur of aortic stenosis and the comparative loudness of the stenotic and regurgitation murmurs to be of limited help, and they must be considered together with evidence obtained by other methods of examination, especially cardiac catheterization and angiocardiography.

AORTIC REGURGITATION. — The murmur can, of course, enable one to make the diagnosis, but peripheral signs of aortic regurgitation and cardiac size are more valuable when one is making the decision regarding the severity of the condition and the need for operation. If the peripheral signs of aortic regurgitation are marked, the importance of a loud systolic murmur should be minimized. Cardiac catheterization and angiocardiography are of most value.

CHAPTER 13

Arteriosclerosis and Ischemic Heart Disease

ARTERIOSCLEROSIS IS UBIQUITOUS and produces well-known changes in the heart and the arterial system. It may involve predominantly the aorta and large arteries or it may be more marked in specialized areas, notably in the coronary artery system. The physical findings, and especially auscultatory phenomena, vary with the different types of involvement. An attempt will be made to separate these into their clinical categories.

General Arteriosclerosis

Arteriosclerosis may involve only the aorta and large vessels but often encroaches on the aortic ring and valve cusps. The proximal aorta is often dilated. This may result in accentuation of the aortic closure sound and basal systolic murmurs in the absence of hemodynamic obstruction. Apical systolic murmurs are much less frequent but may present a diagnostic problem. The following differential points are helpful:

1. Many apical systolic murmurs are transmitted from the aortic region. If the quality and timing of the murmurs are similar in the two regions, the murmur should be considered as arising at the aortic valve. This may be true even if the murmur is loudest at the apex because the sounds in the aortic region in older persons are diminished by an increase in the diameter of the chest or by emphysema (or both).

2. Many apical systolic murmurs are of rheumatic origin. The patient may admit, on questioning, that he has known about a murmur for many years. It is impressive how often a systolic murmur, previously unheard in an older person, turns out on autopsy to have been due to mild mitral involvement, often of rheumatic origin. These murmurs are usually high pitched and, if loud, can be recognized as being pansystolic. Less intense murmurs may not sound pansystolic.

3. The murmur should be carefully checked to see if it is actually of maximum intensity at the apex. Sometimes the murmur will be of maximum intensity midway between the apex and the sternal border. Such a murmur may be produced, like the innocent murmurs, by some changes in flow rather than by valvular involvement.

4. Arteriosclerotic involvement of the mitral valve or mitral annulus may sometimes be a cause of an apical systolic murmur. Calcification of the mitral annulus and base of the valve cusp occurs especially, though not exclusively, in elderly females. On occasion, it may be extremely marked. In some of these patients, marked mitral regurgitation with a loud harsh murmur is present. The murmur resembles that of aortic stenosis in quality but is pansystolic, maximum at the apex and widely transmitted.

Involvement of branches from the aortic arch results in systolic bruits heard over the subclavian arteries (supraclavicular fossae) or the carotids. Vertebral artery bruits occur rarely. Occasionally, carotid or subclavian bruits may be audible in high-flow states where obstruction is modest or inconsequential.

The abdominal aorta may be involved such that systolic bruits occur because of narrowing in its main portion, in the renal arteries, at the ileofemoral branchings, and less commonly in other branches such as the celiac or splenic arteries. These bruits are usually best heard in the epigastrium; rarely, renal artery stenosis may be best heard below the costal margins laterally and ileofemoral obstruction in the lower quadrants.

An unusual auscultatory phenomenon in arteriosclerosis is that due to stenosis of a large surface coronary artery; these murmurs are usually diastolic, rarely continuous, and are almost always best heard at the upper left sternal border or at the apex. They may be heard in the absence of clinical symptoms and are often accompanied by visible calcifications on roentgenography.

Acute Myocardial Ischemia

Arteriosclerotic obstruction of the coronary arteries results in the most common type of clinical heart disease. Its extreme prevalence has brought it under close scrutiny as a result of coronary care units and much has been added to our knowledge of the hemodynamic changes induced by ischemia and the auscultatory phenomena that reflect them. It is significant that auscultation, aided by palpation and other simple bedside methods, has attained a striking accuracy in this crucial area.

Ischemia is segmental and involves a variable portion of the myocardium. Hemodynamic changes invariably accompany ischemia; they include a reduction in contractile force, a decreased stroke volume, an increased enddiastolic volume, frequently an increased enddiastolic pressure, and usually a slight reduction in ejection time often accompanied by a prolonged isovolumic contraction time.

By far the most common of all auscultatory abnormalities present in acute ischemia is a fourth heart sound. This sound follows atrial contraction but precedes the onset of ventricular ejection and reflects the reduced compliance of the ischemic left ventricle. This sound has been shown to arise within the left ventricle and its origin is discussed in Chapter 5. It is often accompanied by a transient palpable presystolic impulse at the apex (this is determined by palpation at the apex and over a carotid artery simultaneously).

The fourth sound behaves in a characteristic fashion as follows:

1. During an episode of ischemia, the sound may appear or become prominent.

2. It may become clearly audible with little change throughout the respiratory cycle, whereas in the absence of an ischemic episode it tends to be maximal in expiration.

3. Its intensity with relation to the first sound may increase, and the interval between the fourth and first sounds may lengthen.

4. When the ischemic episode has subsided, the fourth sound may recede.

5. Because of the extremely low frequency of the fourth heart sound, it may at times be palpable when inaudible.

In acute ischemia, the first heart sound is reduced in both intensity and frequency, giving it a characteristic muffled quality. This results from the decreased contractility and the altered position of the mitral cusps (due to increased ventricular volume at the time of maximum tension).

The intensity of the first sound is difficult to judge but a change in its quality is common.

In acute ischemia, a *transient* apical systolic murmur of variable quality and duration may occur due to altered mitral valve function. It is most often due to papillary muscle dysfunction, or it may result from simple architectural disproportion between the mitral valve and the left ventricle when this chamber is suddenly dilated during an ischemic episode. The resulting murmur may be late crescendo or it may be pansystolic; its quality is often harsh and its radiation depends upon its loudness as well as upon the leaflet involved. When the posterior leaflet is abnormally positioned, the murmur may radiate anteriorly and be well heard at the left sternal border and even at the cardiac base. When the anterior mitral valve leaflet is involved, the murmur may be well transmitted to the left axilla and posterior chest. The appearance and disappearance of these murmurs can be striking. Their association with a late systolic click is a point of controversy. Clicks are definitely heard in this situation although a direct relationship can only be assumed (see the following section on acute myocardial infarction).

It is of interest that the first heart sound may be normal or increased, rather than decreased, in company with mitral systolic murmurs due to papillary muscle abnormalities. Thus, these murmurs are somewhat unique in that they may appear in conjunction with a prominent fourth sound and a loud first sound.

On rare occasions during an ischemic episode the second heart sound may be paradoxically split due to delayed emptying of the left ventricle. Another change that may occur in the second heart sound is accentuation of the pulmonic closure sound, reflecting myocardial failure.

Acute Myocardial Infarction

During the very early stage of myocardial infarction, auscultatory phenomena may be identical with those described for myocardial ischemic episodes. They tend, of course, to be of longer duration and in some cases permanent.

A paradoxical impulse may be visible and palpable anteriorly much more prominently than the paradoxical impulse present in a transient ischemic episode; this impulse reflects the infarcted segment, usually of the anterior wall. The greater the compliance of this segment, the more prominent it becomes. It is invariably accompanied by signs of myocardial dysfunction, that is, a fourth heart sound, a reduced intensity of the first sound, and occasionally a third sound. Short, nondescript and circumscribed systolic murmurs may also be present due to this noncontracting segment.

A pericardial friction sound is common. Indeed myocardial infarction is the most common cause of this auscultatory phenomenon. It is often evanescent, varying even from hour to hour, and is most common in the first three days. Friction sounds may occur with any site of myocardial infarction, although more commonly with anterior infarcts. These sounds are unmistakable as a rule, varying with respiration, having a scratchy, "superficial" quality, and when fully developed exhibiting three components (presystolic, systolic and early diastolic).

Papillary muscle dysfunction results in apical systolic murmurs of mitral valve origin (see Fig 7–4). They are somewhat more common with inferior myocardial infarction but may occur with infarction at any site. They are occasionally present in the acute stage, improving with healing of the infarct. When this murmur is pansystolic with the acute episode, it suggests more severe mitral regurgitation and is more likely to remain as a permanent finding. When it occurs as a late systolic crescendo murmur in the acute stage, it is more likely to disappear with time. If, on the other hand, the myocardium is extensively damaged and congestive heart failure supervenes, an initially late crescendo murmur may become pansystolic.

Infrequently, a late systolic click accompanies these murmurs. We have noted the murmurs and associated clicks to appear and disappear in the presence of acute myocardial infarctions, most notably in inferior myocardial infarction, and we have assumed a causal relationship. Authoritative opinion is divided on this subject and we concede that it is at least uncommon. However, the pathoanatomic relationship in the typical click-murmur syndrome and that seen in papillary muscle dysfunction do not seem disparate. Thus, it would appear almost inevitable that an occasional click will be detected in papillary muscle dysfunction if frequent auscultation is carried out. We cannot, of course, state categorically that a click-murmur phenomenon was not previously present in all these patients.

In recent years, it has become increasingly evident that apical systolic murmurs due to papillary muscle dysfunction may first appear during the convalescent period. In this setting, the murmurs most likely reflect change in the left ventricle resulting from healing of the infarct. Less often, congestive heart failure or reinfarction is causative.

Papillary muscle rupture is a dramatic event, producing a sudden loud systolic murmur that is widely transmitted. When this occurs, the posterior papillary muscle is involved more frequently than the anterior papillary muscle. The murmur is maximum at the apex and is accompanied by obvious signs of left ventricular failure. An accompanying thrill is not uncommon.

Perforation of the interventricular septum is also a dramatic event, most often developing abruptly and producing severe pulmonary vascular engorgement. The murmur is maximum to the left of the lower sternal edge and is high pitched with a varying degree of harshness. The clinical course of the patient will vary with the size of the shunt. There is usually a systolic thrill. The lesion occurs most commonly with anteroseptal myocardial infarction.

Perforation of the free wall of the left ventricle due to myocardial infarction is the most dramatic event of all. It may be accompanied by a harsh systolic murmur, although few of these murmurs are appreciated. They are, by definition, quite short lived since the patient's course is one of rapid deterioration, culminating in early death.

In the chronic stage of survivors of myocardial infarctions, certain auscultatory findings are common, if not characteristic. A fourth heart sound is almost invariable although it may diminish in intensity after the acute stage and move closer to the first sound. The first sound may resume a more normal character. With exercise or during acute ischemic episodes, the fourth sound will increase in intensity and move away from the first sound, and the first sound may again become muffled. Apical systolic murmurs may persist; they may be present at rest or may be heard only with exercise or during an ischemic episode. They may remain pansystolic and even be accompanied by a third heart sound. Nondescript systolic murmurs may be heard over an area of palpable akinesis (aneurysm) and are usually quite short, early or midsystolic in time, and generally unchanged by exercise.

CHAPTER 14

Auscultatory Phenomena in Various Conditions

Myocardial Failure

WHEN CONGESTIVE HEART FAILURE occurs, the cardinal features include chamber dilatation (an abnormal degree of fiber stretch); an elevated enddiastolic volume and pressure while stroke volume is reduced; usually an increased heart rate; and finally, a raised venous pressure. Important auscultatory phenomena result (Fig 14–1):

1. A fourth heart sound is almost invariable and a third sound is very common. These may be produced on the left side, the right side or both sides. With heart rates in excess of 100 beats per minute a summation sound is usually heard. When both sounds are present at a somewhat slower rate, they may separate in time and give the impression of a middiastolic murmur.

2. The first sound usually becomes diminished in intensity and muffled in character.

3. The pulmonic second sound increases in intensity and may become louder than the aortic second sound. Paradoxical splitting of the second sound may occasionally occur.

4. The murmur of mitral regurgitation may develop as a consequence of dilatation of the left ventricle and papillary muscle misalignment.

5. The systolic murmur of tricuspid regurgitation can occur as a result of right ventricular dilatation.

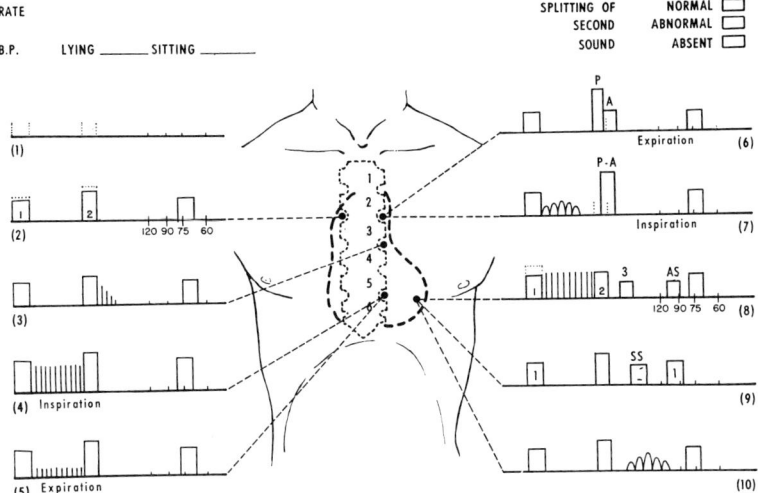

Fig 14–1.—Auscultatory findings in myocardiopathies and myocardial failure. The following features are shown:

　a. A third heart sound *(8)* at the apex and often in the mesocardiac area.

　b. An atrial sound at the apex *(8)*.

　c. A summation sound when the rate is rapid *(9)*.

　d. A high-pitched systolic murmur due to mitral regurgitation *(8)*. This may be a presenting sign with a primary myocardiopathy.

　e. Accentuation of the pulmonic second sound due to an increase in pulmonary artery pressure resulting from left ventricular failure *(6)*.

　f. Paradoxical splitting of the second heart sound *(6) (7)*. Left ventricular systole is, at times, prolonged because of myocardial weakness.

　g. A high-pitched, systolic murmur due to tricuspid regurgitation. This is louder in inspiration *(4)* than in expiration *(5)*.

　h. An apical middiastolic murmur may be heard occasionally *(10)*.

　i. A faint, early diastolic murmur of pulmonic regurgitation is heard on occasion *(3)*.

6. Rarely, an early diastolic murmur of pulmonic regurgitation may develop when pulmonary artery pressures are markedly elevated.

7. In some patients with a large left ventricle, an apical middiastolic murmur may be heard.

Cardiac Tumors

Involvement of the heart with tumor is uncommon. With the exception of intracardiac myxomas, none exhibits helpful auscultatory findings.

LEFT ATRIAL MYXOMA. — 1. Middiastolic and presystolic murmurs quite similar to those of mitral stenosis usually occur. Although the first sound is not accentuated, an early diastolic sound with the same timing as an opening snap of the mitral valve occurs in many cases ("tumor plop"); thus, left atrial myxoma is often mistaken for mitral stenosis.

2. A variation in the intensity of the murmurs in different positions and at different times may be striking and when present is virtually diagnostic. Unfortunately, this variation is not always present.

3. Occasionally only a systolic murmur is present and is due to extension of the tumor through the mitral valve.

RIGHT ATRIAL MYXOMA. — A tricuspid systolic murmur is more frequent than a diastolic murmur, but either or both may be heard. Unlike left atrial tumors, right atrial tumors do not usually produce auscultatory findings that mimic tricuspid stenosis.

Often, myxomas of either side, but especially of the right atrium, may produce murmurs that are strikingly unlike any murmur one may expect to hear, that is, systolic and diastolic or even continuous. These peculiar and "different" sounding murmurs should always suggest the diagnosis.

Cardiomyopathy

Regardless of the underlying cause, cardiomyopathy consists of an abnormality of cardiac muscle which results in decompensation, conduction defects, dysrhythmias and valvular dysfunction. Diastolic sounds with variable changes in the first sound as well as apical systolic murmurs of mitral origin occur even in the absence of cardiomegaly. The diagnosis of cardiomyopathy in the absence of a fourth sound is almost untenable. Third heart sounds occur somewhat less frequently, but both sounds are often present and may persist over long periods of time.

Hypertension and Hypertensive Heart Disease

The increased peripheral vascular resistance results in left ventricular hypertrophy and dilatation of the proximal aorta including the aortic valve ring. In addition, it is commonly associated with accelerated arteriosclerosis. These changes produce several abnormal auscultatory features:

1. The aortic second sound becomes accentuated (p. 43).

2. A fourth heart sound is common (p. 56).

3. Abdominal bruits may be heard due to luminal narrowing of the aorta or its branches or due to primary renal artery stenosis (p. 210).

4. With dilatation of the aorta and with arteriosclerotic involvement of the aortic valve, an aortic systolic murmur may occur (p. 114).

5. An early diastolic murmur of aortic regurgitation may be heard. This may come and go and vary in intensity with the degree of blood pressure elevation (p. 139).

6. A murmur of mitral regurgitation may result from left ventricular enlargement.

7. Rarely, an aortic ejection sound is present (p. 66).

8. With the appearance of decompensation, the findings are those of myocardial failure (p. 216).

Marfan's Syndrome

This inherited disorder of connective tissue involves primarily the elastic fibers of the aorta and results in cystic necrosis of the media. Less frequently, the mitral valve is affected, producing incompetence.

1. Aortic regurgitation may develop, often very rapidly, and the murmur may be maximal to the right of the sternum rather than to the left.

2. An accentuated aortic second sound may be present due to dilatation of the aorta and the more rapid closure of the aortic valve associated with the aortic regurgitation (p. 45).

3. When the mitral valve is involved, the resulting murmur is invariably that of regurgitation. Although most often pansystolic and slightly harsh, it may be the late crescendo systolic murmur more characteristic of leaflet prolapse, occasionally accompanied by a click.

Other connective tissue disorders, such as Ehlers-Danlos, pseudoxanthoma elasticum, and osteogenesis imperfecta, are rarely associated with aortic and mitral valvular abnormalities similar to that seen in Marfan's syndrome.

Pectus Excavatum and Straight Back Syndrome

This anatomical defect produces a systolic murmur, which may be confused with one due to organic disease, as well as a change in the first and second heart sounds and occasionally the appearance of diastolic filling sounds.

1. The pulmonic second sound is often increased. Expiratory splitting of the second sound may occasionally be heard, while inspiratory splitting may be exaggerated.

2. A rough, systolic murmur, maximum in the left second interspace but at times lower down the left border of the sternum, is common. Small pressure gradients across the right ventricular outflow tract have been measured in several cases.

3. The first sound may be increased in loudness at the lower end of the sternum.

4. A right-sided fourth sound may be present.

Thyrotoxicosis

Hyperthyroidism produces distinct effects on the heart and circulation. These are direct results of hypermetabolism, which increases heat production, and the specific effects of the increased concentration of circulating hormone. There is a diminished vascular resistance (especially in the skin and skeletal muscle, together constituting the largest vascular supply in the human body) and certain effects that appear to enhance myocardial contractility. The underlying mechanisms are not completely resolved, but the clinical results are an increased stroke volume, tachycardia, and a consequent increase in cardiac output.

In addition to arrhythmias, notably atrial fibrillation and ventricular premature contractions, cardiocirculatory influences produce these common auscultatory findings:

1. The first heart sound is usually accentuated and together with the tachycardia produces a "tick-tock" rhythm.

2. A third heart sound is not uncommon, especially in young adults, and a fourth sound is occasionally present.

3. A rough, scratchy, basal, systolic murmur is frequently present and may be due to increased flow in the aorta and pulmonary artery (Lerman-Means scratch).

4. An arterial systolic bruit over the thyroid gland is more often mentioned than heard.

5. A venous hum is frequently present in the neck.

6. Occasionally, a middiastolic flow murmur may be heard at the apex or mesocardiac area.

Cardiovascular Syphilis

The infection involves the ascending aorta; initially there is calcification, which is followed in about half the cases by the gradual development of one or more of the three important pathologic changes constituting "complicated" cardiovascular syphilis. These are ascending aortic aneurysm, stenosis of the coronary ostia and involvement of the aortic valve ring producing aortic regurgitation. Auscultatory features which commonly occur are:

1. A tympanitic and accentuated aortic second sound occasionally accompanied by an ejection systolic murmur is heard with aortic dilatation alone.

2. The diastolic murmur of aortic regurgitation results from dilatation of the aortic ring and widening of the commissures. This murmur may become extremely loud and is often maximal to the right of the sternum.

3. With marked aortic regurgitation, a systolic murmur is present in the aortic region. This murmur is produced by the dilatation of the aorta and the increased velocity of the blood flow through the aortic valve. The murmur may be loud and suggests the murmur of aortic stenosis.

4. A middiastolic and presystolic murmur may be heard at the apex (Austin Flint; p. 141).

5. An apical systolic murmur is usually present and may be transmitted from the aortic region or be the result of a relative mitral regurgitation.

6. A loud, very musical diastolic murmur occurs in some patients in whom an aortic cusp becomes retroverted.

7. The first heart sound may be diminished due to early closure of the mitral valve.

The auscultatory findings in some patients with cardiovascular syphilis may be indistinguishable from those heard in patients with rheumatic heart disease with combined mitral and aortic involvement.

Endocarditis

Endocarditis, regardless of the specific agent, is an invasion of the superficial tissues of the endocardium of the heart, especially of the valves. Mitral and aortic valves are most often involved, in that order, with tricuspid less and pulmonic valves least often affected. The process most often superimposes itself upon abnormal endocardium, notably chronic rheumatic valvulitis, less often congenital anomalies, and occasionally completely normal tissue. Therefore, auscultatory features usually include preexisting abnormalities. The following are common features:

1. In most patients there is evidence of valvular involvement as indicated by murmurs, but in older patients there may, at least for a while, be no murmurs.

2. The murmurs may show a variation in intensity from day to day, although more important is the development of new murmurs under observation. Occasionally, very loud aortic or mitral murmurs may develop as a result of valve leaflet perforation or chordal rupture.

3. If cardiac failure occurs, as it commonly does, its characteristic features are superimposed upon those of both the infectious process and any underlying pathology.

Pulmonary Embolism

Small pulmonary emboli may produce no auscultatory changes. Patients with massive embolism often show important changes which may appear abruptly and last for several days. The following points are helpful:

1. The pulmonic second sound is increased in intensity due to the elevation of the pulmonary artery pressure. This phenomenon is very helpful when present; however, for reasons not entirely clear, it is occasionally normal in the presence of significant pulmonary arterial obstruction. On occasion, right ventricular output may be so diminished that pulmonary artery pressures also fall, resulting in a pulmonic closure that is not accentuated.

2. Splitting is unpredictable. As indicated in Chapter 4 (p. 48), splitting depends primarily on the duration of right ventricular systole; if this period is reduced, reflecting a decreased stroke volume, then splitting may be narrow or ab-

sent. If right ventricular systole is maintained at a normal or increased duration, splitting may be normal or abnormally wide, failing to close on expiration (persistent splitting). Thus, while accentuation of pulmonic closure is dependent on pulmonary arterial pressure, splitting reflects the ability of the right ventricle to maintain its active state (which means that its systolic "effort" is normal, whether or not its stroke volume is normal).

3. A right-sided fourth sound may be heard.

4. A rough, systolic murmur may occur in the pulmonic area; rarely, a continuous murmur may be heard.

5. A faint to moderately loud murmur of tricuspid regurgitation is occasionally heard.

6. In addition to a pleural friction rub, a pericardial friction rub may occasionally be present.

Carcinoid Syndrome

Carcinoid tumors arise in argentaffine tissue, producing and releasing into the circulation excessive amounts of serotonin (5-hydroxytryptamine) and kallikreins. It is likely that as yet unidentified substances are involved as well. They arise primarily in the ileum, appendix and jejunum, although they have been known to arise in almost any segment of the gastrointestinal tract and even in ovarian and bronchial tissue. Except for the latter two, liver metastases appear necessary for the production of symptoms. A clear-cut relationship between the known chemical products and the cardiac lesions has not been proved.

Cardiac involvement consists of an intense inflammatory fibrosis of the endocardium. Presumably because the chemical products are altered or filtered out by the pulmonary circulation, the right side of the heart is affected almost exclusively. Thus, murmurs of tricuspid and pulmonic valvular origin typically occur.

The most common cardiac findings are a pansystolic murmur varying with respiration at the lower left sternal edge and a harsh, sometimes rough, ejection murmur at the left base. Less frequently, there may be a middiastolic murmur of tricuspid stenosis or the early diastolic murmur of pulmonic regurgitation. The latter may be low pitched or even rough, reflecting the minimal pulmonary arterial-right ventricular gradient.

Rarely, a high cardiac output state occurs, resulting in basal systolic murmurs due to turbulence. Congestive heart failure is rather common and may reduce the intensity of the murmurs and abolish the respiratory variation of the tricuspid murmur.

Ankylosing Spondylitis

Aortitis and aortic valvulitis with fibrosis of the leaflets and widening of the commissures occur in this disease (which is probably not related to rheumatoid arthritis). The resulting early diastolic murmur of aortic regurgitation is heard in a small percentage of patients, although autopsy findings are present in a much higher number. Other valves are not affected.

Rheumatoid Arthritis

Involvement of the heart at autopsy is extremely common in patients with rheumatoid arthritis, although lesions specific to this disease are as yet not clearly defined. Rheumatoid granulomas, which may occur in virtually any part of the heart, appear to be the only pathologic change exclusive to rheumatoid arthritis. Other abnormalities seen include: (1) pericarditis, (2) vasculitis, (3) aortic and rarely mitral valvular deformities and (4) myocarditis.

The lesions producing common auscultatory abnormalities are pericarditis and aortic valvular deformity. Pericarditis produces the typical scratchy, superficial friction sounds common to all types of pericardial inflammation.

The most frequent valvular manifestation is aortic stenosis, due to either or both granulomatous involvement and endocarditis similar to that seen in rheumatic fever. This results in the typical ejection systolic murmur heard at the right base and transmitted into the carotids. Rarely, the early diastolic murmur of aortic regurgitation, the middiastolic murmur of mitral stenosis, or the pansystolic murmur of mitral regurgitation is present.

Systemic Lupus Erythematosus (SLE)

Like rheumatoid arthritis, SLE causes a single cardiac lesion exclusive to itself: the atypical verrucous endocarditis of

Libman and Sacks. These lesions are characterized by degenerative and inflammatory reactions which become nodular or verrucous and involve any portion of the endocardium, notably the chordae tendineae and leaflet tissue of the mitral and tricuspid valves. These changes are detectable at autopsy in one fourth to one half of patients with SLE, but clinically significant valve abnormalities are much less common.

When valvular function is sufficiently compromised, mitral and/or tricuspid regurgitation result with the appearance of pansystolic murmurs appropriate to these abnormalities. Instances of aortic regurgitation have been described. The murmurs may wax and wane with the activity of the underlying autoimmune mechanism, occasionally coincident with the administration of corticosteroids.

Again like rheumatoid arthritis, pericarditis is the most common cardiac lesion seen in SLE, clinically and at autopsy. The associated friction rub(s) have been described in previous sections, there being no distinguishing auscultatory features in any of the etiologic entities. Myocarditis is occasionally found at autopsy.

Other disease entities related pathologically to SLE include scleroderma, polymyositis and polyarteritis nodosa. Unlike SLE, these less common diseases rarely produce specific cardiac lesions and even the nonspecific ones are unusual.

Methysergide-Induced Endocarditis

Methysergide infrequently produces retroperitoneal fibrosis. Endocarditis is a rare accompaniment and is due to an inflammatory type of fibrosis.

Aortic regurgitation is the most common finding although mitral regurgitation is rarely present. Although rare, a patient presenting with symptoms of retroperitoneal fibrosis, a murmur of aortic regurgitation, and a history of taking methysergide may benefit from stopping the medication, since the lesions tend to regress.

Vascular murmurs may be present over the abdomen. This is due to stenosis of arteries involved in the fibrosis and may affect mesenteric or renal vessels.

CHAPTER 15

Postsurgical Sounds

WITH THE ADVENT of cardiovascular surgery, marked alteration in physical findings may be effected in patients with cardiovascular disease. It is essential for the clinician to become familiar with many of these changes.

A pericardial friction rub invariably occurs following open heart surgery and may persist for days and sometimes weeks. A friction rub may recur weeks or months after surgery as a part of the "postpericardiotomy syndrome," including fever, malaise and pericardial effusion. This is believed to be a type of autoimmune reaction identical with the postmyocardial infarction syndrome of Dressler.

Prosthetic Valves

While all four heart valves may be replaced by prosthetic devices, the aortic and mitral valves are most commonly replaced, with tricuspid valve replacement far less common, and pulmonic valve replacement most unusual. A large number of prosthetic devices have been introduced and many of them subsequently abandoned. A detailed discussion of all devices is beyond the scope of this book.

Prosthetic devices can be characterized into four basic types (Fig 15–1): (1) ball in cage—e.g., Starr-Edwards, Cutter-Smelloff; (2) floating disc—e.g., Beall, Kay-Shiley; (3) tilting disc—e.g., Björk-Shiley; and (4) homografts and heterografts.

Ball valves, tilting disc valves, and homografts have been used in all valve positions, whereas the floating disc devices

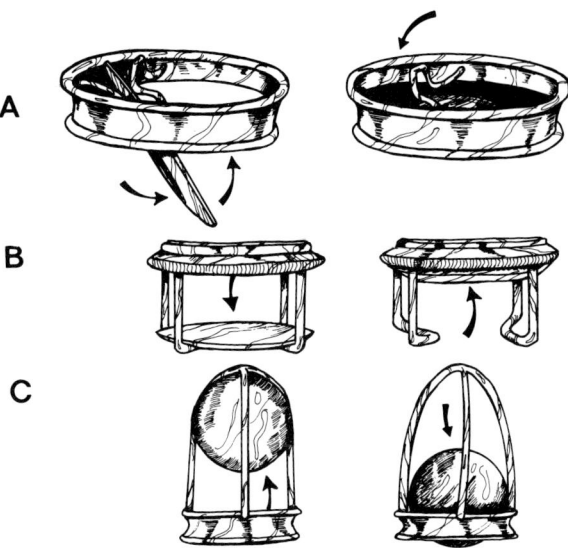

Fig 15–1.—Prosthetic heart valves. Open position on the left and closed position on the right. **A,** Björk-Shiley tilting disc valve. Note that in opening the occluder pivots around a steel strut but strikes nothing at the point of maximum excursion. The opening sound of this valve is consequently relatively quiet. **B,** Beall floating lenticular valve. The excursion of the occluder is limited by two steel struts in the open position and by the valve ring when closed. **C,** Starr-Edwards ball valve. The ball is limited in its excursion by the steel struts and the valve ring. In the process of opening, especially when in the aortic position, the ball may "bounce" at the apex of the cage, producing multiple clicking sounds in addition to a systolic murmur. All valves are shown without their cloth sewing rings.

are reserved for the mitral or tricuspid areas. Homografts and heterografts have no characteristic auscultatory findings and are indistinguishable from normal valves on physical examination. Postoperative development of regurgitant murmurs is not uncommon with these valves however.

In the aortic position, ball valves and tilting disc valves have an opening sound which frequently obscures the first sound, and a closing sound which replaces the aortic component of the second sound. These prosthetic sounds are far more prominent with the ball than with the disc-type devices. In both instances the sounds are sharp and of high frequency. They are generally described as "crisp" and "clicking," and may be audible at the bedside without the aid of a stethoscope. Ball valves are frequently audible at a considerable distance from the patient. The opening sound of a ball valve in the aortic area usually consists of multiple vibrations of the ball in the apex of the cage at the onset of ejection. The closing sound is sharp and usually single. A loud, harsh, midsystolic murmur is usually present, especially with ball-type prostheses.

In the mitral and tricuspid areas the opening sound of a prosthetic valve corresponds in timing to an opening snap (Fig 15–2). The closing sound coincides with the first heart sound.

Regurgitation through a prosthetic valve may occur through the valve ring due to malfunction of the occluder or, with dehiscence of the suture line, around the valve ring (paravalvular). These regurgitant murmurs generally have the same auscultatory characteristics of similar murmurs in the native valve, but significant regurgitation has been known to occur with mitral valve dehiscence in the absence of a murmur. The following points should lead one to suspect valve dysfunction: the development of a murmur when none was present, a change in the character of an existing murmur, the muffling or loss of one or more of the components of the prosthetic sounds, or inconstancy of prosthetic sounds in a patient in sinus rhythm. More grave signs include the develop-

Fig 15–2. – Sounds produced by a prosthetic (Starr-Edwards) mitral valve. The closing sound *(CS)* and opening sound *(OS)* produced by the valve have a similar quality and are sharp and clicking. The closing sound has the position of the first heart sound. The opening sound corresponds to the opening snap of the mitral valve. Following the opening sound, there is a series of clicking sounds which is apparently produced by the ball bouncing in its cage.

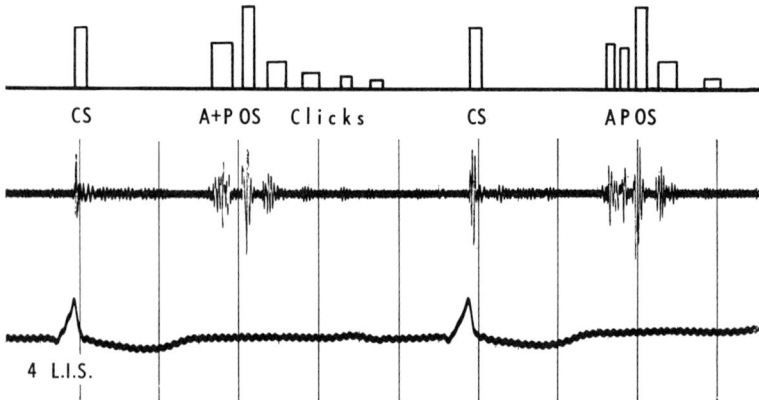

CS   A+P OS   Clicks   CS   AP OS

4 L.I.S.

ment of congestive heart failure, pulmonary edema, severe hemolysis or systemic emboli. Some specific findings reflecting malfunction peculiar to certain valve prostheses have been described. Most of these are relevant to prostheses no longer in common use and will not be detailed here. Likewise, the use of sound spectroscopy has not found wide acceptance in detecting prosthetic valve malfunction.

Pacemakers

Several auscultatory phenomena are associated with implanted cardiac pacemakers. These devices generally are used to stimulate the ventricular myocardium and are consequently associated with wide splitting of the heart sounds due to the wide QRS complex. With right ventricular endocardial pacemakers, a left bundle branch block pattern occurs and the splitting of the second heart sound may be paradoxical. In the presence of atrioventricular dissociation and regular atrial activity, a variable intensity of the first sound will occur due to the varying P-R interval (p. 34), and diastolic atrial sounds may be heard.

Occasionally a clicking sound immediately preceding the first sound is heard, which has been shown to be due to intercostal or diaphragmatic muscle activation and may sometimes be an indication of penetration of the pacing wire through the myocardium. A pericardial friction rub is a common occurrence in the latter situation. Surprisingly, perforation is rarely of serious import and is treated by simple retraction of the pacing wire. Intercostal and diaphragmatic activity is frequently associated with visible and palpable rhythmic twitching of the affected muscle.

A systolic murmur may develop following transvenous pacemaker implantation, which has the characteristics of tricuspid regurgitation and is thought to result from interference with tricuspid valve function by the pacing wire in the ventricle. The development of a systolic murmur, however, does not necessarily indicate the presence of tricuspid regurgitation.

Valve Surgery

Surgical procedures on stenotic mitral valves will generally reduce the intensity and alter the quality of the murmur. It is unusual, however, for mitral valve commissurotomy to completely eliminate a murmur of stenosis or even for it to result in the disappearance of an opening snap. With the advent of cardiopulmonary bypass surgery, commissurotomies done by this method have yielded improved results (p. 206).

A murmur of regurgitation may appear postoperatively as a complication of mitral valvular commissurotomy. Repair of regurgitant valves, usually by an annuloplasty, may diminish or eliminate a murmur of valvular regurgitation of either mitral or tricuspid origin.

Aortic and pulmonic valvular stenosis of congenital origin is occasionally treated by valvulotomy. Postoperatively a systolic murmur of lesser intensity generally persists, and a murmur of valvular regurgitation commonly appears. An ejection click, if present preoperatively, will be diminished or absent after surgery.

Tricuspid regurgitation often results from severe pulmonary hypertension as is commonly seen with long-standing severe mitral stenosis. Following the relief of the latter, the murmur of secondary tricuspid regurgitation tends to disappear over the ensuing weeks. A Graham Steell murmur of pulmonary regurgitation will likewise disappear.

Congenital Heart Surgery

Successful closure of an intra- or extracardiac shunt (ASD, VSD, PDA, etc.) eliminates the murmur associated with these defects (see Chapter 11). The wide, fixed splitting of the second heart sound, associated with an atrial septal defect, moves normally with respiration following surgical repair, although complete closure in expiration may not occur.

A method of surgical treatment of tetralogy of Fallot consists of the establishment of an aortopulmonary anastomosis to increase the pulmonary blood flow. A number of these "shunt procedures" have been introduced, including the Blalock-Taussig technique of anastomosing the left subclavian artery to the left pulmonary artery, and the Pott's procedure of anastomosing the main pulmonary artery to the aorta. In each instance a loud continuous murmur is produced at the site of anastomosis. With the advent of total correction at an early age, shunt procedures have become less popular. Following total

correction, a murmur of some degree of right ventricular outflow obstruction commonly persists.

Following surgical correction of coarctation of the aorta, the
characteristic systolic murmur is eliminated, blood pressure in
the extremities may be normalized, and a brachial-femoral
pulse lag disappears.

Coronary Revascularization

Surprisingly, revascularization procedures using aortocor-
onary saphenous vein grafts, internal mammary grafts, and
internal mammary artery implantations are not generally associated with murmurs, although there have been a few reports
of systolic or continuous murmurs.

Aneurysm Resection

Successful resection of a ventricular aneurysm is generally
associated with a reduction or disappearance of the left precordial paradoxical bulge associated with the aneurysm. The
occasionally associated systolic murmur may disappear.

DISSECTING HEMATOMA (ANEURYSM) OF THE AORTA. — This
grave and commonly fatal event is associated with the abrupt
appearance of physical signs, which may disappear with successful surgical correction. A brief, harsh systolic murmur
heard at the base occasionally reflects turbulent flow into the
"entry site" or intimal tear. Vascular bruits may appear in the
neck, subclavicular areas, abdomen or femoral areas when
peripheral arterial flow is compromised by the dissection. A
blood pressure discrepancy between limbs suggests arterial
compromise of a limb and peripheral pulses may be lost. Occasionally a bisferiens pulse may be felt in one or both femoral
arteries, indicating dissection to this level and probably reflecting a delay in the pulse transmission in the false channel
when compared to the true. Finally, the appearance of a murmur of aortic regurgitation is a very grave sign prognostically,
for it indicates dissection proximally to the level of the aortic
valve and disruption of leaflet function. A pericardial friction
rub and signs of cardiac tamponade are indicative of dissection into the pericardium.

As stated above, surgical correction, involving either oversewing of the aorta or insertion of a graft, usually results in disappearance of vascular bruits, equalization of blood pressure in the limbs, and loss of the systolic murmur. The diastolic murmur may persist unless the aortic valve is repaired, usually by valve replacement.

Idiopathic Hypertrophic Subaortic Stenosis

Recently this entity has been successfully corrected surgically. The postoperative findings have generally been a reduction in the intensity of the systolic murmur and occasionally complete disappearance, even following maneuvers commonly used to elicit the murmur.

Other Prosthetic Devices

A number of other prosthetic devices have been introduced in the management of cardiovascular disorders; one in common use is a counterpulsation technique using an intra-aortic balloon. This is generally introduced via the femoral artery and synchronized with the cardiac cycle so that it expands in diastole, displacing its volume of blood, and collapses in systole. It thereby augments the cardiac output by assisting flow in diastole. On auscultation a prominent "squishing" sound is heard in systole and diastole, which may obscure the heart sounds.

CHAPTER 16

Nonauscultatory Findings in Cardiovascular Disease

MANY SIGNS of cardiovascular disease are easily recognized by examination of the chest wall. A proper study includes inspection for chest wall deformities, abnormal pulsations or movements, palpation for abnormal cardiac or vascular activity, and correlation of these findings with auscultatory events.

CHEST WALL DEFORMITIES. — Those deformities associated with cardiovascular disease include:

1. Precordial prominence as seen in right ventricular overload states, such as atrial septal defect where the prominence is usually predominantly in the left parasternal region, and ventricular septal defect where the prominence is generally more symmetrical.

2. Sternal depression (pectus excavatum; p. 220) is of no clinical significance unless severe, in which case cardiac compression against the thoracic vertebrae can occur, producing murmurs of right ventricular outflow obstruction and symptoms of breathlessness and palpitation. Cardiac output with effort may be reduced and surgical correction may be indicated. On the other hand, marked sternal prominence (pectus carinatum) is of no cardiovascular significance.

3. Examination of the back may reveal absence of the normal kyphotic curve of the upper spine. In conjunction with a narrow anterior posterior diameter of the chest, this may be a clue to the presence of the "straight back syndrome" and can be confirmed by auscultatory and radiographic examination (see p. 220).

233

4. Kyphoscoliosis, when severe, may lead to cor pulmonale.

Following thoracoplasty or pneumonectomy, there is frequently a considerable shift of the mediastinum, obscuring the location of cardiac landmarks. The presence of traumatic and surgical scars on the chest may suggest that unusual vascular sounds are due to an acquired arteriovenous fistula.

CARDIAC PULSATIONS OR MOVEMENTS. — With the patient in the supine position, and preferably with tangential light, a number of pulsations may be visible as well as palpable on the chest wall, especially in the presence of cardiac disease.

Inspection and palpation should begin with a search for the apex beat. The apex beat is usually the point of maximum impulse (PMI). In pathological states, however, an abnormal impulse, more prominent than the apex beat, may be present and may be located elsewhere than over the apex of the heart.

In the normal heart the apex beat is usually detected by light palpation. It is an area 1 – 2 cm in diameter in the left fifth intercostal space at or medial to the midclavicular line. The apex beat moves outward during initial (isovolumic) contraction of the ventricle prior to opening of the aortic valve. If not readily felt in the supine position, the PMI can generally be detected (more laterally) in the left decubitus position. It is a brief, nonsustained and single impulse. In pathological situations a number of alterations may be seen in the apex beat.

With left ventricular hypertrophy without dilatation, the apical impulse becomes more diffuse and sustained. Left ventricular dilatation tends to displace the apical impulse laterally and inferiorly. A diffuse systolic heave adjacent to the sternum, felt best with the palm of the hand, generally denotes right ventricular enlargement. Rarely, dilatation of the left atrium displaces the heart anteriorly and may result in a false impression of a right ventricular heave. Abnormal (dyskinetic) motion involving the anterior left ventricular wall can frequently be felt or seen as an outward systolic movement in the left precordium. Such a finding is common following large anterior wall infarctions and may be seen transiently during ischemic attacks. Following myocardial infarction it frequently disappears in one or two weeks. Its persistence is highly indicative of a left ventricular aneurysm.

Double and sometimes triple apex beats may be felt. A double impulse frequently represents a forceful atrial contraction against a thickened noncompliant ventricle. It is always associated with auscultatory findings of a fourth heart sound and is felt in the same conditions in which the latter is heard (aortic stenosis, systemic hypertension, acute myocardial infarction and cardiomyopathies). Palpable atrial activity, of course, is far less common than is the auscultatory equivalent. A left ventricular filling sound (S_3) may sometimes also be palpated, especially in situations of marked left ventricular dilatation (Fig 16–1).

In muscular subaortic stenosis, systolic ejection consists of a rapid phase followed by a slow phase. As a result there is an initial apical thrust followed by a more diffuse outward movement, giving the impression of a double apical impulse (Fig 16–2). In some situations, however, this double impulse is due to a palpable atrial contraction, as described above.

When the first heart sound is readily palpable separate from the apex beat, it is suggestive of mitral stenosis (Cossio's sign).

Visible and palpable pulsations are common in the left sec-

Fig 16–1.—A palpable summation sound *(SS)*. The patient was a young man with severe cardiomyopathy and congestive heart failure. A kinetocardiogram *(KG)* at the apex records a double outward motion corresponding to a left ventricular thrust in systole and another outward motion in diastole coinciding with the summation sound.

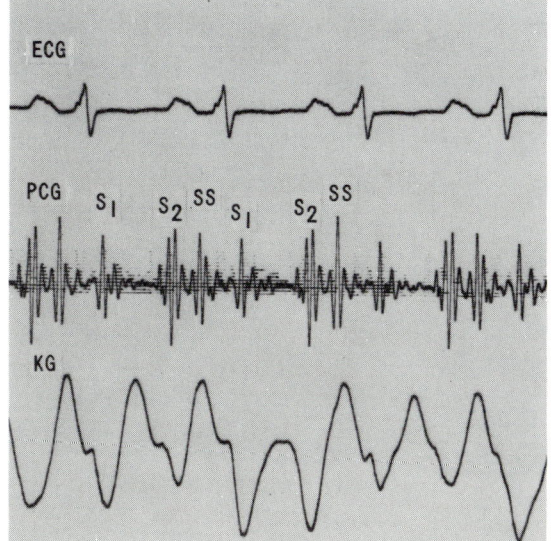

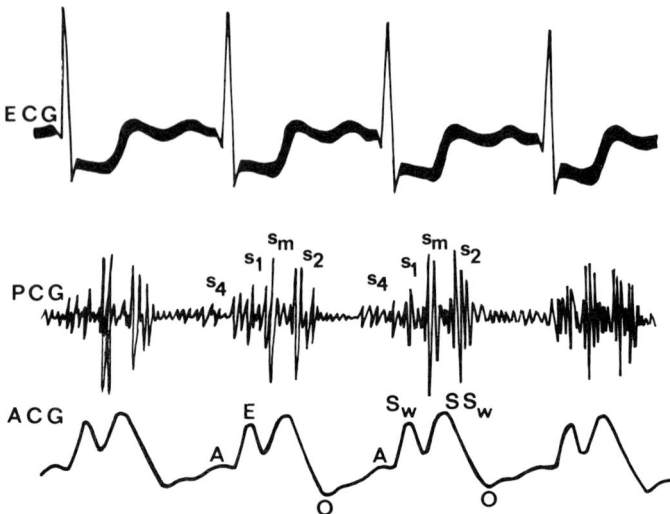

Fig 16–2. — Muscular subaortic stenosis. The apexcardiogram *(ACG)* demonstrates a double impulse. The first systolic wave (S_w) is followed by a
second and broader wave (SS_w). The first of these corresponds to the initial
rapid ejection of blood from the ventricle beginning at the *E* point. Ejection
is suddenly slowed in early systole due to the subvalvular obstruction which
develops as the ventricle contracts, and there is a second outward movement
of the apex béginning at this point.

In other patients, a double impulse appears to be due to a palpable A-
wave associated with forceful atrial contraction, followed by a single ventricular component. *PCG* = phonocardiogram mid-left sternal border; s_m =
systolic murmur; *A* = A-wave; *O* = O point.

ond intercostal space (pulmonic area), especially in young
slender individuals, due to the proximity of the main and left
pulmonary arteries to the chest wall in this area. However,
prominent pulsations in this area in an adult suggest pulmonary artery dilatation due to pulmonary hypertension or high
flow into the pulmonary artery, as seen with left-to-right
shunts. A palpable shock of pulmonic valve closure with a
loud pulmonic second sound helps to confirm a high-pressure
rather than a high-flow state. Pulsation in the aortic area is far
less common but may be seen in the presence of aortic dilatation due to aneurysm of the ascending aorta or in severe aortic
regurgitation.

On rare occasions visible and palpable pulsations may be
detectable in the intercostal arteries, especially along the pos-

terior and lateral thorax, denoting a coarctation of the aorta with marked dilatation of intercostal collateral channels.

Detection of thrills adds very little to what has already been learned from auscultation and will therefore be discussed only briefly. A thrill generally denotes the palpable, lowest-frequency components of very loud murmurs. Consequently even loud murmurs with a few low-frequency components are rarely accompanied by palpable thrills (e.g., aortic, pulmonic or mitral regurgitation). On the other hand, aortic valvular stenosis, especially when severe, is frequently accompanied by a systolic thrill at the upper right sternal border and may be associated with a carotid artery "shudder." The diastolic thrill of mitral stenosis is generally felt medial to the apex beat and is felt best in the lateral decubitus position. The thrill of a ventricular septal defect is most prominent along the lower left sternal border.

When cardiac activity is not detectable by palpation or inspection of the chest wall, light percussion may aid in locating the heart borders.

Blood Pressure and Pulse

Sphygmomanometric measurement of the blood pressure and examination of peripheral pulses are essential parts of every cardiovascular examination.

METHOD OF DETERMINATION.—The ideal cuff is one in which the inflatable bladder almost completely surrounds the limb and extends over two thirds of the proximal portion of the extremity being used. The cuff is rapidly inflated and the bell or diaphragm of the stethoscope is placed over the brachial or popliteal artery. The cuff is slowly deflated and the first appearance of audible Korotkoff sounds is the systolic pressure. As the cuff is further deflated, the sounds abruptly become muffled and then disappear. These latter two events usually occur within 10 mm of each other. It is generally accepted that the complete disappearance of sound best approximates the true diastolic pressure, but when these two events are widely separated it is reasonable to record both in addition to the systolic pressure (e.g., 170/70/40). The position of the patient and the limb used should always be recorded.

The intensity and clarity of the Korotkoff sounds are dependent in part on the capacity and distensibility of the arterial bed distal to the cuff. These factors in turn may be limited by venous trapping in the process of inflating the cuff. Consequently, the sounds may be enhanced by maneuvers designed to limit venous trapping, including elevation of the arm prior to cuff inflation and rapid inflation of the cuff to prevent venous engorgement, which occurs while the cuff exceeds venous pressure and before it attains systolic pressure. When the cuff is deflated to listen for the sounds, it should always be completely deflated prior to repeat inflation, to allow for venous drainage as well as patient comfort. Opening and closing of the hand several times after the cuff pressure exceeds systolic pressure dilates the peripheral arteries and likewise enhances the audibility of the Korotkoff sounds.

Occasionally there is an auscultatory gap between the first few sounds, representing systolic pressure, and the reappearance of the sounds at a lower pressure. This pitfall can be avoided if the pulse is felt while the cuff is inflated, for it must disappear when systolic pressure is exceeded. More rapid inflation of the cuff may also eliminate an auscultatory gap.

In addition to blood pressure recording by direct arterial puncture, other methods of recording the blood pressure include a Doppler technique and the flush method in infants. The latter is performed by wrapping an extremity tightly from distal to proximal portion, and placing the cuff proximally and inflating it. The wrapping is removed and the cuff is slowly deflated. The appearance of a flush to the skin is an approximation of the systolic pressure.

While blood pressure recorded in the legs by the usual methods may reveal a greater pressure than in the arms, this finding is usually artifactual due to improper cuff size and the larger muscle mass in the leg. True blood pressure is normally equal in both the upper and lower extremities. A simpler method of recording blood pressure in the lower legs is to use a standard-size cuff wrapped around the calf and palpating for the pulse in the dorsalis pedis or posterior tibial arteries. By this method only systolic pressure, of course, can be obtained.

Pulses should be searched for and notated in the radial, brachial, carotid, femoral, popliteal, posterior tibial and dorsalis pedis arteries. Those in the feet may be difficult to feel if the pulse volume is small but should be recorded if only for future reference. The dorsalis pedis artery is absent in a small percentage of persons, and a lateral tarsal may be felt instead. A decrease and delay in the femoral pulse, when simultaneously compared with the brachial, strongly suggest coarctation of the aorta.

Changes in the quality of the pulse result from alterations in stroke volume and the degree of peripheral vasoconstriction or vasodilatation present. Such changes are best appreciated in the carotid or femoral arteries which lie nearest the heart. The brachial pulse is less and the radial least sensitive in this respect.

INFORMATION OBTAINED. — In addition to detecting the presence of hypertension or hypotension, a considerable amount of additional information may be obtained from sphygmomanometry. The normal pulse pressure (difference between systolic and diastolic pressure) is 30–60 mm mercury, and the presence of an unusually wide or narrow pulse pressure may be a strong clue to a number of disease entities. In the presence of significant aortic regurgitation, there is virtually always a widening of the pulse pressure and when diastolic pressure is below 70 mm mercury it indicates significant disease. The peripheral signs of widened pulse pressure, such as capillary pulsation, head nodding, and Duroziez's sign, provide little additional information.

In some of these patients, sounds may be heard over the artery with the cuff pressure at 0, and therefore the muffling of the sounds more closely approximates true diastolic pressure. The same phenomenon associated with a wide pulse pressure and bounding pulse is sometimes seen in hyperkinetic states, e.g., after exercise and in association with anemia, thyrotoxicosis, high fever, pregnancy, systemic arteriovenous fistulas, and the so-called idiopathic hyperkinetic state thought to be a forerunner of essential hypertension. Wide pulse pressures, generally with normal diastolic pressures, are seen in patients with generalized atherosclerosis and decreased compliance of the aortic wall.

Conversely, a narrow pulse pressure associated with a thready pulse is occasionally a forerunner of circulatory collapse, in which case the systolic and diastolic blood pressures approach each other before a drop in both. A rising diastolic pressure, in the presence of a normal systolic pressure, may be an early sign of cardiac tamponade.

A small pulse with a delayed rise is characteristic of aortic valvular stenosis. This results from prolonged ejection of blood through a narrowed orifice and it correlates with the severity of stenosis. A high systolic pressure is rarely associated with significant aortic stenosis. On rare occasions a deflection can be felt on the upstroke of the pulse and is more easily demonstrated by intra-arterial pressure recording. This is called an *anacrotic notch*. In typical aortic stenosis, the pulse usually only confirms what one hears on auscultation. The character of the pulse assumes greater importance in two specific situations where left ventricular outflow obstruction is under consideration. In the patient terminally ill with aortic stenosis, a systolic murmur may become soft or actually inaudible due to severe congestive heart failure and diminished flow. A narrow pulse pressure with slow rise may alert the physician to check for other signs of tight aortic stenosis, such as left ventricular hypertrophy on electrocardiogram or calcification in the aortic valve on fluoroscopy. In the other instance, the murmur of aortic stenosis may be confused with that of idiopathic hypertrophic subaortic stenosis (IHSS). A slow, small pulse indicates valvular stenosis, whereas a pulse with rapid rise and collapse tends to favor IHSS (see Fig 7 – 12).

In some normal individuals the systolic blood pressure while standing is slightly lower than while supine, whereas in others this difference may be marked and may actually lead to syncope. Marked postural hypotension is seen in hypovolumic states, cardiogenic shock, hypersensitive carotid sinus syndrome, after use of ganglionic blocking agents or vasodilators, and in most patients after prolonged bed rest.

With failure of the left ventricle there is commonly the development of pulsus alternans and this phenomenon is frequently more easily detected by observing the Korotkoff sounds at systolic pressure where alternate sounds are audible than by palpation of the pulse.

Pulsus paradoxus is a term describing the exaggerated fall in systolic pressure during inspiration, occurring most typically in cardiac tamponade and pericardial constriction. It is actually found most commonly, however, in patients with chronic obstructive lung disease and cor pulmonale. With the cuff inflated to just greater than systolic pressure, the pressure is reduced slowly. The sounds will be audible during normal expiration but not during inspiration for as much as 10 mm below peak systolic pressure in normal individuals, and for 20 or more millimeters of mercury in patients demonstrating pulsus paradoxus. It is clear that the phenomenon is not at all paradoxical but is simply an exaggeration of a normal process.

Blood pressure recorded in both arms is generally quite similar. However, a marked discrepancy in blood pressure between the arms is found in a number of conditions and may be a clue to the diagnosis. Coarctation of the aorta most commonly occurs just beyond the origin of the left subclavian artery. If it occurs proximal to the left subclavian, it results in a lower blood pressure (15 mm or more systolic) in the left arm. Aortic dissection may occlude one or the other subclavian artery, resulting in marked discrepancy in blood pressure between the arms. Atherosclerotic occlusion of one or the other subclavian, commonly at the origin, will give rise to a marked discrepancy in blood pressure between arms; this may be accompanied by a subclavian "steal" syndrome, whereby flow in the vertebral artery on that side is reversed and supplies the subclavian via the circle of Willis. The runoff of blood from the cerebral circulation may result in neurologic signs and symptoms greatly exacerbated by exercising the respective arm. Pulse differences may result from a peculiar form of arteritis affecting the great vessels, resulting in a loss of pulses and pressures in one or the other extremity (Takayasu's or pulseless disease). Thoracic outlet syndrome, systemic embolus, and vascular trauma are other causes of a marked difference in blood pressure between the arms.

Abnormally low or absent blood pressure in the legs is seen in coarctation of the aorta, dissecting hematoma of the aorta, Leriche syndrome, atherosclerotic occlusive disease of the femoral arteries, and saddle embolism to the aortic bifurcation.

Venous Pressure and Pulsations

Inspection of the jugular venous pressure is an indispensable part of the cardiac examination. To study the jugular pulsations properly, the lighting must be good and a backrest provided which can be tilted to the desired angle. The ideal position (between 30 and 90 degrees) is one that allows observation of the oscillating top of the column of blood in the internal jugular vein. Since this vein freely communicates with the superior vena cava and right atrium, its pressure level accurately reflects that in the right atrium at all stages in the cardiac cycle.

The location of the internal jugular pulse is anterior to the sternomastoid muscle, where it may be confused with the carotid pulse. It differs from the arterial pulse by showing (1) a venous wave pattern (described below), by (2) a tendency to collapse on inspiration, by (3) easy obliteration with gentle finger pressure at the base of the neck, and by a (4) rise in pressure on abdominal compression especially in pathologic states. Both sides of the neck should be examined since a rise on one side may occur from localized, external obstruction of that vein.

Two main observations are usually possible from neck vein examination: the level of venous pressure and the primary type of venous wave pattern. The sternal angle (the transverse ridge between manubrium and body of the sternum) provides a useful reference point for measuring the venous pressure. The center of the right atrium lies about 5 cm below the sternal angle whether the subject is upright or horizontal. The distance between the top of the oscillating venous column and the sternal angle plus 5 cm will therefore represent the peak central venous pressure. Normally this figure does not exceed 8 cm.

Elevation of the venous pressure usually means an increase in right atrial pressure. In turn, this finding indicates an abnormality of the tricuspid or pulmonary valve, pulmonary hypertension or right ventricular failure. If the venous pressure exceeds 20 cm, the internal jugular vein will be maximally distended and visible at the angle of the jaw with the patient sitting upright, and the normal fluctuations will not be visible at this level. Absence of any detectable venous pulse in any position is a finding associated with circulatory collapse due to hypovolemia. Obstruction of the superior vena cava by clot or tumor may produce marked elevations of jugular venous pressure, usually without much pulsation, and must be distinguished from an elevated central venous pressure.

ECG

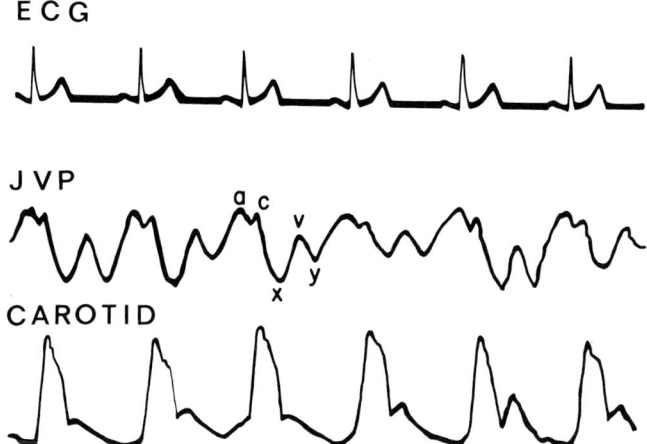

Fig 16–3.—A normal jugular venous pulse, taken simultaneously with a carotid pulse.

The normal venous pulsations consist of an a, a c, and a v-wave (Fig 16–3). Right atrial contraction produces the a-wave, which disappears in atrial fibrillation. The c-wave is thought to result from forceful closure of the tricuspid valve during systole. It appears to have little clinical significance. The v-wave is thought to result from a small increase in right atrial pressure during ventricular ejection. The downward slope that follows the a-wave is called the x-descent and that occurring after the v-wave is the y-descent. With rapid heart rate and less than ideal conditions, recognition of the waves is quite difficult and of limited value.

The a-wave can be recognized by listening to the apex beat and palpating the carotid artery. It occurs just before the first heart sound or carotid pulse and has a sharp rise and fall. The v-wave occurs just after the arterial pulse and has a slower, undulating pattern.

Pathologic states alter these waves in characteristic fashion. A large a-wave occurs with tricuspid stenosis, elevated right ventricular pressure from pulmonary stenosis or right ventricular failure, or from long-standing pulmonary hypertension.

When there is dissociation between atrial and ventricular contraction, some of the atrial contractions occur when the tricuspid valve is closed during ventricular systole. This produces a markedly accentuated a-wave, which has been called a *giant* or *cannon a-wave*. Irregular cannon a-waves may occur with slow heart rates (complete heart block) or with rapid rates due to ventricular tachycardia. Regularly occurring cannon waves with each heart beat result from junctional rhythms which may be rapid or slow (see Table 10–1).

Prominent v-waves develop mainly when congestive heart failure, usually with pulmonary hypertension, is present. They are most apparent with atrial fibrillation. They also occur with tricuspid regurgitation and become more prominent on inspiration. In the latter instance, the large v-waves are an invaluable sign and may be present when the characteristic murmur is absent. With more advanced degrees of tricuspid regurgitation, transmitted venous waves produce pulsations in the liver, in the superficial veins, in the extremities, and even in the orbits.

Pericardial effusion with tamponade or pericardial constriction is also likely to elevate the jugular venous pressure during inspiration (Kussmaul's sign).

A rapid *y*-descent, or diastolic collapse of the venous pulse, is characteristic of constrictive pericarditis. The opposite, an unusually slow *y*-descent, occurs with tricuspid stenosis.

CHAPTER 17

Use of Physiologic and Pharmacologic Maneuvers in Auscultation

PHYSIOLOGIC AND PHARMACOLOGIC MANEUVERS alter auscultatory findings by inducing changes in venous return, chamber size, arterial pressure, heart rate, stroke volume, systemic or pulmonary flow, and contractility.

Physiologic maneuvers such as respiration, Valsalva, postural changes, and exercise have been described in previous chapters dealing with specific entities. They will be reviewed only briefly in this chapter.

Pharmacologic intervention may be very informative in situations in which murmurs are present and where their hemodynamic origin and pathologic significance are uncertain.

Physiologic Maneuvers

QUIET RESPIRATION. — Auscultation with attention to respiration makes use of the phasic changes in resistance of the pulmonary vascular bed. During inspiration, pulmonary vascular resistance decreases and produces an increase in flow through the right atrium and ventricle while decreasing pulmonary venous flow into the left heart. The reverse occurs in expiration. The mechanism can best be understood by remembering that it is in the *pulmonary vascular bed*, not in the right heart, where resistance is primarily reduced during inspiration.

In the presence of congestive heart failure phasic changes in flow are greatly reduced and auscultatory changes with respiration are less evident and may be absent altogether.

The sounds influenced by respiration are as follows:

1. Splitting of the second sound is an important auscultatory phenomenon and is discussed in Chapter 4.

2. The ejection sound in pulmonic stenosis tends to move closer to the first sound during inspiration due to the augmented diastolic volume and increased rate of contraction of the right ventricle.

3. The systolic click associated with mitral leaflet prolapse tends to occur earlier in systole during inspiration than during expiration.

4. The maximum intensities of third and fourth heart sounds coincide with the time of maximum myocardial "stretch." Right-sided third and fourth sounds are therefore best heard at or just following the end of inspiration. Left-sided filling sounds are of course much more common and are best heard (often *only* heard) during expiration. These responses coincide with the periods of greatest venous return to the respective ventricle (see Fig 5–3). This phenomenon is especially valuable in evaluation of left ventricular function in ischemic states.

5. In congestive heart failure, these sounds are influenced little, if at all.

The murmurs influenced by respiration are as follows:

1. Murmurs of tricuspid regurgitation and stenosis are increased in intensity during inspiration.

2. The murmur of pulmonic regurgitation is often augmented during inspiration but to a lesser degree.

3. The murmur of pulmonic valvular stenosis is less influenced.

4. The murmur in mitral leaflet prolapse tends to increase in intensity during expiration, while the click moves later in systole. Only the increased intensity of the murmur is often noted.

VALSALVA MANEUVER. — This maneuver is well known and consists of forced expiratory effort against a closed glottis (or into a manometer system to a pressure of about 40 mm mercury) for approximately 10 seconds. Its physiologic consequences are rather striking and are separated into four phases. Phase I occurs immediately, consists of an increase in arterial pressure, and is very brief. Phase II begins as venous return and stroke volume drop sharply and is characterized by a progressive fall in mean arterial pressure and especially pulse pressure. During this interval, due to reduced pulse pressure, reflex constriction occurs. Phase III is a small further drop in arterial pressure on release of the expiratory effort. Phase IV exhibits a dramatic increase in arterial pressure due to sudden increase in venous return and consequent increased stroke volume being pumped into a constricted arterial bed; the abrupt increase in pulse pressure induces a reflex bradycardia. The whole may last 20 – 30 seconds. Auscultatory evaluation is directed mainly to phase II.

With two exceptions, *all* murmurs are decreased. This reflects the decrease in venous return and stroke volume on both sides of the heart. The two exceptions are the systolic murmurs heard in asymmetrical septal hypertrophy (IHSS) and mitral valve leaflet prolapse (click-murmur syndrome).

In asymmetric septal hypertrophy, the systolic murmur usually increases due to decreased chamber size and narrowing of the left ventricular outflow tract. During phase IV, when there is increased peripheral resistance and increased chamber size, the murmur may diminish below the average level.

With mid to late systolic mitral murmurs, especially those with clicks, the change is usually evident and consists of the murmur becoming more nearly pansystolic and the click moving closer to the first sound. The murmur may not become louder, thus attention should be directed to its duration and the position of the click. In some patients with a loud click but no murmur, the maneuver may bring out the full-blown complex. The same changes occur on having the patient sit or stand but are usually less dramatic.

With Valsalva the first sound does not change significantly, and the response of the second sound splitting is described in Chapter 4.

Diastolic filling sounds (third and fourth sounds) may diminish or disappear altogether during phase II, only to become louder during phase IV.

CHANGES IN BODY POSITION. — Various simple postural maneuvers are commonly used in auscultation. The standard position for optimal auscultation is recumbency, but the patient may be asked to sit, stand, turn in the left lateral position, squat, assume the standing-flexion position, or even support himself on hands and knees in order to clarify some sound or murmur.

The recumbent position equalizes hydrostatic pressure, resulting in increased venous return, increased diastolic volume and chamber radius, increased stroke volume, variable slight increase in arterial pressure and decrease in heart rate. This position is the most fruitful one since the great majority of sounds and murmurs are most prominent under these circumstances. Third and fourth sounds are most significantly altered and may be heard only with recumbency. Almost all murmurs are increased, both systolic and diastolic. Two notable exceptions are asymmetric septal hypertrophy and the click-murmur syndrome.

The sitting or standing position produces the opposite effects; third and fourth heart sounds may diminish or disappear. The majority of murmurs will become a grade or two softer. The systolic murmurs of asymmetric septal hypertrophy and the click-murmur syndrome will increase in intensity. The latter may become holosystolic with the click moving closer to the first sound and occasionally fusing with it.

The left lateral position is known to maximize the diastolic rumble in mitral stenosis. The act of turning induces an increase in heart rate which may be out of proportion to the effort involved, while the transmission of the murmur is enhanced by moving the left ventricular apex closer to the chest wall. Diastolic filling sounds and palpable presystolic impulses (A-waves) are often best appreciated in this position as well. As previously noted, venous hums are usually diminished or obliterated by recumbency.

The sitting and leaning forward position will enhance the murmur of aortic regurgitation and pericardial friction sounds.

The standing-flexion position may be used as a suitable substitute for both the left lateral and leaning forward positions and is especially convenient in conjunction with upright exercise (see Fig 2–3).

Abrupt squatting produces a prompt rise in venous return, stroke volume and arterial pressure. The increases in intracardiac volume and arterial resistance combine to decrease or eliminate altogether the systolic murmur in muscular subaortic stenosis (asymmetric septal hypertrophy).

Various positions, assumed abruptly, may result in dramatic changes in murmurs and sounds due to intracardiac masses (myxomas and ball-valve thrombi). Obviously, they should be carried out with caution in patients who have a history of sudden appearance of symptoms related to position change.

EXERCISE. — Muscular activity, dynamic and isometric, increases heart rate, cardiac output and contractility, and generally augments cardiac work. Dynamic exercise usually decreases vascular resistance whereas isometric exercise tends to increase it, sometimes markedly.

Common types of dynamic exercise readily done during physical examination include running in place, sit-ups, and bicycle or treadmill exercises. The single easily available and standardized form of isometric exercise is the handgrip. With the latter, the patient maintains vigorous handgrip for ½–1 minute.

In all forms of exercise auscultation is carried out before, after, and frequently during the activity.

The augmented flow and contractility increase most murmurs, especially aortic and pulmonic stenosis, ventricular septal defect, patent ductus arteriosus, mitral stenosis, tricuspid stenosis and tricuspid regurgitation. It is therefore most valuable when these murmurs are faint or atypical.

Dynamic exercise may increase the murmur of asymmetric septal hypertrophy due to the decreased peripheral resistance, but with the increased venous return the opposing influence is also present and thus the response is variable. Isometric exercise increases peripheral resistance significantly and the murmur of asymmetric septal hypertrophy is usually decreased.

Exercise tends to increase the intensity of the first heart sound and may result in appearance or augmentation of a fourth sound and occasionally a third sound. When cardiac function is compromised, the fourth sound becomes loud and persists throughout the respiratory cycle while the first sound diminishes in intensity and frequency. A third sound may appear as well and rarely a summation sound is transiently heard.

The pulmonic closure sound may be accentuated.

In the exercise testing of ischemic heart disease, auscultation can be extremely valuable but is infrequently utilized.

This type of testing is the most frequent use of exercise in medical evaluation and false positives and false negatives are distressingly common. Supporting evidence from auscultation often renders it more reliable. During exercise, and for a variable period after its termination, the following features may be present with ischemic heart disease:

1. A fourth sound may appear; if present at rest, it may become louder and vary little or not at all with respiration. On occasion, it exceeds the first sound in intensity.

2. The first sound may become "mushy," that is, reduced in both intensity and frequency.

3. Apical systolic murmurs, due to papillary muscle abnormality induced by ischemia, may appear.

4. In addition to cardiac auscultatory changes, auscultation of the lung bases may reveal interstitial edema by a change in the quality of the breath sounds from the normal to a distinctly harsh or coarse quality. Less often, moist rales may appear.

5. Areas of dyskinesis may be detected by palpation (these are very often visible as well).

An infrequent but striking auscultatory finding is the rather prompt disappearance of an apical systolic murmur (and often a palpable dyskinetic area) with the administration of nitroglycerin to patients having angina, whether spontaneous or exercise induced.

Pharmacologic Maneuvers

If the ideal drug were available (which it is not) it would produce an immediate but transient response, leave no residual ill effect, be easily administered at the bedside, be safe at all ages, and yield results that are informative and reproducible in various circulatory states. In fact, only two types of drugs are commonly helpful: a pure alpha stimulator (phenylephrine, methoxamine and angiotensin) and a potent vasodilator (primarily amyl nitrite).

ALPHA STIMULATORS (PHENYLEPHRINE, METHOXAMINE, ANGIOTENSIN)

Alpha stimulators produce an elevation of arterial pressure and a reflex bradycardia. They may be given in a single intravenous dose or by continuous drip sufficient to induce a 15–25 mm mercury rise in arterial pressure with accompanying reduction of heart rate. An important secondary change is a slight decrease in cardiac output roughly proportional to the decreased heart rate and the degree of rise of systemic mean pressure. The pulmonary vasculature is much less affected than the systemic.

The use of these agents is contraindicated in elderly persons or in patients where the myocardium may poorly tolerate the added burden.

The effects on murmurs are:

1. The elevated peripheral resistance tends to increase the murmur of aortic regurgitation as well as that of rheumatic mitral regurgitation, while changing the murmurs of aortic and pulmonic stenosis little, if at all.

2. Because of the lesser pulmonary vascular response, the murmur of ventricular septal defect without pulmonary hypertension will increase, sometimes sharply.

3. The diastolic component of the murmur of patent ductus arteriosus may be brought out or augmented; that is, it may produce a continuous murmur where only a systolic murmur was previously heard. However, with large shunts at any level and elevated pulmonary pressures due to high flow, the effect is less predictable and may be confusing.

4. Mitral regurgitation due to leaflet prolapse responds differently than that due to rheumatic involvement. Enddiastolic volume is often increased with phenylephrine. Thus, the click-murmur complex may fade, with the murmur and click occurring later in systole.

VASODILATORS (AMYL NITRITE)

Amyl nitrite is the potent vasodilator best suited for bedside use and is by far the most common agent used in auscultatory evaluation. Its vasodilating effect produces a sharp decrease in blood pressure, increase in heart rate, and generalized flushing within seconds; 30–60 seconds later there is an increased cardiac output due to augmented venous return. Pulmonary artery pressure is very mildly affected, if at all. Various murmurs and sounds change during one or both of these phases.

TECHNIQUE OF THE AMYL NITRITE TEST.—The patient

should be instructed to breathe somewhat more deeply and rapidly than normally and should be reassured regarding the innocuousness of the test. He is told that an ampule will be broken which will release a substance with a pungent odor, which he is to inhale. After it is broken, the ampule is held close to the patient's nose and he inhales the amyl nitrite somewhat deeply for 20–30 seconds, by which time there is usually a marked tachycardia and flush. During this time and for 2–3 minutes afterward, any changes in the murmurs and sounds are noted, preferably by recording them.

During the initial phase, the following effects are noted:

1. A decrease in the intensity of the murmur of mitral regurgitation due to enhanced left ventricular-aortic flow with a resultant decrease in regurgitant flow.

2. A decrease in the intensity of the murmur of ventricular septal defect for similar reasons (Fig 17–1).

3. A decrease in the intensity of the murmur of patent ductus arteriosus due to a decrease in the aortic-pulmonary artery pressure gradient.

4. A decrease in the intensity of the murmur of aortic regurgitation due to a decrease in the aortic-diastolic left ventricular pressure gradient.

5. A decrease or disappearance of an Austin Flint murmur coincident with the decrease in the murmur of aortic regurgitation and for the same reasons. This is a simple way of distinguishing between the Austin Flint murmur and that of organic mitral stenosis, since the latter is increased or unaffected by amyl nitrite (p. 256).

6. An increase, sometimes sharp, in the systolic murmur of muscular subaortic stenosis (asymmetric septal hypertrophy) in the initial phase due to the abrupt fall in peripheral resistance. This effect may or may not extend through the second phase since during this interval there is competition between the effects of the decreased peripheral resistance and increased venous return.

7. The occurrence earlier in systole of the click and systolic murmur in the click-murmur syndrome due to a decrease in average left ventricular dimensions. Since the murmur itself is more dependent on structural factors than on the volume of retrograde flow, it is influenced little by changes in cardiac output which occur with amyl nitrite.

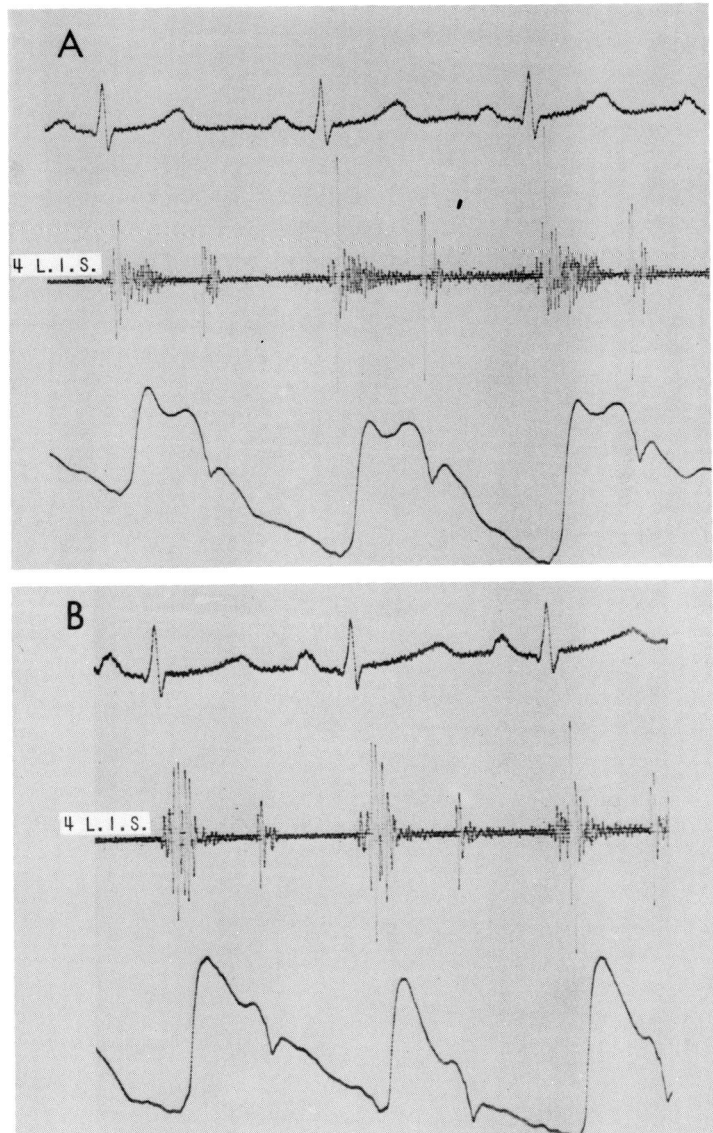

Fig 17–1.—A, a young woman with a small ventricular septal defect. Murmur is harsh, decrescendo and present in early and midsystole. **B,** following inhalation of amyl nitrite, the murmur has almost disappeared.

The second phase of the amyl nitrite effect begins 30 seconds after the beginning of inhalation and lasts for about 1 minute. The effects are due to increased venous return and an increased cardiac output. Any murmur due to obstruction will be increased, and the following effects are noted: (1) an increase in the murmur of pulmonary stenosis; (2) an increase in the murmur of aortic stenosis (this is usually not as clear cut as the change in the murmur of pulmonary stenosis); (3) an increase in the murmur of tricuspid stenosis, whether the stenosis is organic or relative; (4) an increase in the murmur of mitral stenosis; and (5) usually an increase in the murmur of tricuspid regurgitation, since this murmur is sensitive to the degree of filling of the right ventricle (p. 108).

SITUATIONS IN WHICH DRUG EFFECTS MAY HELP DIFFERENTIATE MURMURS

DIFFERENTIATION OF MODERATELY SEVERE PULMONARY STENOSIS WITH AN INTACT SEPTUM FROM A MILD, ACYANOTIC TETRALOGY OF FALLOT. — In *pulmonary stenosis with an intact septum,* there is an *increased loudness* of the pulmonary systolic murmur during the second phase of amyl nitrite action. In *tetralogy of Fallot,* the right-to-left shunt increases because amyl nitrite lowers the left ventricular systolic pressure during the first phase of its action; this decreases right ventricular pressure and pulmonary artery flow, resulting in a *decreased intensity* of the murmur. The pulmonic second sound may become more evident in pulmonary stenosis because of the increased closing pressure, and may become less evident in tetralogy because of the decreased pulmonary artery pressure. Depending upon the size of the ventricular septal defect and the grade of stenosis, the expected results, however, may not always occur.

DIFFERENTIATION OF VENTRICULAR SEPTAL DEFECT FROM MILD PULMONARY STENOSIS OR INFUNDIBULAR STENOSIS WITH INTACT SEPTUM. — The auscultatory findings in these conditions may be very similar. Amyl nitrite decreases the murmur of ventricular septal defect (see Fig 17–1) during its first phase of action, and increases the murmur of pulmonary stenosis during the second phase; it can thus be effective in differentiating these conditions when they are both mild. If the ventricular septal defect is large, the amyl nitrite may not affect it. Vasoconstrictor drugs increase the murmur of ventricular septal defect and do not affect the murmur of pulmonary stenosis significantly.

RECOGNITION OF THE MURMUR OF PATENT DUCTUS ARTERIOSUS WHEN THE MURMUR IS IN THE USUAL LOCATION BUT NOT CLASSICAL. — Amyl nitrite decreases the length of the murmur and makes it less intense, whereas vasopressor drugs increase the intensity and duration of the murmur. This is also true for other arteriovenous shunts. It is not true for the continuous murmur heard with severe pulmonary stenosis or atresia and dilated bronchial arteries.

DIFFERENTIATION OF INNOCENT SYSTOLIC MURMURS FROM THE MURMUR OF A SMALL VENTRICULAR SEPTAL DEFECT. — Amyl nitrite increases innocent systolic murmurs. It decreases the murmur of ventricular septal defect. Vasoconstrictor drugs increase the murmur of ventricular septal defects and may or may not change the intensity of an innocent systolic murmur.

DIFFERENTIATION OF THE MURMUR OF AORTIC STENOSIS FROM THE MURMUR OF MITRAL REGURGITATION AT THE APEX. — The problem is the detection of the murmur of mitral regurgitation when the systolic murmur of an associated aortic stenosis is transmitted to the apex. This problem has already been discussed on page 113. If one listens at the apex, or possibly just lateral to the apex, after administering amyl nitrite, the murmur of mitral regurgitation will show a decrease in intensity at the end of the first 20 seconds and then return to normal intensity. On the other hand, the murmur of aortic stenosis is slightly decreased, or not changed, during the first 20 seconds, and then increases following the first 25 seconds to reach a peak somewhere around 45–60 seconds; it may be accentuated for as long as 2 minutes. If, therefore, the murmur fades first, there is an associated mitral regurgitation. This may be difficult to determine in the presence of atrial fibrillation; with a very tight aortic stenosis one may actually get a misleading result, in that the left ventricular pressure does not fall enough to affect the mitral regurgitation murmur. No change, or only a slight change, may occur in one third to one half of the cases, and the difficulty is increased if one uses auscultation alone without phonocardiography.

If a vasoconstrictor is given, the murmur of mitral regurgitation increases and the murmur of aortic stenosis is variably affected. With a fairly marked degree of aortic stenosis, an effect on the mitral regurgitation may not be evident.

DIFFERENTIATION OF THE MURMUR OF AORTIC REGURGI-TATION FROM THE MURMUR OF PULMONARY REGURGITA-TION. — As noted on page 146, this may be difficult or impossible on an auscultatory basis alone. Drugs may help, but there is some difference of opinion as to how clear-cut the changes are. The murmur of aortic regurgitation should decrease in loudness during the first phase of amyl nitrite action. The murmur of pulmonary regurgitation should not be affected. With a vasopressor drug, the murmur of aortic regurgitation should be increased and that of pulmonary regurgitation not affected. Serotonin has been used to differentiate these murmurs. With this drug the pulmonary resistance is increased and pulmonary pressure is elevated; thus, the murmur of pulmonary regurgitation is said to be increased, whereas that of aortic regurgitation is unchanged.

DIFFERENTIATION OF TRICUSPID REGURGITATION FROM MITRAL REGURGITATION. — With amyl nitrite, the murmur of mitral regurgitation decreases in intensity, and the tricuspid regurgitation murmur increases. The former occurs early in the first period and the latter in the second period. Phenylephrine increases the murmur of mitral regurgitation and does not affect the murmur of tricuspid regurgitation.

DIFFERENTIATION OF MITRAL STENOSIS FROM THE AUSTIN FLINT MURMUR. — As noted, amyl nitrite increases the murmur of mitral stenosis and decreases the Austin Flint murmur. This is due to the decreased resistance to forward flow and reduction of the diastolic aortic-left ventricular gradient.

Phenylephrine may "uncover" an opening snap on occasion and usually diminishes the murmur of mitral stenosis, although not markedly. It will increase the Austin Flint murmur due to the raised aortic-left ventricular gradient in diastole, which augments the volume of aortic regurgitation.

DIFFERENTIATION OF MUSCULAR SUBAORTIC STENOSIS (ASYMMETRIC SEPTAL HYPERTROPHY) FROM MITRAL REGUR-GITATION. — Amyl nitrite, due to its vasodilating effect, intensifies the murmur of muscular subaortic stenosis and decreases the murmur of mitral regurgitation. The effect on both, especially on the former, is sometimes striking. Phenylephrine has the opposite effect; i.e., it will decrease the murmur of muscular subaortic stenosis while increasing the murmur of mitral regurgitation due to its vasoconstricting action.

INOTROPIC AGENTS (BETA STIMULATORS)

These agents act centrally by increasing myocardial contractility, while their peripheral alpha-inhibiting effect is less potent and variable. They are infrequently used, since they often yield confusing results and are not as safe as the purely peripherally acting drugs. The most common diagnostic use is the administration of isoproterenol to induce a gradient (and a systolic murmur) across the left ventricular outflow tract in muscular subaortic stenosis. It is given by continuous intravenous drip while the patient is closely monitored and ideally is carried out only in the catheterization laboratory.

Since digitalis glycosides are inotropic, the left ventricular outflow obstruction in muscular subaortic stenosis may be increased when they are administered. The well-known increase in loudness of the systolic murmur and worsening of symptoms result.

CHAPTER 18

Eponyms

Austin Flint murmur. — A middiastolic and presystolic murmur heard at the apex in patients with aortic regurgitation but without mitral stenosis (p. 141).

Carey-Coombs murmur — A middiastolic murmur heard at the apex in patients with acute rheumatic fever (p. 142).

Carvallo's sign. — Accentuation of the murmur of tricuspid regurgitation with inspiration (p. 108).

Corrigan's pulse. — A water-hammer or collapsing arterial pulse in severe aortic regurgitation.

Cossio's sign. — A palpable first heart sound distinct from the apex beat, in mitral stenosis (p. 235).

Duroziez's sign. — The double murmur, systolic and diastolic, produced by moderate compression of a peripheral artery, such as the femoral or the brachial artery (p. 157).

Erb's point or area. — The 3d left intercostal space at the sternal margin. The murmur of aortic regurgitation is usually heard best in this area.

Gallavardin phenomenon. — The occurrence in severe aortic stenosis of a very harsh murmur in the aortic area, and a less harsh and mainly high-pitched murmur at the apex (p. 111).

Gibson murmur. — The continuous murmur of patent ductus arteriosus (p. 171).

Graham Steell murmur. — The high-pitched, early diastolic murmur of pulmonary regurgitation. It is often heard in pulmonary hypertension associated with mitral stenosis (p. 145).

HAMMAN'S SIGN. — A systolic "crunching" sound heard over the precordium due to free air in the mediastinum (p. 150).

KOROTKOFF SOUNDS. — The sounds heard over a peripheral artery when blood pressure is being taken by a blood pressure cuff. The sounds are heard with the stethoscope over the artery immediately distal to the cuff (p. 237).

KUSSMAUL'S SIGN. — Inspiratory elevation of the jugular venous pulse seen with pericardial constriction or tamponade (p. 244).

LERMAN-MEANS SCRATCH. — A scratchy systolic murmur heard in the pulmonary area in patients with thyrotoxicosis (p. 220).

QUINCKE'S SIGN. — Pulsations of capillary beds, especially the nail beds, in severe aortic regurgitation (p. 239).

ROGERS' MURMUR. — The holosystolic murmur heard in interventricular septal defects of mild to moderate size (p. 177).

STILL'S MURMUR. — The innocent systolic murmur heard in the apicosternal area (p. 121).

VALSALVA MANEUVER. — Forced expiration against a closed glottis.

Selected Bibliography

Stethoscopes, Graphic Representation, Sound Production and Transmission

Constant, J., and Lippschutz, E. J.: Diagramming and grading heart sounds and murmurs, Am. Heart J. 70:326, 1965.

Ertel, P. Y., *et al.*: Acoustic differences among stethoscopes, Univ. Mich. Med. Cent. J. 32:35, 1966.

Faber, J. J., and Burton, A. C.: Spread of heart sounds over chest wall, Circ. Res. 11:96, 1962.

Faber, J. J., and Burton, A. C.: Biophysics of heart sounds and its application to clinical auscultation, Can. Med. Assoc. J. 91:120, 1964.

Feinstein, A.: Acoustic distinctions in cardiac auscultation, Arch. Intern. Med. 121:209, 1968.

Fergulio, G. A.: Intracardiac phonocardiography: A new departure in cardiac catheterization. Recent advances, Acta Cardiol. 19:372, 1964.

Groom, D.: Comparative efficiency of stethoscopes, Am. Heart J. 68:220, 1964.

Hollins, P. J.: The stethoscope—Some facts and fallacies, Br. J. Hosp. Med. 5: 509, 1971.

Latimer, K. E.: How to test stethoscopes, Med. Res. Eng. 10:19, 1971.

Leatham, A.: An improved stethoscope, Lancet 1:463, 1958.

Luisada, A. A., MacCanon, D. M., and Slodki, S. J.: Intracardiac phonocardiography: Description of a new simplified system, Circulation 32:563, 1965.

McKusick, V. A.: Spectral phonocardiography, Am. J. Cardiol. 4:200, 1959.

Rappaport, M. B., and Sprague, H. B.: Physiologic and physical laws that govern auscultation, and their clinical application: The acoustic stethoscope and the electrical amplifying stethoscope and stethograph, Am. Heart J. 21: 257, 1941.

Ravin, A., Craddock, L. D., and de la Fuente, L. M.: The standing-flexion position for auscultation of the heart, J.A.M.A. 192:60, 1965.

Ravin, A., and Frame, F. K.: *International Bibliography of Cardiovascular Auscultation and Phonocardiography,* American Heart Association Monograph, no. 31 (New York: American Heart Association, Inc., 1971).

Rushmer, R. F., and Morgan, C.: Meaning of murmurs, Am. J. Cardiol. 21:722, 1968.

Segall, H. N.: A simple method for graphic description of cardiac auscultatory signs, Am. Heart J. 8:533, 1933.

Segall, H. N.: Evolution of graphic symbols for cardiovascular sounds and murmurs, Br. Heart J. 24:1, 1962.

Segall, H. N.: On learning about cardiovascular sound. Comments on clinical clues to the physiology of first sound and the Korotkoff sounds, Manitoba Med. Rev. 47:503, 1967.

Shah, P. M., MacCanon, D. M., and Luisada, A. A.: Spread of the "mitral" sound over the chest: A study of five subjects with the Starr-Edwards valve, Circulation 28:1102, 1963.

Shah, P. M., Slodki, S. J., and Luisada, A. A.: A revision of the "classic" areas of auscultation of the heart: A physiologic approach, Am. J. Med. 36:293, 1964.

Heart Sounds

Abbott, J. A., and Whipple, G. H.: Paradoxic splitting of the second heart sound in systemic hypertension. The role of myocardial competence, Dis. Chest 46:304, 1964.

Adolph, R. J., and Fowler, N. O.: The second heart sound: A screening test for heart disease, Mod. Concepts Cardiovasc. Dis. 39:91, 1970.

Adolph, R. J., Stephens, J. F., and Tanaka, K.: The clinical value of frequency analysis of the first heart sound in myocardial infarction, Circulation 41:1003, 1970.

Aygen, M. M., and Braunwald, E.: The splitting of the second heart sound in normal subjects and in patients with congenital heart disease, Circulation 25:328, 1962.

Beck, W., Schrire, V., and Vogelpoel, L.: Splitting of the second heart sound in constrictive pericarditis, with observations on the mechanism of pulsus paradoxus, Am. Heart J. 64:765, 1962.

van Bogaert, A., et al.: Modifications du premier bruit du coeur dans la bloc de branche: Etude clinique et expérimentale, Arch. Mal. Coeur 56:1253, 1963.

Burggraf, G. W., and Craige, E.: The first heart sound in complete heart block, Circulation 50:17, 1973.

Cossio, P., Dambrosi, R. G., and Warnford-Thomson, H. F.: The first heart sound in auricular and ventricular extrasystoles, Br. Heart J. 9:275, 1947.

Craige, E.: On the genesis of heart sounds: Contributions made by echocardiographic studies, Circulation 53:207, 1976.

Dickerson, R. B., and Nelson, W. P.: Paradoxical splitting of the second heart sound: An informative clinical notation, Am. Heart J. 67:410, 1964.

Dock, W.: Further evidence for the purely valvular origin of the first and third heart sounds, Am. Heart J. 30:332, 1945.

Gould, L., Ettinger, S. J., and Lyon, A. F.: Intensity of the first heart sound and arterial pulse in mitral insufficiency, Dis. Chest 53:545, 1968.

van der Hauwaert, L. G.: The effect of the Valsalva maneuver on the splitting of the second sound, Acta Cardiol. 19:518, 1964.

Heintzen, P.: The genesis of the normally split first heart sound, Am. Heart J. 62:332, 1961.

Kusukawa, R., Bruce, D. W., Sakamoto, T., MacCanon, D. M., and Luisada, A. A.: Hemodynamic determinants of the amplitude of the second heart sound, J. Appl. Physiol. 21:938, 1966.

Leatham, A.: The second heart sound key to auscultation of the heart, Acta Cardiol. 19:395, 1964.

Leon, D. F., and Shaver, J. A. (eds.): Physiologic Principles of Heart Sounds and Murmurs, American Heart Association Monograph, no. 46 (New York: American Heart Association, Inc., 1975).

Luisada, A. A.: The second heart sound in normal and abnormal conditions, Am. J. Cardiol. 28:150, 1971.

Luisada, A. A., MacCanon, D. M., Kumar, S., and Feigen, L. P.: Changing views on the mechanism of the first and second heart sounds, Am. Heart J. 88:503, 1974.

Luisada, A. A., and Shah, P. M.: Controversial and changing aspects of auscultation. I. Areas of auscultation: A new concept. II. Normal and abnormal first and second sounds, Am. J. Cardiol. 11:774, 1963.

Rappaport, M. B., and Sprague, H. B.: The graphic registration of the normal heart sounds, Am. Heart J. 23:591, 1942.

Ravin, A., and Bershof, E.: The intensity of the first heart sound in auricular fibrillation with mitral stenosis, Am. Heart J. 41:539, 1951.

Rytand, D. A.: The variable loudness of the first sound in auricular fibrillation, Am. Heart J. 37:187, 1949.

Schrire, V., and Vogelpoel, L.: The role of the dilated pulmonary artery in abnormal splitting of the second heart sound, Am. Heart J. 63:501, 1962.

Schwab, L., Smiley, G. L., and Meyn, W. P.: Xiphosternal crunch: An analysis of 106 cases among 3,224 army separatees, Ann. Intern. Med. 31:228, 1949.

Shah, P. M., et al.: Hemodynamic correlates of the various components of the first heart sound, Circulation Res. 12:386, 1963.

Shah, P. M., and Slodki, S. J.: The Q-II interval: A study of the second heart sound in normal adults and in systemic hypertension, Circulation 29:551, 1964.

Shaver, J. A., Nadolny, R. A., O'Toole, J. D., Thompson, M. E., Reddy, P. S., Leon, D. F., and Curtiss, E. I.: Sound pressure correlates of the second heart sound, Circulation 49:316, 1974.

Shearn, M. A., Tarr, E., and Rytand, D. A.: The significance of changes in amplitude of the first heart sound in children with A-V block, Circulation 7:839, 1953.

Sutton, G., Harris, A., and Leatham, A.: Second heart sound in pulmonary hypertension, Br. Heart J. 30:743, 1968.

Wolferth, C. C., and Margolies, A.: The influence of auricular contraction on the first heart sound and the radial pulse, Arch. Intern. Med. 46:1048, 1930.

Yurchak, P. M., and Gorlin, R.: Paradoxical splitting of the second heart sound in coronary heart disease, N. Engl. J. Med. 269:741, 1963.

Abnormal and Extra Heart Sounds

Arevalo, F., et al.: Hemodynamic correlates of the third heart sound, Am. J. Physiol. 207:319, 1964.

Barlow, J. B.: Some observations on the atrial sound, S. Afr. Med. J. 34:887, 1960.

Benchimol, A., and Dimond, E. G.: The apex cardiogram in ischaemic heart disease, Br. Heart J. 24:581, 1962.

Coulshed, N., and Epstein, E. J.: Third heart sound after mitral valve replacement, Br. Heart J. 34:301, 1972.

Crevasse, L., et al.: The mechanism of the generation of the third and fourth heart sounds, Circulation 25:635, 1962.

Dock, W.: The genesis of diastolic heart sounds, Am. J. Med. 50:178, 1971.

Epstein, E. J., et al.: Cineradiographic studies of the early systolic click in aortic valve stenosis, Circulation 31:842, 1965.

Evans, W.: Triple heart rhythm, Br. Heart J. 5:205, 1943.

Fowler, N. O., and Adolph, R. J.: Fourth sound gallop or split first sound? Am. J. Cardiol. 30:441, 1972.

Goldblatt, A., Aygen, M. M., and Braunwald, E.: Hemodynamic-phonocardiographic correlations of the fourth heart sound in aortic stenosis, Circulation 26:92, 1962.

Grant, C., Greene, D. G., and Bunnell, I. L.: The valve-closing function of the right atrium: A study of pressures and atrial sounds in patients with heart block, Am. J. Med. 34:325, 1963.

Grayzel, J.: Gallop rhythm of the heart. I. Atrial gallop, ventricular gallop and systolic sounds, Am. J. Med. 28:578, 1960.

Grayzel, J.: Gallop rhythm of the heart. II. Quadruple rhythm and its relation to summation and augmented gallops, Circulation 20:1053, 1959.

Harris, W. S., Rodin, P., and Tabatznik, B.: Modification of the atrial sound by the cold pressor test, carotid sinus massage, and the Valsalva maneuver, Circulation 28:1128, 1963.

Harvey, W. P., and Stapleton, J.: Clinical aspects of gallop rhythm with particular reference to diastolic gallops, Circulation 18:1017, 1958.

Kincaid-Smith, P., and Barlow, J.: The atrial sound in hypertension and ischaemic heart disease, with reference to its timing and mode of production, Br. Heart J. 21:479, 1959.

Kontos, H. A., Shapiro, W., and Kemp, V. E.: Observations on the atrial sound in hypertension, Circulation 28:877, 1963.

Leatham, A., and Vogelpoel, L.: The early systolic sound in dilatation of the pulmonary artery, Br. Heart J. 16:21, 1954.

Leonard, J. J., Weissler, A. M., and Warren, J. V.: Modification of ventricular gallop rhythm induced by pooling of blood in the extremities, Br. Heart J. 20:502, 1958.

Leonard, J. J., Weissler, A. M., and Warren, J. V.: Observations on the mechanism of atrial gallop rhythm, Circulation 17:1007, 1958.

Luisada, A. A., and Shah, P. M.: Controversial and changing aspects of auscultation. III. Diastolic sounds. IV. Intervals. V. Systolic sounds, Am. J. Cardiol. 13:243, 1964.

Minhas, K., and Gasul, B. M.: Systolic clicks: A clinical phonocardiographic, and hemodynamic evaluation, Am. Heart J. 57:49, 1959.

Mounsey, P.: The opening snap of mitral stenosis, Br. Heart J. 15:135, 1953.

Nixon, P. G. F.: The genesis of the third heart sound, Am. Heart J. 65:712, 1963.

Oriol, A., et al.: Prediction of left atrial pressure from the second sound-opening snap interval, Am. J. Cardiol. 16:184, 1965.

Parry, E., and Mounsey, P.: Gallop sounds in hypertension and myocardial ischaemia modified by respiration and other manoeuvres, Br. Heart J. 23:393, 1961.

Proctor, M. H., et al.: The phonocardiogram in mitral valvular disease: A correlation of Q-1 and 2-OS intervals with findings at catheterization of the left side of the heart and at mitral valvuloplasty, Am. J. Med. 24:861, 1958.

Reid, J. V. O.: Midsystolic clicks, S. Afr. Med. J. 35:353, 1961.

Rodin, P., and Tabatznik, B.: The effect of posture on added heart sounds, Br. Heart J. 25:69, 1963.

Sakamoto, T., Kaito, G., and Ueda, H.: Electrocardiographic and phonocardiographic studies in hypertension. Part I. Electrocardiographic study with special reference to the P-wave. Part II. Phonocardiographic study with special reference to the atrial sound and "Q-1" interval, Jpn. Heart J. 1:198, 1960.

Spodick, D. H.: Fourth heart sound gallop or split first heart sound? Am. J. Cardiol. 31:530, 1973.

Tavel, M. E.: The fourth heart sound—a premature requiem? (editorial), Circulation 49:4, 1974.

Vogel, J. H. K., and Blount, S. G., Jr.: Clinical evaluation in localizing level of obstruction to outflow from left ventricle: Importance of early systolic ejection click, Am. J. Cardiol. 15:782, 1965.

Wagner, G. R.: Some observations on ejection sounds, Australas. Ann. Med. 10:33, 1961.

Systolic Murmurs

Allen, H., Harris, A., and Leatham, A.: Significance and prognosis of an isolated late systolic murmur: A 9-to-22 year follow-up, Br. Heart J. 36:525, 1974.

Barlow, J. B.: Conjoint clinic on the clinical significance of late systolic murmurs and nonejection clicks, J. Chronic Dis. 18:665, 1965.

Barlow, J. B., Bosman, C. K., Pocock, W. A., and Marchand, P.: Late systolic murmurs and nonejection ("mid-late") systolic clicks, Br. Heart J. 30:203, 1968.

Barlow, J. B., and Pocock, W. A.: The significance of aortic ejection systolic murmurs, Am. Heart J. 64:149, 1962.

Bruns, D. L.: A general theory of the causes of murmurs in the cardiovascular system, Am. J. Med. 27:360, 1959.

Bruns, D. L., and van der Hauwaert, L. G.: The aortic systolic murmur developing with increasing age, Br. Heart J. 20:370, 1959.

Burch, G. E., and Phillips, J. H.: Murmurs of aortic stenosis and mitral insufficiency masquerading as one another, Am. Heart J. 66:439, 1963.

Cohen, L. S., Mason, D. T., and Braunwald, E.: Significance of an atrial gallop sound in mitral regurgitation. A clue to the diagnosis of ruptured chordae tendineae, Circulation 35:112, 1967.

Counihan, T. B., Rappaport, M. B., and Sprague, H. B.: Physiologic and physical factors that govern the clinical appreciation of cardiac thrills, Circulation 4:716, 1951.

DeBusk, R. F., and Harrison, D. C.: The clinical spectrum of papillary muscle disease, N. Engl. J. Med. 281:1458, 1969.

deMonchy, C., van der Hoeven, G. M. A., and Benekin, J. E. W.: Studies on innocent praecordial vibratory murmurs in children. III: Follow-up study of children with an innocent praecordial vibratory murmur, Br. Heart J. 35: 685, 1973.

Dillon, J. C., Haine, C. L., Chang, S., and Feigenbaum, H.: Use of echocardiography in patients with prolapsed mitral valve, Circulation 43:503, 1971.

Fontana, M. E., Wooley, C. F., Leighton, R. F., and Lewis, R. P.: Postural changes in left ventricular and mitral valvular dynamics in the systolic click-late systolic murmur syndrome, Circulation 51:165, 1975.

Freeman, A. R., and Levine, S. A.: The clinical significance of the systolic murmur: A study of 1,000 consecutive "non-cardiac" cases, Ann. Intern. Med. 6:1371, 1933.

Goodwin, J. F.,: ?IHSS. ?HOCM. ?ASH. A plea for unity, Am. Heart J. 89:269, 1975.

Hancock, E. W., and Cohn, K.: The syndrome associated with midsystolic click and late systolic murmur, Am. J. Med. 41:183, 1966.

Hansing, C. E., and Rowe, G. G.: Tricuspid insufficiency. A study of hemodynamics and pathogenesis, Circulation 45:793, 1972.

Henke, R. P., March, H. W., and Hultgren, H. N.: An aid to identification of the murmur of aortic stenosis with atypical localization, Am. Heart J. 60: 354, 1960.

Howell, T. H.: Cardiac murmurs in old age: A clinico-pathological study, J. Am. Geriatr. Soc. 15:509, 1967.

Jeresaty, R. M.: Mitral valve prolapse — click syndrome, Prog. Cardiovasc. Dis. 15:623, 1973.

Karliner, J. S., O'Rourke, R. A., Kearney, D. J., and Shabetai, R.: Haemodynamic explanation of why the murmur of mitral regurgitation is independent of cycle length, Br. Heart J. 35:397, 1973.

Keenan, T. J., and Schwartz, M. J.: Tricuspid whoop, Am. J. Cardiol. 31:642, 1973.

Kelly, D. T., Wulfsberg, E., Rowe, R. D.: Discrete subaortic stenosis, Circulation 46:309, 1972.

Leatham, A.: Auscultation of the heart, Lancet 2:703, 757, 1958.

Leatham, A.: Systolic murmurs, Circulation 17:601, 1958.

Leatham, A., Segal, B., and Shafter, H.: Auscultatory and phonocardiographic findings in healthy children with systolic murmurs, Br. Heart J. 25:451, 1963.

Leon, D. F., et al.: Effect of respiration on pansystolic regurgitant murmurs as studied by biatrial intracardiac phonocardiography, Am. J. Med. 39:429, 1965.

McKusick, V. A., et al.: Musical murmurs, Bull. Johns Hopkins Hosp. 97:136, 1955.

Nellen, M., Gotsman, M. S., Vogelpoel, L., Beck, W., and Schrire, V.: Effect of prompt squatting on the systolic murmur in idiopathic hypertrophic obstructive cardiomyopathy, Br. Med. J. 3:140, 1967.

Pansegrau, D. G., Kioshos, J. M., Durnin, R. E., and Kroetz, F. W.: Supravalvular aortic stenosis in adults, Am. J. Cardiol. 31:635, 1973.

Perloff, J. K.: Clinical recognition of aortic stenosis. The physical signs and differential diagnosis of the various forms of obstruction to left ventricular outflow, Prog. Cardiovasc. Dis. 10:323, 1968.

Perloff, J. K., and Harvey, W. P.: Auscultatory and phonocardiographic manifestations of pure mitral regurgitation, Prog. Cardiovasc. Dis. 5:172, 1962.

Perry, L. W.: Innocent murmurs, Clin. Proc. Children's Hosp. Washington, D.C. 24:67, 1968.

Phillips, J. H., Burch, G. E., and De Pasquale, N. P.: The syndrome of papillary muscle dysfunction: Its clinical recognition, Ann. Intern. Med. 59:508, 1963.

Reddy, P. S., Shaver, J. A., and Leonard, J. J.: Cardiac systolic murmurs: Pathophysiology and differential diagnosis, Prog. Cardiovasc. Dis. 14:1, 1971.

Rios, J. C., Massumi, R. A., Breesmen, W. T., and Sarin, R. K.: Auscultatory features of acute tricuspid regurgitation, Am. J. Cardiol. 23:4, 1969.

Rivero Carvallo, J. M.: A new diagnostic sign of tricuspid insufficiency, Am. Heart J. 33:728, 1947.

Roberts, W. C.: Anomalous left ventricular band. An unemphasized cause of a precordial musical murmur, Am. J. Cardiol. 23:735, 1969.

Roberts, W. C., and Perloff, J. K.: Mitral valvular disease, Ann. Intern. Med. 77:939, 1972.

Ronan, J. A., Perloff, J. K., and Harvey, W. P.: Systolic clicks and the late systolic murmur: Intracardiac phonocardiographic evidence of their mitral valve origin, Am. Heart J. 70:319, 1965.

Schrire, V.: The relation of the apical systolic murmur to mitral valve disease, Am. Heart J. 68:305, 1964.

Simon, M. A., and Liu, S. F.: Calcification of the mitral valve annulus and its relation to functional valvular disturbance, Am. Heart J. 48:497, 1954.

Diastolic Murmurs

Craige, E., and Millward, D. K.: Diastolic and continuous murmurs, Prog. Cardiovasc. Dis. 14:38, 1971.

Criley, J. M., and Hermer, A. J.: Crescendo presystolic murmur of mitral stenosis with atrial fibrillation, N. Engl. J. Med. 285:1284, 1971.

Dack, S., et al.: Mitral stenosis: Auscultatory and phonocardiographic findings, Am. J. Cardiol. 5:815, 1960.

Fortuin, N. J., and Craige, E.: On the mechanism of the Austin Flint murmur, Circulation 45:558, 1972.

Harvey, W. P.: Silent Valvular Heart Disease, in Brest, A. N. (ed.): *Valvular Heart Disease*, Cardiovascular Clinics, vol. 5, no. 2 (Philadelphia: F. A. Davis Co., 1973), p. 77.

Harvey, W. P., Corrado, M. A., and Perloff, J. K.: "Right-sided" murmurs of aortic insufficiency. (Diastolic murmurs better heard to the right of the sternum rather than to the left), Am. J. Med. Sci. 245:533, 1963.

Reddy, P. S., Curtiss, E. I., Salerni, R., O'Toole, J. D., Griff, F. W., Leon, D. F., and Shaver, J. A.: Sound pressure correlates of the Austin Flint murmur, Circulation 53:210, 1976.

Sangster, J. F., and Oakley, C. M.: Diastolic murmur of coronary artery stenosis, Br. Heart J. 35:840, 1973.

Segal, J. P., Harvey, W. P., and Corrado, M. A.: The Austin Flint murmur: Its differentiation from the murmur of rheumatic mitral stenosis, Circulation 18:1025, 1958.

Toutouzas, P., Koidakis, A., Velimezis, A., and Avgoustakis, D.: Mechanism of diastolic rumble and presystolic murmur in mitral stenosis, Br. Heart J. 36:1096, 1974.

Pericardial Friction Rub, Venous Hum, Extracardiac Auscultation and Arrhythmias

Allen, N.: The significance of vascular murmurs in the head and neck, Geriatrics 20:525, 1965.

Burchell, H. B.: Peripheral auscultation: Prospecting with a stethoscope, Heart Bull. 12:81, 1963.

Buttross, D.: The venous hum: History, pathogenesis, incidence, recognition and significance, Am. Pract. Digest Treat. 6:342, 1955.

Crevasse, L.: Carotid artery murmurs: Clinical and pathophysiologic correlation, Neurology 11 (pt. 2):100, 1961.

Dressler, W.: Effect of respiration on the pericardial friction rub, Am. J. Cardiol. 7:130, 1961.

Fisher, C. M.: Augmentation bruit of the vertebral artery, J. Neurol. Neurosurg. Psychiatry 29:343, 1966.

Fowler, N. O., and Gause, R.: The cervical venous hum, Am. Heart J. 67:135, 1964.

Gilroy, J., and Meyer, J. S.: Auscultation of the neck in occlusive cerebrovascular disease, Circulation 25:300, 1962.

Haber, E., and Leatham, A.: Splitting of heart sounds from ventricular asynchrony in bundle branch block, ventricular ectopic beats, and artificial pacing, Br. Heart J. 27:691, 1965.

Harvey, W. P.: Auscultatory findings in diseases of the pericardium, Am. J. Cardiol. 7:15, 1961.

Harvey, W. P., and Corrado, M. A.: Multiple sounds in paroxysmal ventricular tachycardia, N. Engl. J. Med. 257:325, 1957.

Harvey, W. P., and Ronan, J. A., Jr.: Bedside diagnosis of arrhythmias, Prog. Cardiovasc. Dis. 8:419, 1966.

Holldack, K., Heller, A., and Groth, W.: The pericardial friction rub in the phonocardiogram, Am. J. Cardiol. 4:351, 1959.

Kelly, J. V., and Bonnet, G.: Studies of the uterine souffle, Obstet. Gynecol. 25:56, 1965.

Moser, R. J., Jr., and Caldwell, J. R.: Abdominal murmurs, an aid in the diagnosis of renal artery disease in hypertension, Ann. Intern. Med. 56:471, 1962.

Neporent, L. M.: Atrial heart sounds in atrial fibrillation and flutter, Circulation 30:893, 1964.

Ravin, A.: Disorders of the heart beat, Rocky Mt. Med. J. 43:468, 1946.

Rowe, G. G., et al.: The mechanism of the production of Duroziez's murmur, N. Engl. J. Med. 272:1207, 1965.

Schrire, V., and Vogelpoel, L.: The clinical and electrocardiographic differentiation of supraventricular and ventricular tachycardias with regular rhythm, Am. Heart J. 49:162, 1955.

Tabatznik, B., Randall, T. W., and Hersch, C.: The mammary souffle of pregnancy and lactation, Circulation 22:1069, 1960.

Wales, R. T., and Martin, E. A.: Arterial bruits in anaemia, Br. Med. J. 2:1444, 1963.

Zuckerman, R.: Der Herzchall bei Arrhythmien und Leitungsstörungen, Z. Kreislaufforsch. 50:395, 1961.

Congenital Heart Disease

Barritt, D. W., Davies, D. H., and Jacob, G.: Heart sounds and pressures in atrial septal defect, Br. Heart J. 27:90, 1965.

Bousvaros, G., and Palmer, W.: Phonocardiographic features of the systolic murmur in pulmonary artery stenosis, Br. Heart J. 27:374, 1965.

Braunwald, E., et al.: Congenital aortic stenosis. I. Clinical and hemodynamic findings in 100 patients. II. Surgical treatment and the results of operation, Circulation 27:426, 1963.

Braunwald, E., and Morrow, A. G. (eds.): Idiopathic Hypertrophic Subaortic Stenosis, American Heart Association Monograph, no. 10 (New York: American Heart Association, Inc., 1964). (First appeared as Suppl. 4 to Circulation 30:1964.)

Daoud, G., et al.: Auscultatory findings of pure infundibular stenosis, Am. J. Dis. Child. 108:73, 1964.

Dimond, E. G., and Benchimol, A.: Phonocardiography in atrial septal defect: Correlation between hemodynamics and phonocardiographic findings, Am. Heart J. 58:343, 1959.

Dimond, E. G., and Benchimol, A.: Phonocardiography in pulmonary stenosis: Special correlation between hemodynamics and phonocardiographic findings, Ann. Intern. Med. 52:145, 1960.

Fishleder, B. L.: El fonocardiograma en la enfermedad de Ebstein, Arch. Inst. Cardiol. Mex. 32:205, 1962.

Forster, J. W., and Humphries, J. O.: Right ventricular anomalous muscle bundle, Circulation 43:115, 1971.

Gamboa, R., Hugenholtz, P. G., and Nadas, A. S.: Accuracy of the phonocardiogram in assessing severity of aortic and pulmonic stenosis, Circulation 30:35, 1964.

van der Hauwaert, L., and Nadas, A. S.: Auscultatory findings in patients with a small ventricular septal defect, Circulation 23:886, 1961.

Hollman, A., *et al*.: Auscultatory and phonocardiographic findings in ventricular septal defect: A study of 93 surgically treated patients, Circulation 28:94, 1963.

Hultgren, H. N., Reeve, R., Cohn, K., and McLeod, R.: The ejection click of valvular pulmonic stenosis, Circulation 40:631, 1969.

Karnegis, J. N., and Wang, Y.: The phonocardiogram in idiopathic dilatation of the pulmonary artery, Am. J. Cardiol. 14:75, 1965.

Kumar, S., and Luisada, A. A.: The second heart sound in atrial septal defect, Am. J. Cardiol. 28:168, 1971.

Leatham, A., *et al*.: Discussion on the significance of cardiac murmurs in the first few days of life, Proc. R. Soc. Med. 52:75, 1959.

Leatham, A., and Segal, B.: Auscultatory and phonocardiographic signs of ventricular septal defect with left-to-right shunt, Circulation 25:318, 1962.

Linhart, J. W., and Razi, B.: Late systolic murmur: A clue to the diagnosis of aneurysm of the membranous ventricular septum, Chest 60:285, 1971.

Macieira-Coelho, E., and Coelhoe, E.: Auscultatory and phonocardiographic diagnosis of Fallot-type complex, Cardiologia 41:193, 1962.

Menges, M., Jr., Brandenburg, R. O., and Brown, A. L., Jr.: The clinical, hemodynamic, and pathologic diagnosis of muscular subvalvular aortic stenosis, Circulation 24:1126, 1961.

Neill, C., and Mounsey, P.: Auscultation in patent ductus arteriosus, with a description of two fistulae simulating patent ductus, Br. Heart J. 20:61, 1958.

Neufeld, H. N., *et al*.: Aorticopulmonary septal defect, Am. J. Cardiol. 9:12, 1962.

Perloff, J. K., Lebauer, E. J.: Auscultatory and phonocardiographic manifestations of isolated stenosis of the pulmonary artery and its branches, Br. Heart J. 31:314, 1969.

Rowe, R. D., and Lowe, J. B.: Auscultation in the diagnosis of persistent ductus arteriosus in infancy: A study of 50 patients, N. Z. Med. J. 63:195, 1964.

Schrire, V., *et al*.: Atrial septal defect. Part II: Endocardial-cushion defects, S. Afr. Med. J. 37:839, 1963.

Shapiro, W.: Unusual experiences with precordial continuous murmurs, Am. J. Cardiol. 7:511, 1961.

Spencer, M. P., Johnston, F. R., and Meredith, J. H.: The origin and interpretation of murmurs in coarctation of the aorta, Am. Heart J. 56:722, 1958.

Vogelpoel, L., and Schrire, V.: Auscultatory and phonocardiographic assessment of Fallot's tetralogy, Circulation 22:73, 1960.

Vogelpoel, L., and Schrire, V.: Auscultatory and phonocardiographic assessment of pulmonary stenosis with intact ventricular septum, Circulation 22:55, 1960.

Wells, B.: The sounds and murmurs in transposition of the great vessels, Br. Heart J. 25:748, 1963.

Auscultation in Various Diseases

Aronow, W. S., Uyeyama, R. R., Cassidy, J., and Nebolon, J.: Resting and post-exercise phonocardiogram and electrocardiogram in patients with angina pectoris and in normal subjects, Circulation 43:273, 1971.

Barlow, J., Fuller, D., and Denny, M.: A case of right atrial myxoma with special reference to an unusual phonocardiographic finding, Br. Heart J. 24:120, 1962.

Barlow, J., and Kincaid-Smith, P.: The auscultatory findings in hypertension, Br. Heart J. 22:505, 1960.

Bashour, F. A.: Mitral regurgitation following myocardial infarction. The syndrome of papillary mitral regurgitation, Dis. Chest 48:113, 1965.

Bland, E. F., and Jones, T. D.: The delayed appearance of heart disease after rheumatic fever, J.A.M.A. 113:1380, 1939.

Bland, E. F., Jones, T. D., and White, P. D.: Disappearance of the physical signs of rheumatic heart disease, J.A.M.A. 107:569, 1936.

Bland, E. F., White, P. D., and Jones, T. D.: Development of mitral stenosis in young people, with discussion of frequent misinterpretation of middiastolic murmur at cardiac apex, Am. Heart J. 10:995, 1935.

de Leon, A. C., Jr., et al.: The straight back syndrome: Clinical cardiovascular manifestations, Circulation 32:193, 1965.

de Leon, A. C., Perloff, J. K., Twigg, H. L., and Majd, M.: The straight back syndrome: Clinical cardiovascular manifestation, Circulation 32:193, 1965.

Evans, W.: The heart in sternal depression, Br. Heart J. 8:162, 1946.

Feinstein, A. R.: The stethoscope: A source of diagnostic aid and conceptual errors in rheumatic heart disease, J. Chronic Dis. 11:91, 1960.

Graham, J., Suby, H. I., LeCompte, P. R., and Sadowsky, N. L.: Fibrotic disorders associated with methysergide therapy for headache, N. Engl. J. Med. 274:359, 1966.

Gremmel, H., Loogen, F., and Vieten, H.: Kardiovaskuläre Befunde beim Marfan-Syndrom, Fortschr. Geb. Röentgenstr. Nuklearmed. 100:612, 1964.

Harvey, W. P., and Perloff, J. K.: The auscultatory findings in primary myocardial disease, Am. Heart J. 61:199, 1961.

Holloway, D. H., Whalen, R. E., and McIntosh, H. D.: Systolic murmur developing after myocardial ischemia or infarction: Differential diagnosis, J.A.M.A. 191:888, 1965.

Kluss, C. O.: Auskultatorische Alarmsymptome beim Myokardinfarkt, Münch. Med. Wochenschr. 103:2463, 1961.

Najmi, M., and Segal, B. L.: Auscultatory and phonocardiographic findings in patients with prosthetic ball valves, Am. J. Cardiol. 16:794, 1965.

Nellen, M., Maurer, B., and Goodwin, J. F.: Value of physical examination in acute myocardial infarction, Br. Heart J. 35:777, 1973.

Puchner, T. C., Huston, J. H., and Hellmuth, G. A.: Heart sounds and murmurs in arterial hypertension, Am. J. Cardiol. 6:630, 1960.

Reusch, C. S.: Hemodynamic studies in pectus excavatum, Circulation 24:1143, 1961.

Roberts, W. C., and Buchbinder, N. A.: Right-sided valvular infective endocarditis, Am. J. Med. 53:7, 1972.

Roberts, W. C., Dangel, J. C., and Bulkley, B. H.: Nonrheumatic Valvular Cardiac Disease: A Clinico-pathologic Survey in 27 Different Conditions Causing Valvular Dysfunction, in Brest, A. N. (ed.): Valvular Heart Disease, Cardiovascular Clinics, vol. 5, no. 2 (Philadelphia: F. A. Davis Co., 1973), p. 333.

Schrire, V., and Barnard, C. N.: The pre-operative assessment of mitral-valve disease, S. Afr. Med. J. 38:721, 1964.

Siegel, J. S., and Schechter, E.: The straight back syndrome, Am. J. Med. 42:309, 1967.

Titus, J. L.: Rheumatic and Collagen Involvement of the Heart, in Brest, A. N. (ed.): Clinical-Pathologic Correlations, Cardiovascular Clinics, vol. 4, no. 2 (Philadelphia: F. A. Davis Co., 1972), p. 307.

Ueda, H., et al.: Phonocardiographic study of hyperthyroidism, Jpn. Heart J. 4:509, 1963.

Wassermil, M., Warkentin, D. L., and Ravin, A.: Myxoma of the left atrium: Phonocardiographic study of three cases, Circulation 25:50, 1962.

Waller, B. F., Knapp, W. S., and Edwards, J. E.: Marantic valvular vegetations, Circulation 48:644, 1973.
Yoshimura, S., et al.: Phonocardiographic study on the acute rheumatic carditis, Jpn. Heart J. 2:28, 1961.
Zilli, A., and Gamna, G.: Evolution of murmurs in early rheumatic heart disease, Am. J. Med. 17:775, 1954.

Postsurgical Findings

Bonicort, O. W., Bristow, J. D., Starr, A., and Griswold, H. E.: A phonocardiographic study of patients with multiple Starr-Edwards prosthetic valves, Br. Heart J. 28:531, 1966.
Dock, W.: Heart sounds from Starr-Edwards valves, Circulation 31:801, 1965.
Gianelly, R. E., Popp, R. L., and Hultgren, H. H.: Heart sounds in patients with homograft replacement of the mitral valve, Circulation 42:309, 1970.
Harris, A.: Pacemaker "heart sound," Br. Heart J. 24:608, 1967.
Leachman, R. D., and Cokkinos, D. V. P.: Absence of opening click in dehiscence of mitral-valve prosthesis, N. Engl. J. Med. 281:461, 1969.
Misra, K. P., Korn, M., Ghahramani, M. D., and Samet, P.: Auscultatory findings in patients with cardiac pacemakers, Ann. Intern. Med. 74:245, 1971.
Nachnani, G. H., Gooch, A. S., and Hsu, I.: Systolic murmurs induced by pacemaker catheters, Arch. Intern. Med. 124:202, 1969.

Nonauscultatory Findings

Beiser, G. D., Epstein, S. E., Stampfer, M., Goldstein, R. E., Noland, S. P., and Levitsky, S.: Impairment of cardiac function in patients with pectus excavatum, with improvement after operative correction, N. Engl. J. Med. 287:267, 1972.
Berry, M. R.: The mechanism and prevention of impairment of auscultatory sounds during determination of blood pressure of standing patients, Proc. Staff Meeting Mayo Clinic, 15:699, 1940.
Bordley, J., III, Connor, C. A. R., Hamilton, W. F., Kerr, W. J., and Wiggers, C. J.: Recommendations for human blood pressure determinations by sphygmomanometers, Circulation 4:503, 1951.
Bramwell, C.: The arterial pulse in health and disease, Lancet 2:239, 301, 366, 1937.
Davies, H.: Chest deformities in congenital heart disease, Br. J. Dis. Chest 53: 151, 1959.
Editorial: Standardization of methods of measuring the arterial blood pressure, Br. Heart J. 1:261, 1939.
Fleming, P. R.: The mechanism of the pulsus bisferiens, Br. Heart J. 19:519, 1957.
Lovibond, J. L.: Diagnosis of clubbed fingers, Lancet 1:363, 1938.
Perloff, J. K.: Diagnostic inferences drawn from observation and palpation of the precordium with special reference to congenital heart disease, Adv. Cardiopulm. Dis. 4:13, 1969.
Ragan, C., and Bordley, J., III: The accuracy of clinical measurements of arterial blood pressure, Bull. Johns Hopkins Hosp. 69:504, 1941.
Rebuck, A. S., and Pengelly, L. D.: Development of pulsus paradoxus in the presence of airways obstruction, N. Engl. J. Med. 288:66, 1973.
Reich, L. L., and Tavel, M. E.: The origin of the jugular C-wave, N. Engl. J. Med. 284:1309, 1971.
Stafford, R. W., Kronenberg, M. W., Dunbar, J. D., and Wooley, C. F.: Contin-

uous precordial murmur due to internal mammary artery fistulas, Am. J. Cardiol. 24:414, 1969.

Wachtel, F. W., Ravitch, M. W., and Grishman, A.: The relation of pectus excavatum to heart disease, Am. Heart J. 52:121, 1956.

Wood, P.: *Diseases of the Heart and Circulation* (3d ed.; Philadelphia: J. B. Lippincott Co., 1968).

Effect of Drugs

Barlow, J., and Shillingford, J.: The use of amyl nitrite in differentiating mitral and aortic systolic murmurs, Br. Heart J. 20:162, 1958.

Beck, W., et al.: Hemodynamic effects of amyl nitrite and phenylephrine on the normal human circulation and their relation to changes in cardiac murmurs, Am. J. Cardiol. 8:341, 1961.

Bousvaros, G. A.: Effect of norepinephrine on the phonocardiographic, auscultatory and hemodynamic features of congenital and acquired heart disease, Am. J. Cardiol. 8:328, 1961.

Crevasse, L.: The use of a vasopressor agent as a diagnostic aid in auscultation, Am. Heart J. 58:821, 1959.

Dohan, M. C., and Criscitiello, M. G.: Physiological and pharmacological manipulations of heart sounds and murmurs, Mod. Concepts Cardiovasc. Dis. 39:121, 1970.

Endrys, J., and Bártová, A.: Pharmacological methods in the phonocardiographic diagnosis of regurgitant murmurs, Br. Heart J. 24:207, 1962.

Rautenburg, H. W., and Menner, K.: Der Amylnitrit-Test zur Differential Diagnose angeborener und erworbener Angiokardiopathien im Kindesalter, Arch. Kreislaufforsch. 47:73, 1965.

Schrire, V., et al.: The effects of amyl nitrite and phenylephrine on the intracardiac murmurs of small ventricular septal defects, Am. Heart J. 62:225, 1961.

Vogelpoel, L., et al.: The use of amyl nitrite in the differentiation of Fallot's tetralogy and pulmonary stenosis with intact ventricular septum, Am. Heart J. 57:803, 1959.

Vogelpoel, L., et al.: The use of amyl nitrite in the diagnosis of systolic murmurs, Lancet 2:810, 1959.

Vogelpoel, L., et al.: The use of phenylephrine in the differentiation of Fallot's tetralogy from pulmonary stenosis with intact ventricular septum, Am. Heart J. 59:489, 1960.

Vogelpoel, L., et al.: The atypical systolic murmur of minute ventricular septal defect and its recognition by amyl nitrite and phenylephrine, Am. Heart J. 62:101, 1961.

Vogelpoel, L., et al.: Variations in the response of the systolic murmur to vasoactive drugs in ventricular septal defect, with special reference to the paradoxical response in large defects with pulmonary hypertension, Am. Heart J. 64:169, 1962.

General

Butterworth, J. S., Chassin, M. R., and McGrath, R.: *Cardiac Auscultation* (2d ed.; New York: Grune & Stratton, Inc., 1960).

Feruglio, G. A.: *Intracardiac Auscultation and Phonocardiography (Techniques and Clinical Applications)* (Turin, Italy: Panminerva Medica, 1964).

Harvey, W. P.: Some newer or poorly recognized findings on clinical auscultation, Mod. Concepts Cardiovasc. Dis. 37:85, 89, 1968.

Levine, S. A., and Harvey, W. P.: *Clinical Auscultation of the Heart* (2d ed.; Philadelphia: W. B. Saunders Co., 1959).

Luisada, A. A.: *From Auscultation to Phonocardiography* (St. Louis: C. V. Mosby Co., 1965).

McKusick, V. A.: *Cardiovascular Sound in Health and Disease* (Baltimore: Williams & Wilkins Co., 1958).

Ongley, P. A., *et al.*: *Heart Sounds and Murmurs, a Clinical and Phonocardiographic Study* (New York: Grune & Stratton, Inc., 1969).

Orias, O., and Braun-Menéndez, E.: *The Heart-Sounds in Normal and Pathological Conditions* (London: Oxford University Press, 1939).

Ravin, A., and Frame, F. K.: *International Bibliography of Cardiovascular Auscultation and Phonocardiography.* American Heart Association Monograph, no. 31 (New York: American Heart Association, Inc., 1971).

Ravin, A., Tucker, C. E., and Craddock, L. D.: An instrument for simulating heart sounds and murmurs, Am. J. Cardiol. 18:622, 1966.

Rovelli, F., *et al.*: *Testo Atlante di Fonocardiografia* (Turin, Italy: Minerva Medica, 1965).

Segal, B. L., and Likoff, W.: *Auscultation of the Heart* (New York: Grune & Stratton, Inc., 1965).

Segal, B. L., Likoff, W., and Moyer, J. H. (eds.): *The Theory and Practice of Auscultation* (Philadelphia: F. A. Davis Co., 1964).

Ueda, H., Kaito, G., and Sakamoto, T.: *Auscultation of the Heart Using Heart Sound Record and Illustrated by Phonocardiograms* (Tokyo: Nanzando Co., Ltd., 1960).

Zuckermann, R.: *Herzauskultation* (Leipzig: Georg Thieme, 1963).

Index

A

Aged: sinus arrhythmia of, 169–170
Alpha stimulators, 250–251
Amyl nitrite, 251–257
  to differentiate murmurs,
      254–257
  in murmur of ventricular septal
      defect, 253
  test, technique of, 251–254
Anacrotic notch, 240
Aneurysm resection: sounds after,
      231–232
Angiotensin, 250–251
Ankylosing spondylitis, 224
Aorta
  coarctation of, 185–186
  descending, murmurs in,
      156–157
  hematoma of, dissecting,
      postsurgical sounds, 231–232
Aortic
  ejection sounds (see Sounds,
      ejection, aortic)
  regurgitation (see Regurgitation,
      aortic)
  stenosis (see Stenosis, aortic)
  valve
    deformity, systolic murmur of
        (see Murmurs, systolic, of
        aortic valvular deformity)
    in rheumatic fever, 205
    stenosis (see Stenosis, aortic)
Aortopulmonary septal defect:
    differentiated from patent

ductus arteriosus, 175–176
Apicosternal region (see Murmurs,
    systolic, innocent, in
    apicosternal region)
Arrhythmia, 158–170
  examination
    clinical setting, 161
    exercise and, 161
  jugular venous pulse in, 160–161
  physical signs of, 159
  sinus, 166
    of aged, 169–170
  sounds in
    first, intensity of, 160
    splitting of, 160
  Valsalva maneuver in, 161
Arteries
  murmurs over (see Murmurs,
      arterial)
  pressure, influencing loudness of
      second heart sound, 44–45
  pulmonary, dilatation, idiopathic,
      184
Arteriosclerosis, 209–211
  murmur associated with, basal
      systolic, 114–115
Arteriosclerotic heart disease
  rhythm in, quadruple or
      cogwheel, 79
  summation sound in, 79
Arteriovenous fistula: causing
      arterial murmurs, 152–153
Arthritis: rheumatoid, 224
Atheromatous changes: causing
      arterial murmurs, 152

273

Atresia: tricuspid, 191
Atrial
    contractions, premature, 166–168
    fibrillation (*see* Fibrillation)
    flutter (*see* Flutter)
    gallop (*see* Sounds, fourth)
    murmur, systolic, 59
    myxoma, 218
    septal defects (*see* Septal defects,
        atrial)
    sound (*see* Sounds, fourth)
    tachycardia (*see* Tachycardia,
        atrial)
Atrioventricular
    canal, persistent, 183
    conduction, delayed, and fourth
        heart sound, 62
    valve position, and intensity of
        first heart sound, 33–37
Auscultation
    areas, 4
    exercise and, 249–250
    extracardiac, 152–157
    graphic recording of, 19–26
        alternative method for, 24–26
        chest diagram used for, 22–23
        symbols used in, 20
    pharmacologic maneuvers in,
        250–257
    physiologic maneuvers in,
        245–250
    postural maneuvers in, 247–249
    respiration and, quiet, 245–246
    Valsalva maneuver in, 246–247
Austin Flint murmur, 258
    aortic regurgitation and, 143
    differentiation from mitral
        stenosis, drugs used, 256
AV (*see* Atrioventricular)

B

Back: straight back syndrome, 220
Basal systolic murmur: associated
        with arteriosclerosis and/or
        hypertension, 114–115
Beall floating lenticular valve, 227
Beta stimulators, 257
Björk-Shiley tilting disc valve, 227
Block
    2:1, with sinus or atrial
        tachycardia, 165
    3:1, atrial flutter with, 165

4:1, atrial flutter with, 165
bundle branch
    left, splitting of first heart
        sound in, 38
    left, splitting of second heart
        sound in, 47–48
    right, splitting of first heart
        sound in, 38
    right, splitting of second heart
        sound in, 47
complete, 166
    sounds in, first, intensity of, 34,
        35
    sounds in, fourth, 62
partial, 166
second-degree, Wenckebach type
    of, 168
Blood
    flow increase causing arterial
        murmurs, 152
    pressure (*see* Cardiovascular
        disease, blood pressure and
        pulse in)
Bradycardia: sinus, 166
Bruit, 155
Bundle branch block (*see* Block,
    bundle branch)

C

Calcification: of mitral annulus
        fibrosis, causing mitral
        regurgitation, 102
Carcinoid syndrome, 223–224
Cardiomyopathy, 218
Cardiopulmonary murmur, 125
Cardiovascular disease
    blood pressure and pulse in,
        237–241
    information obtained, 239–241
    method of determination,
        237–239
    cardiac pulsations or movements
        in, 234–237
    chest wall deformities in,
        233–234
    nonauscultatory findings in,
        233–244
Cardiovascular syphilis, 221
Carditis (*see* Rheumatic carditis)
Carey-Coombs murmur, 258
Carotid sinus massage
    in arrhythmias, 161

in differentiation of
   supraventricular tachycardias,
   164
Carvallo's sign, 258
Chest wall
   deformities in cardiovascular
      disease, 233–234
   thickness, and intensity of first
      heart sound, 32
Chordae
   elongation causing click-murmur
      syndrome, 105
   rupture causing mitral
      regurgitation, 106
Click
   -murmur syndrome, 68
      chordae elongation causing, 105
      echo of, 104
      mitral regurgitation due to,
         103–106
   systolic, 67–69
      in atrial septal defect, 67
Coarctation of aorta, 185–186
Commissurotomy
   finger fracture, 71
   mitral, in rheumatic fever,
      207
   tricuspid, in rheumatic fever, 207
Conduction: delayed
      atrioventricular, and fourth
      heart sound, 62
Contractions
   atrial premature, 166–168
   ventricular
      premature, 166–168
      premature, splitting of first
         heart sound in, 38
      rate of, and intensity of first
         heart sound, 37–38
Coronary revascularization: sounds
   after, 231
Corrigan's pulse, 258
Cossio's sign, 258

D

Deformities
   aortic valve (see Murmurs,
      systolic, of aortic valvular
      deformity)
   chest wall, in cardiovascular
      disease, 233–234
Diastolic murmurs (see Murmurs,
      diastolic)
Diastolic overload, 48
Drugs (see Pharmacologic
      maneuvers)
Duroziez's sign, 157, 258

E

Ebstein's disease, 191
Echocardiogram
   of aortic regurgitation and Austin
      Flint murmur, 143
   of mitral stenosis, 130–131
   mitral valve
      normal, 28
      in subaortic stenosis, 119
Eisenmenger's complex, 180
Ejection
   murmurs, 85
      discussion of term, 87–88
   sounds (see Sound(s), ejection)
Elderly: sinus arrhythmia of,
      169–170
Embolism: pulmonary, 222–223
Emphysema: and intensity of first
      heart sound, 32–33
Endocardial cushion defect, 183
Endocarditis, 222
   methysergide–induced, 225
Erb's point (area), 258
Exercise
   arrhythmia examination and, 161
   auscultation and, 249–250
   effect on murmurs, 93
      diastolic, of mitral stenosis, 133

F

Fallot's tetralogy (see Tetralogy of
      Fallot)
Fever (see Rheumatic fever)
Fibrillation, atrial, 168–169
   intensity of first heart sound in,
      36
   with mitral stenosis, intensity of
      first heart sound in, 36–37
Fibrosis: mitral annulus,
      calcification of, causing mitral
      regurgitation, 102
Finger fracture commissurotomy, 71
First heart sound, 28–39
   description of, 28–32
   intensity of

First heart sound *(cont.)*
  in arrhythmias, 160
  atrial fibrillation and, 36
  atrioventricular valve position and, 33–37
  cardiac factors influencing, 33–38
  changes in, 32–38
  chest wall thickness and, 32
  emphysema and, 32–33
  extracardiac factors influencing, 32–33
  in heart block, complete, 34, 35
  mitral stenosis with atrial fibrillation affecting, 36–37
  pericardial fluid and, 33
  P-R interval change and, 34, 36
  tachycardia and, ventricular, 36
  valve changes influencing, pathologic, 37
  loudness of *(see* intensity of *above)*
  masking of, 38
  splitting of, abnormal, 38–39
  in tricuspid regurgitation, 108
  variation in, in different locations, 30
Fistula: arteriovenous, causing arterial murmurs, 152–153
Flutter, atrial
  with block, 3:1 or 4:1, 165
  carotid sinus massage in, 164
  Valsalva maneuver in, 164
Friction rub: pericardial, 148–150

G

Gallavardin phenomenon, 258
Gallop
  atrial *(see* Sounds, fourth)
  presystolic *(see* Sounds, fourth)
  rhythm, 53
  summation *(see* Sounds, summation)
  systolic *(see* Clicks, systolic)
Gibson murmur, 258
Graham Steell murmur, 145–147, 258

H

Hamman's sign, 259
Head: murmurs in, 154–156

Heart
  block *(see* Block)
  disease
    arteriosclerotic *(see* Arteriosclerotic heart disease)
    congenital, 171–191
    congenital, apical diastolic murmur of, 143–144
    hypertensive, 218–219
    rheumatic, 192–208
    rheumatic, inactive, with mitral regurgitation, murmur in, 144–145
  factors influencing intensity of first heart sound, 33–38
  failure, arteriosclerotic, summation sound in, 79
  lesions, congenital, 190–191
  movements, in cardiovascular disease, 234–237
  pulsations, in cardiovascular disease, 234–237
  sounds *(see* Sounds)
  surgery, congenital, sounds after, 230–231
  tumors, 217–218
Hematoma: of aorta, dissecting, postsurgical sounds, 231–232
Hum, venous, 150–151, 157
  patent ductus arteriosus differentiated from, 175
Hypertension, 218–219
  murmur associated with, basal systolic, 114–115
  pulmonary
    patent ductus arteriosus with, 174
    primary, 183
    pulmonary ejection sounds in, 64
    in rheumatic fever, 200–203
  systemic, fourth sound in, 60
Hypertensive heart disease, 218–219

I

Infarction: acute myocardial, 213–215
Inotropic agents, 257
Intercostal space: second left, innocent systolic murmurs in, 124
Ischemia: myocardial, acute, 211–212

J

Jugular venous pulse, 243
 in arrhythmias, 160–161

K

Korotkoff sounds, 259
Kussmaul's sign, 259

L

Lactation: mammary souffle of, 157
Leatham stethoscope, 8
Lerman-Means scratch, 259
Littman stethoscope, 8
Lung (*see* Pulmonary)
Lupus erythematosus: systemic,
 224–225

M

Mammary souffle: of pregnancy and
 lactation, 157
Marfan's syndrome, 219
Masking
 of first heart sound, 38
 of second heart sound, 45
Massage (*see* Carotid sinus
 massage)
Methoxamine, 250–251
Methysergide–induced
 endocarditis, 225
Mitral
 annulus fibrosis calcification
 causing mitral regurgitation,
 102
 commissurotomy, effect on mitral
 murmurs in rheumatic fever,
 207
 regurgitation (*see* Regurgitation,
 mitral)
 stenosis (*see* Stenosis, mitral)
 valve
 normal, echocardiogram
 of, 28
 opening snap of, 69–74
 prosthetic, sounds produced by,
 228
 in rheumatic fever (*see under*
 Rheumatic fever)
 stenosis (*see* Stenosis, mitral)
Murmurs, 82–95
 accidental (*see* Murmurs, systolic,
 innocent *below*)
 in aorta, descending, 156–157
 of aortic regurgitation,
 differentiation from murmur
 of pulmonary regurgitation,
 drugs used, 256
 of aortic stenosis, differentiated
 from murmur of mitral
 regurgitation, drugs used,
 255–256
 arterial
 arteriovenous fistulae causing,
 152–153
 atheromatous changes causing,
 152
 blood flow increase causing,
 152
 murmurs produced in heart,
 152
 pressure gradient across an
 obstruction causing, 153–154
 pressure with stethoscope or
 finger causing, 152
 production of, 152–154
 transmission of, 152
 augmentation, 155
 Austin Flint (*see* Austin Flint
 murmur)
 cardiopulmonary, 125
 Carey-Coombs, 258
 click-murmur syndrome (*see*
 Click, -murmur syndrome)
 collision, 84
 crescendo, 85
 crescendo-decrescendo, 85
 decrescendo, 85
 description of, 85–93
 diamond-shaped, 85
 diastolic (*see below*)
 drugs to differentiate, 254–257
 duration of, 85–88
 ejection, 85
 discussion of term, 87–88
 exercise affecting, 93
 flow, 85, 92
 functional (*see* Murmurs, systolic,
 innocent *below*)
 Gibson, 258
 Graham Steell, 145–147, 258
 in head, 154–156
 holosystolic, 85
 intensity of, 88–90
 middiastolic, of mitral
 regurgitation, 144–145

Murmurs, *(cont.)*
  mitral, in rheumatic fever, effect
      of mitral commissurotomy on,
      207
  of mitral regurgitation,
      differentiated from murmur of
      aortic stenosis, drugs used,
      255–256
  musical, 92
  in neck, 154–156
  pansystolic, 85
  pansystolic regurgitant, 85
  of patent ductus arteriosus,
      171–177
      drugs used to recognize, 255
  physiologic (*see* Murmurs,
      systolic, innocent *below*)
  pitch of, 90–93
  point of maximum intensity of
      factors influencing location of,
          93–94
      factors influencing transmission
          of murmur from, 94
  production of, 82–84
  of pulmonary regurgitation,
      differentiated from murmur of
      aortic regurgitation, drugs
      used, 256
  of pulmonary stenosis
      infundibular, 180
      valvular, 180
  quality of, 90–93
  relation to thrills, 94–95
  Roger's, 259
  rough, 92
  Still's, 259
  systolic (*see below*)
  timing of, 85–88
  transmission of, 93–94
      quality of murmur and, 94
  of ventricular septal defect, 178
Murmurs, diastolic, 126–147
  of aortic regurgitation, 136–140
      area of transmission, 137, 138
      duration of, 136
      heart sound changes and, 139
      intensity of, maximum, point of,
          137
      intensity of, relation to severity
          of lesion, 139
      occurrence of, 139
      pitch of, 136–137
      position of patient and, 137
      quality of, 136–137

  timing of, 136
  apical, 140–145
      of aortic regurgitation, 141–142
      of congenital heart disease,
          143–144
      differentiation, 141–145
      occurrence of, 141–145
      of rheumatic carditis, acute,
          142–143
      in rheumatic heart disease,
          inactive, with mitral
          regurgitation, 144–145
      in ventricular enlargement, left,
          145
  causes of, 147
  cooling, 93
  duration of, 88
  of mitral stenosis, 126–134
      area of transmission, 127–130
      differentiation, 134
      duration of, 126–127, 134
      exercise and, 133
      heart sound changes and,
          132–133
      intensity of, maximum,
          127–130
      intensity of, relation to severity
          of lesion, 133–134
      pitch of, 130–132
      position of patient and, 132
      quality of, 130–132
      respiration and, 132
      timing of, 126–127
  of pulmonary regurgitation,
      145–147
  timing of, 88
  of tricuspid stenosis, 134–135
Murmurs, systolic, 96–125
  of aortic stenosis, 109–114
      area of transmission, 110–112
      differentiation, 113–114
      duration of, 109
      heart sound changes and, 112
      intensity of, maximum, point of,
          110–112
      intensity of, relation to severity
          of lesion, 112–113
      occurrence of, 113
      pitch of, 109–110
      position of patient and, 112
      quality of, 109–110
      timing of, 109
  of aortic valvular deformity,
      109–114

area of transmission, 110–112
differentiation, 113–114
duration of, 109
heart sound changes and, 112
intensity of, maximum, point of,
  110–112
intensity of, relation to severity
  of lesion, 112–113
occurrence of, 113
pitch of, 109–110
position of patient and, 112
quality of, 109–110
timing of, 109
atrial, 59
of atrial septal defects, 181
basal, associated with
  arteriosclerosis and/or
  hypertension, 114–115
division of, basis for, 86
duration of, 85–88
innocent, 121–124
innocent, in apicosternal region,
  121–124
  area of transmission, 121
  differentiation, 124
  duration of, 121
  heart sound changes and,
    123–124
  loudness of, 123
  pitch of, 121–123
  position of patient and, 123
  quality of, 121–123
  respiration and, 123
  timing of, 121
innocent, differentiated from
  atrial septal defect, 184
innocent, in intercostal space,
  second left, 124
innocent, of ventricular septal
  defect, 179–180
of mitral regurgitation, 96–102
  area of transmission, 98–100
  differentiation, 106–107
  duration of, 96–98
  heart sound changes and, 101
  holosystolic character of, 97
  intensity of, maximum, point of,
    98–100
  intensity of, relation to degree
    of regurgitation, 101–102
  pitch of, 100
  position of patient and, 100
  quality of, 100
  respiration affecting, 100

timing of, 96–98
of subaortic stenosis, 117–120
of tetralogy of Fallot, 190
timing of, 85–88
of tricuspid regurgitation,
  107–109
  differentiation, 108
  heart sounds in, first, 108
  pitch of, 108
  point of maximum intensity,
    107
  quality of, 108
  respiration affecting, 108
Muscle dysfunction: papillary,
  causing mitral regurgitation,
  99, 102–103
Myocardial
  failure, 216–217
  infarction, acute, 213–215
  ischemia, acute, 211–212
Myocardiopathies: fourth heart
  sounds in, 61
Myxoma: atrial, 218

N

Neck: murmurs in, 154–156

O

Opening snap
  of mitral valve, 69–74
  of tricuspid valve, 74
Ostium primum: persistent, 183

P

Pacemakers, 229
Papillary muscle dysfunction:
  causing mitral regurgitation,
  99, 102–103
Patent ductus arteriosus, 171–177
  differentiation, 175–177
    from aortopulmonary septal
      defect, 175–176
    from ventricular septal defect,
      175
    from tetralogy, 176
    from venous hum, 175
  murmurs of, 171–177
    drugs used to recognize, 255
  pulmonary hypertension and,
    174
Pectus excavatum, 220

Pericardial fluid: and intensity of
    first heart sound, 33
Pericardial friction rub, 148–150
Pericarditis: constrictive, third heart
    sound in, 78
Pharmacologic maneuvers
    in auscultation, 250–257
    to differentiate murmurs,
        254–257
Phenylephrine, 250–251
Phonocardiography, 10–11
    intracardiac, 11
    spectral, 11
Physiologic maneuvers: in
    auscultation, 245–250
Postsurgical sounds, 226–232
Pregnancy: mammary souffle of, 157
Pressure
    arterial, effect on loudness of
        second heart sound, 44–45
    in cardiovascular disease (see
        Cardiovascular disease, blood
        pressure and pulse in)
    gradient across an obstruction
        causing arterial murmur,
        153–154
    venous, 241–244
P-R interval change: and intensity
    of first heart sound, 34, 36
Prosthetic devices: and postsurgical
    sounds, 232
Prosthetic valves, 226–229
    Beall floating lenticular, 227
    Björk-Shiley tilting disc, 227
    mitral, sounds produced by, 228
    Starr-Edwards ball, 227
Pseudoparadoxical splitting, 73
Pulmonary
    aortopulmonary septal defect
        differentiated from patent
        ductus arteriosus, 175–176
    artery dilatation, idiopathic, 184
    cardiopulmonary murmur, 125
    ejection sounds (see Sounds,
        ejection, pulmonary)
    embolism, 222–223
    hypertension (see Hypertension,
        pulmonary)
    regurgitation (see Regurgitation,
        pulmonary)
    stenosis (see Stenosis, pulmonary)
    venous drainage, anomalous, 183
Pulse
    cardiac, in cardiovascular disease,

        234–237
    in cardiovascular disease (see
        Cardiovascular disease, blood
        pressure and pulse in)
    Corrigan's, 258
    venous, 241–244
    jugular, 243
    jugular, in arrhythmias,
        160–161
Pulseless disease, 156
Pulsus paradoxus, 240–241

Q

Quincke's sign, 259

R

Regurgitation, 84–85
    aortic
        aortic ejection sound in, 66, 67
        murmur of, Austin Flint, 143
        murmur of, diastolic (see under
            Murmurs, diastolic)
        murmur of, differentiated from
            murmur of pulmonary
            regurgitation, drugs used, 256
        in rheumatic fever, surgery for,
            208
    functional, 85
    mitral
        calcification of mitral annulus
            fibrosis causing, 102
        chordae rupture causing, 106
        click-murmur syndrome
            causing, 103–106
        conditions producing, 102–107
        differentiation from muscular
            subaortic stenosis, drugs
            used, 256–257
        differentiation from tricuspid
            regurgitation, drugs used, 256
        murmur of, differentiated from
            murmur of aortic stenosis,
            drugs used, 255–256
        murmur of, middiastolic,
            144–145
        murmur of, systolic (see
            Murmurs, systolic, of mitral
            regurgitation)
        papillary muscle dysfunction
            causing, 99, 102–103
        in rheumatic fever (see
            Rheumatic fever, mitral

regurgitation in)
rheumatic heart disease with,
   murmur in, 144–145
stethoscope usage in, 14, 15
ventricular dilatation causing,
   left, 103
organic, 85
relative, 85
tricuspid
   differentiation from mitral
      regurgitation, drugs used, 256
   first heart sound in, 108
   murmur of, systolic (see
      Murmurs, systolic, of
      tricuspid regurgitation)
   in rheumatic fever, 201–203
Respiration
   effect on murmurs
      diastolic, of mitral stenosis, 132
      systolic, in apicosternal region,
         123
      systolic, of mitral regurgitation,
         100
      systolic, of tricuspid
         regurgitation, 108
   effect on sounds, second, 41
   quiet, effect on auscultation,
      245–246
Revascularization: coronary, sounds
   after, 231
Rheumatic carditis, acute, 192–193
   murmur of, apical diastolic,
      142–143
   regression of acute phase, 193
   subsequent course of, 193
Rheumatic fever
   aortic regurgitation in, surgery
      for, 208
   aortic stenosis in, surgery for,
      207–208
   aortic valve involvement in, 203–
      206
   carditis due to (see Rheumatic
      carditis)
   commissurotomy in
      mitral, 207
      tricuspid, 207
   heart disease due to, 192–208
   inactive, with mitral
      regurgitation, murmur in,
      144–145
   mitral regurgitation in, 102
      combined with mitral stenosis,
         196–198

severe, 195–196
   mitral stenosis in
      combined with mitral
         regurgitation, 196–198
      tight, 198–200
      tight, with early pulmonary
         hypertension, 200–201
      tight, with pulmonary
         hypertension and tricuspid
         regurgitation, 201–203
   mitral valve involvement in,
      193–203
   surgery for, 206–207
   valvular involvement in, surgery
      for, 206–208
Rheumatoid arthritis, 224
Rhythm
   cogwheel, 81
      in arteriosclerotic heart disease,
         79
   gallop, 53
   irregular
      absolutely, 168–170
      rhythmically, with normal heart
         rate, 166–168
      transiently, with normal heart
         rate, 166–168
      transiently, with rapid heart
         rate, 168
      transiently, with slow heart
         rate, 168
   quadruple, 81
      in arteriosclerotic heart disease,
         79
   regular
      with normal heart rate, 165
      with rapid heart rate, 161–
         164
      with slow heart rate, 166
   supraventricular, 161–164
   triple, 55
   ventricular, 161–164
Roger's murmur, 259
Rub: pericardial friction, 148–150
Rupture: chordae, causing mitral
   regurgitation, 106

S

Second heart sound, 39–51
   description of, 39–43
   loudness of, 43–45
      arterial pressure influencing,
         44–45

Second heart sound *(cont.)*
  valve changes and, pathologic, 45
  valve ring structural changes and, 45
  vessel changes and, great, 45
  masking of, 45
  respiration affecting, 41
  splitting of, 45–51
    in aortic stenosis, congenital, 48
    in bundle branch block, right, 47
    paradoxical, 48
    ventricular emptying time increase and, left, 50–51
    ventricular emptying time increase and, right, 48–50
Septal defects
  aortopulmonary, differentiated from patent ductus arteriosus, 175–176
  atrial, 180–184
    click in, systolic, 67
    mitral stenosis differentiated from, 184
    murmur differentiated from, innocent systolic, 184
    murmur of, systolic, 181
    stethoscope usage and, 14, 15
  ventricular, 177–180
    differentiation of, drugs used, 254–255
    murmur of, 178
    murmur of, innocent, 179–180
    patent ductus arteriosus differentiated from, 175
Sick sinus syndrome, 170
Sign of Duroziez, 157, 258
Sinus
  arrhythmia, 166
    of aged, 169–170
  bradycardia, 166
  carotid *(see* Carotid sinus massage)
  sick sinus syndrome, 170
  tachycardia *(see* Tachycardia, sinus)
SLE, 224–225
Souffle
  mammary, of pregnancy and lactation, 157
  uterine, 157
Sound(s), 1–4, 27–52
  abnormal, 53–81

atrial *(see* fourth *below)*
changes, effect on murmurs
  diastolic, of aortic regurgitation, 139
  diastolic, of mitral stenosis, 132–133
  systolic, of aortic stenosis, 112
  systolic, of aortic valvular deformity, 112
  systolic, innocent, in apicosternal region, 123–124
  systolic, of mitral regurgitation, 101
duration of, 3
ejection, 63–67
ejection, aortic, 66–67
  in aortic regurgitation, 66, 67
  in aortic stenosis, congenital, 65
  occurrence of, 66–67
ejection, pulmonary, 63–66
  occurrence of, 64–66
  in pulmonary hypertension, 64
extra, 53–81
  table of, 80
first *(see* First heart sound)
fourth, 56–62
  in aortic stenosis, 61
  in atrioventricular conduction, delayed, 62
  in heart block, complete, 62
  in hypertension, systemic, 60
  left-sided, 57–59
  in myocardiopathies, 61
  occurrence of, 60–62
  right-sided, 58
intensity of, 2–3
Korotkoff, 259
loudness of, 2–3
pitch of, 1
postsurgical, 226–232
prosthetic mitral valve producing, 228
quality of, 1–2
second *(see* Second heart sound)
splitting, in arrhythmias, 160
summation, 78–81
  in arteriosclerotic heart disease and failure, 79
  palpable, 235
third, 51–52, 75–78
  description of, 76–77
  occurrence of, 77–78
  in pericarditis, constrictive, 78
  production of, 75–76

timing of, 3, 27–28
transmission of, 3–4
Splitting
  of first heart sound, abnormal,
    38–39
  pseudoparadoxical, 73
  of second heart sound (see
    Second heart sound, splitting
    of)
Spondylitis: ankylosing, 224
Sprague-Bowles stethoscope, 8
Sprague-Rappaport stethoscope, 8
Starr-Edwards ball valve, 227
Stenosis, 85
  aortic
    congenital, aortic ejection
      sound in, 65
    congenital, splitting of second
      in, 48
    murmur of, differentiated from
      murmur of mitral
      regurgitation, drugs used,
      255–256
    murmur of, systolic (see
      Murmurs, systolic, of aortic
      stenosis)
    in rheumatic fever, surgery for,
      207–208
    sounds in, fourth, 61
    subvalvular, discrete, 184–185
    supravalvular, 184–185
    valvular, 184–185
  mitral
    atrial fibrillation and, intensity
      of first heart sound in, 36–37
    atrial septal defect
      differentiated from, 184
    Austin Flint murmur
      differentiated from, drugs
      used, 256
    echocardiogram of, 130–131
    murmur of, diastolic (see
      Murmurs, diastolic, of mitral
      stenosis)
    in rheumatic fever (see
      Rheumatic fever, mitral
      stenosis in)
    stethoscope usage and, 14
  organic, 85
  pulmonary
    differentiation from tetralogy of
      Fallot, drugs used, 254
    differentiation from ventricular
      septal defect, drugs used,
      254–255
    infundibular, differentiated
      from atrial septal defect,
      183–184
    infundibular, murmur of, 180
    peripheral, 189
    valvular, differentiated from
      atrial septal defect, 183–184
    valvular, murmur of, 180
    valvular, with intact ventricular
      septum, 187–189
  subaortic
    idiopathic hypertrophic,
      postsurgical sounds, 232
    mitral valve echocardiogram in,
      119
    murmur of, systolic, 117–120
    muscular, double impulse in,
      236
    muscular, drugs used to
      differentiate from mitral
      regurgitation, 256–257
  tricuspid, diastolic murmur of,
    134–135
Stethoscope, 5–18
  amplifying, 10
  chest pieces, 7–10
    deep bell, illustration of, 9
    illustration of, 8
  ear pieces, 6
  pressure on artery causing arterial
    murmur, 152
  tubes, 6–7
  use of, 11–18
    application of chest piece to
      chest wall, 12–17
    background noise and, 11–12
    listening to the heart, 17–18
    location on chest wall, 17
    position of patient, 12, 13
Still's murmur, 259
Straight back syndrome, 220
Subaortic stenosis (see Stenosis,
  subaortic)
Summation gallop (see Sounds,
  summation)
Summation sounds (see Sounds,
  summation)
Supraventricular rhythm:
  differentiated from
  ventricular rhythm, 161–164
Supraventricular tachycardia:
  differentiation of, 164
Surgery: sounds after, 226–232

Syphilis: cardiovascular, 221
Systolic click, 67–69
  in atrial septal defect, 67
Systolic gallop (*see* Systolic click)
Systolic murmurs (*see* Murmurs,
    systolic)
Systolic overload, 50

T

Tachycardia
  atrial
    block and, 2:1, 165
    carotid sinus massage in, 164
    multifocal, 169
    nodal, carotid sinus massage in,
      164
  sinus
    block and, 2:1, 165
    carotid sinus massage in, 164
    Valsalva maneuver in, 164
  supraventricular, differentiation
    of, 164
  ventricular
    intensity of first heart sound
      and, 36
    splitting of first heart sound in, 39
Tetralogy of Fallot, 189–190
  differentiated from patent ductus
    arteriosus, 176
  mild, acyanotic, differentiation
    from pulmonary stenosis,
    drugs used, 254
  murmur of, systolic, 190
Thrills: relation to murmurs, 94–95
Thyrotoxicosis, 220–221
Transposition of great vessels,
    190–191
Tricuspid
  atresia, 191
  commissurotomy in rheumatic
    fever, 207
  regurgitation (*see* Regurgitation,
    tricuspid)
  stenosis, diastolic murmur of,
    134–135
  valve, opening snap of, 74
Tubes: stethoscope, 6–7
Tumors: cardiac, 217–218
Tycos stethoscope, 8

U

Uterine souffle, 157

V

Valsalva maneuver, 259
  in arrhythmias, 161
  in auscultation, 246–247
  in differentiation of
    supraventricular tachycardias,
    164
Valves
  aortic (*see* Aortic, valve)
  atrioventricular, position, and
    intensity of first heart sound,
    33–37
  changes in
    pathologic, and intensity of first
      heart sound, 37
    second heart sound intensity
      and, 45
  mitral (*see* Mitral, valve)
  prosthetic (*see* Prosthetic valves)
  in rheumatic fever
    mitral regurgitation due to, 102
  surgery and, 206–208
  ring structural changes and
    intensity of second heart
    sound, 45
  surgery of, sounds after, 229–230
  tricuspid (*see* Tricuspid)
Vasodilators, 251–254
Venous
  drainage, anomalous pulmonary,
    183
  hum, 150–151, 157
    patent ductus arteriosus
      differentiated from, 175
  pressure, 241–244
  pulse (*see* Pulse, venous)
Ventricle
  atrioventricular (*see*
    Atrioventricular)
  contractions (*see* Contractions,
    ventricular)
  left
    dilated, causing, mitral
      regurgitation, 103
    emptying time increase, and
      splitting of second heart
      sound, 50–51
    enlargement, apical diastolic
      murmur in, 145
    rhythm, 161–164
  right, emptying time increase,
      and splitting of second heart
      sound, 48–50

septal defects (*see* Septal defects, ventricular)

tachycardia (*see* Tachycardia, ventricular)

Vessels
  (*See also* Cardiovascular)
  great
    structural changes in, and loudness of second heart sound, 45

transposition of, 190–191

W

Wenckebach type of second-degree block, 168

X

Xiphosternal crunch, 32